The
Medical Staff
in the
Modern Hospital

The Medical Staff *in the* Modern Hospital

Edited by

C. WESLEY EISELE, M.D.

Associate Professor of Medicine

Associate Dean for Postgraduate Medical Education

University of Colorado School of Medicine

THE BLAKISTON DIVISION

McGRAW-HILL BOOK COMPANY

NEW YORK   TORONTO   SYDNEY   LONDON

THE MEDICAL STAFF IN THE MODERN HOSPITAL

Library of Congress Catalog Card Number: 67–11206

19118

2345–CO–987

Acknowledgment

I am deeply indebted to Mrs. Toma C. Wilson for her editorial assistance in the preparation of this volume.

Preface

This volume is the outgrowth of several postgraduate conferences conducted by the University of Colorado School of Medicine for the medical staff leaders in community hospitals. The need for a forum to assist staff leaders in acquiring a better understanding of their roles and a better knowledge of their duties, responsibilities, and opportunities has become apparent in recent years. But in the plethora of meetings, conferences, and postgraduate courses, there often seems to be little opportunity for exchange of information—and for inspiration—in this complex and critical area.

The need for conferences for medical staff leaders and for this volume has been demonstrated by the extraordinary response to several postgraduate courses offered by the University of Colorado School of Medicine. The first of these, "A Postgraduate Course on the Internal Medical Audit," was held in Denver, August 10th through 12th, 1960. It was anticipated that perhaps as many as 100 registrants would attend, but there were 210 participants from 37 states and Canada. The enthusiasm of the registrants was gratifying. There was a similar response to the "Chief of Staff Conference" held October 22nd through 24th, 1964, at the Humphreys Postgraduate Center of the University of Colorado School of Medicine in Denver. Again, it was anticipated that about 100 registrants would attend, but there were 337 from 43 states, Canada, and Puerto Rico. Many expressed the opinion that conferences of this nature should be held on a regional basis so that more hospital staff leaders could participate—a concept we strongly support. In 1965 two consecutive conferences were held—"The Hospital Medical Staff Conference," October 11th through 13th and "The Conference on Medical Education in the Hospital," October 14th through 16th. These conferences were held at the YMCA Conference Center in Estes Park, Colorado, to provide larger meeting facilities and a "cultural island" where participants and leaders could live together, away from urban distractions. Several hospital groups sent a number of their medical and administrative staffs—in one instance, ten individuals; and they had the added benefit of a "retreat" to consider together some of their own hospital problems without the usual distractions. The combined attendance at these two conferences was 586 people, many of whom attended both conferences; and they came from 45 states, Canada, and Puerto Rico.

In all these conferences, the need was repeatedly voiced for wider dissemination of the material discussed. Regional conferences may have begun with the one conducted by the Jefferson Medical College at Hershey, Pennsylvania, April 5th through 8th, 1966, entitled "The Community Hospital: Its Organization and Medical Staff in a Changing Era." Others will doubtless follow. The fourth University of Colorado conference, "The Medical Staff Conference," will be held October 3rd through 7th, 1966, again in Estes Park.

The material in this volume is based to a considerable extent upon the three conferences presented by the University of Colorado School of Medicine in 1960, 1964, and 1965. However, the volume does not represent proceedings of these meetings. Earlier versions of some of the chapters were presented at the first "Chiefs of Staff Conference" in October of 1964 and were later published in *Hospital Progress.** A few chapters contain material which will be presented at the conference to be held in October, 1966. Other chapters containing material which was presented at the University of Colorado conferences but which was published elsewhere have acknowledgments listed in the chapter itself.

Two phenomena recur through the volume, and in some respects they may be considered divergent. First several authors state and restate the same principles from different viewpoints. Second, it is apparent that there is no one right way to organize many staff functions or to solve particular staff problems.

Certain principles or themes reiterated in this volume include the acknowledgment of the major role of the director of medical education in the continuing education of the staff; the growing recognition of the need for full-time service chiefs, especially if the hospital is engaged in the education of house staff; the importance of longer tenure for staff officers; the need for a medical director (full-time chief of staff) in larger hospitals to lead and administer staff functions; the vital necessity of medical staff systemic review of medical care; and the importance of bylaw provisions that cover every staff function, with amendments and frequent revisions to keep pace with the dynamic nature of the hospital and its medical staff. A few authors use a phrase coined by Dr. Kenneth Williams at the 1964 "Chiefs of Staff Conference." He referred to the "gauze curtain" that sometimes separates the medical staff from the administration. Several writers have referred to the concept of "fragmentation" of hospital structure and organization, of the hospital's public image, and even of the care rendered.

The chapters in this volume should be evaluated from the viewpoint of each author and the situation in which he works. The author's discussion is usually based largely upon his own experience in one hospital, and it is not intended to infer that this is the only right way. To assist

* Hospital Progress, 46:65–128 (Jan.) 1965.

the reader, brief biographic notes on the author and, where it is appropriate, data on his hospital and community are given in each chapter.

Because reference is made in many chapters to the Joint Commission on Accreditation of Hospitals, an appendix to this volume listing the policies and standards of this organization has been provided by the director, Dr. John Porterfield.

There is a universal need for an authoritative approach to medical staff organization and function. Confusion in nomenclature and title is frequently compounded by indistinct definitions of function and organization. An example is the confusion regarding the titles and the roles of the chief of staff and the president of the staff in hospitals where one or the other or both are present and their relation to each other, the medical director, the governing board, and the executive committee. The impact of research in the field of staff organization and function upon the quality of medicine practiced in this country will likely far exceed that of most of the laboratory investigations which are now so handsomely supported by various foundations and grants. It is hoped that the material presented in this book will stimulate study and discussion which will bring clarity to some of these issues.

C. WESLEY EISELE, M.D.

Contents

Part II. *Clinical Services of the Hospital Staff*

Part III. *Administrative Functions of the Medical Staff*

Part IV. *Perplexing Situations for the Medical Staff*

Part V. *Graduate Medical Education and the Hospital*

Part VI. *Continuing Education of the Staff Physician*

Part VII. *Internships and Residencies*

Part I

Medical Staff Organization and Functions

1

Medical Staff Organization

By Anthony J. J. Rourke, M.D.

Anthony J. J. Rourke is a hospital consultant in New Rochelle, New York, and is a frequent contributor to the hospital literature. He received the M.D. degree from the University of Michigan. He was active in hospital administration from 1937 to 1952 at Columbia Presbyterian Medical Center, the University of Michigan Hospital, then at Stanford University Hospital. He was the director of the Hospital Council of Greater New York from 1952 to 1954. Dr. Rourke is a past president of the American Hospital Association and also served on their Board of Trustees. He was a founding commissioner of the Joint Commission on Accreditation of Hospitals from 1951 to 1954. He is a diplomate of the American Board of Preventive Medicine.

Success in any activity depends largely upon motivation. If physicians are not well motivated in the creation of a good medical staff organization, the result of their efforts will be mediocre. What should be the proper motivation? An objective answer would be, to bring the best possible care to the patient at the least possible cost. This of course places the motivation in a very worthy, patient-centered perspective.

Added to this, however, are other reasons for a good medical staff organization, and I quote from two sources:

In the Report on Physician-Hospital Relations, published by the American Medical Association, the following statement is found:

> The medical profession and the hospitals, cognizant of a growing interdependence, have voluntarily collaborated to institute a system of "self-government" which provides for an organized, departmentalized staff with specific lines of authority and areas of responsibility under an officer and committee structure, all designed to achieve and

maintain high standards of medical care. *Such voluntary controls have proved adequate when effectively applied.* However, survey findings and third-party comments stress that voluntary controls are not being uniformly applied and that, in fact, many medical staffs are not functioning properly.

Responsible leaders of the medical profession stress that voluntary controls need rigorous application if the principle of "self-government" is to be retained.[1]

Dr. Edwin L. Crosby, president of the National Health Council, in his paper to the National Voluntary Health Conference of the American Medical Association held in Chicago, September 17–18, 1964, concluded as follows:

> Let me say that voluntary organizations cannot remain voluntary unless they are free of government controls. Let me also say that they cannot remain voluntary unless they are responsible. This, as you clearly recognize, requires that voluntary organizations must establish their own effective controls. The two words "freedom" and "responsibility" convey what I mean. These words are not antithetical but complementary. To be responsible, a voluntary organization must be free: to be free, it must also be responsible.[2]

Adequate motivation for the establishment of a good medical staff organization exists in abundance. Motivation may be in the interest of the patient's care and his economics or it may be in the interests of the doctor's and hospital's desire for freedom of action and self-government. Further justification would be redundant, but every staff should recognize that without well identified motivation what should be an easy process becomes a painful chore.

THE BLUEPRINT

Medical staff bylaws (see Chap. 2 for additional discussion of bylaws, rules, and regulations) are the blueprints from which are constructed good or bad medical staff organizations. A fuzzy set of bylaws results in a fuzzy staff organization with constant indecision, buck-passing, and discontent. Clear-cut bylaws should leave nothing ambiguous, but should clearly define the methods, the responsibilities, the powers, and the channels of delegation and feed-back. This will help to avoid conflict and to promote a greater degree of success.

To be specific, I believe that every section of a set of bylaws which deals with a committee should clearly state:

The name of the committee.
How it is created—by appointment, by election, or by virtue of position.
If appointed, by whom.

Eligibility for membership—active, associate, and courtesy staff.

Number of members.

Tenure of appointment.

If ex officio member, with or without vote.

How the committee gets its chairman and secretary—by presidential appointment, by vote of committee membership, by seniority, or by virtue of some other office.

Requirements for specified meetings.

How it may be called in emergency session.

Its charge and its powers.

To whom it reports and how often.

Its status if successors fail to be appointed at expiration of the hospital year.

Its form of agenda.

Requirements of recorded minutes, recording of attendance, quorum, and required signature to minutes.

At the risk of having bulky bylaws, it is well to word each section so that it is complete in itself with a minimum of references to other sections. As an illustration, some bylaws have a single statement that the chairmen of all standing committees shall be members of the active attending staff, and it is not repeated again. If this is repeated in the bylaws for each committee, it is possible for the chief of staff, at the beginning of his year, to duplicate that section of the bylaws pertaining to a specific committee. He can then go over it with the new committee chairman without having to leaf back and forth through the complete bylaws.

For guidance in developing bylaws, there are numerous models and numerous requirements and recommendations created by the Joint Commission on Accreditation of Hospitals and other national bodies. For this reason details will not be discussed here. I merely stress the need for a well written, clear set of bylaws.

CHIEF OF STAFF OR PRESIDENT OF THE STAFF

Some hospital staffs use one title, some use the other, and some have two positions and use both titles. In any event, the physician occupying the top position of responsibility for quality care and medical staff cooperation is the keystone to good organization. Appointment or election to such a post should not be considered a reward for previous work, nor should it be based upon a popularity contest. It is perhaps the most misunderstood post in the staff organization and is frequently discounted in importance by the physician who occupies it. On several occasions, I have had an opportunity to sit down with several chiefs of staff from a system of hospitals, and I have asked the question, "What is your job as chief of staff?" These are some of the answers:

"I don't know."
"I make a decision when there is a controversy."
"They bring their problems to me."
"To keep the hospital in line."
"To keep the doctors in line."
"To be available to the administrator for advice."
"No one else would take it so I agreed, but I'm just a rubber stamp."

My next question, "Did you read the bylaws before the year started?" got these answers:

"Do we have bylaws?"
"Why should I?"
"We don't have bylaws."
"We only look at them when some one wants to amend them."

The physicians I met with were all fine men who gave their time to attend a conference to learn something of their new assignments. They were not reluctant or unwilling to do the job, but they were woefully unprepared either to recognize the job or to perform it.

No other post in medical staff life requires the same degree of leadership qualities. Many can never develop them, and others do not have the necessary time or interest.

In a recent study at the Graduate School of Business Administration of the University of Michigan, some interesting findings were developed through careful interviews with 66 successful chief executive officers of American industry. Some corollaries may be drawn relating their findings to the hospital chief of staff. Many of the executives interviewed felt that certain personal qualities or skills became more important as careers progressed. The percentage of various responses is as follows:

Understanding and working with other people . .38 per cent
Reasoning, objectivity, analytical abilities . . . . .17 per cent
Decision-making abilities . . . . .11 per cent

They listed the following special skills which improve performance:

General communication ability . . . . .18 per cent
Public speaking ability . . . . .17 per cent
Understanding and handling people . . . . .17 per cent

The time has come when each medical staff should attack the problem of setting criteria to be met in electing its chief of staff. Business techniques are foreign to the day-to-day life of the physician, and so they should be. However, staff operation is becoming so complex that better leadership must be developed. Within our profession are physicians who have inherent qualities of leadership. We all know doctors who work well with others, are objective and analytical, make wise decisions without pain, and communicate well in both writing and speaking.

Minimum Standards To Be Met by a Chief of Staff. No one, to my knowledge, has listed any such standards, and I would like to suggest the following for no other reason than to stimulate thought and discussion.

1. The largest portion of his hospital practice shall be in the hospital where he is being considered for chief of staff.
2. He shall have been a member of the active staff for not less than five years.
3. He shall be not less than 40 years or more than 62 years of age.
4. He shall have served for at least three years as a member of one or more of the standing committees.
5. He shall have served for at least one year as the chairman of one of the standing committees.
6. He shall have served his county medical society in some capacity for at least one year.
7. He shall have participated in some community health activity for at least one year (Community Chest, Red Cross, United Hospital Fund, Blood Bank, Visiting Nurses Association, etc.).
8. He shall have public speaking ability and shall have presented at least three papers at local, state, regional, or national medical meetings.
9. He shall have professional attributes, including respect for his brother staff physicians.
10. He shall have administrative skills as demonstrated by his ability to get things done in his day-to-day hospital practice, such as prompt completion of medical records, consultations, orders, and regular attendance at meetings.
11. He shall have deep interest in the hospital and a willingness to serve as chief of staff if selected.
12. He shall be able to free sufficient time to carry out the responsibilities of the post.
13. He shall be capable of disagreeing without being disagreeable and willing to tackle the unpleasant tasks as they come along.
14. He shall be willing to relinquish his post as chief of a clinical service if he occupies one during his tenure of office.

You will probably say no such physician exists, and perhaps you are correct; but is this any reason for not attempting to set standards? Let each hospital establish its own standards, reducing requirements to a minimum where men are available for consideration. This procedure

would improve the image of the position and would allow each chief
to contribute substantially to his peers, to his hospital, and to thousands of
hospitalized patients.

Tenure. With the careful selection of the chief of staff, applying minimal standards, greater evidence of faith should be demonstrated by
making appointments for three-year periods and not for a single year.
Annual appointments to such posts are a vestige of the past. If they do
not apply to governing boards, then why should they apply to physicians?

ADVISORY COUNCIL TO THE CHIEF OF STAFF

It has been said in jest, that "There is nothing deader than a past
president." This, in fact, is all too true. As an adjunct to a new program
which sets minimum standards for the chief of staff, each hospital should
develop a nucleus of experienced men who have gone through the
chairs and who meet quarterly to advise and consult with the current
chief. Recognition of their abilities and experience should be written
into the bylaws.

POSITIVE PROGRAMS

The "planning ahead" technique is more frequently absent than
present among hospital medical staffs. This may be most evident in the
helter-skelter activity that takes place in each hospital a few months
before the visit of a surveyor from the Joint Commission on Accreditation of Hospitals. If a qualified chief of staff were giving leadership to
the staff, the last report from the Joint Commission would be in his top
drawer, and he would look at it at least monthly to be sure that the
areas needing attention were getting it.

He would not treat the instances of poor medical judgment as isolated incidents to be handled outside the framework of staff organization. Instead, he would relate them properly and with dignity to programming staff meetings and the scientific discussion at executive committee
meetings.

The alert chief of staff would identify sources of irritation, seek out
the causes, and eliminate them where possible. He would seek out the
trouble makers, the unreasonable members, and the malcontents and
motivate them toward the team concept to the end of integrating them
into full staff participation.

He would be ever alert, by reading and by communicating with other
chiefs of staff, to new methods of evaluating the quality of medical care
and methods of keeping his staff abreast of modern trends.

He would represent his medical confreres to the administration and
the lay governing board as an orderly and secure group of physicians

who are anxious to participate in progress that will bring better care to the patients.

He would represent his medical confreres to the nursing staff and paramedical groups as a mature group of physicians who recognize the contribution of nursing and other groups in the care of their patients.

He would try to offset the derogatory remarks about medicine and hospitals which are all too prevalent in the hospital corridors in our present free-wheeling system.

The potential of "chieftainship" encompasses a positive program that minimizes the function of problem-solving and maximizes the value of positive planning and programming. There are those who may feel that this would take a full-time, salaried physician, and perhaps in large hospitals this may be the case. However, one periodically sees this type of chief who carries an active practice and, because of his organizing ability, is able to do all the things mentioned.

NEED FOR SECURITY

Recent years have seen rapid radical changes in hospital medical staffs, many of which occurred because physicians were not content with the status quo. Some changes were traumatic and led to much unhappiness, anxiety, and insecurity.

The general practitioners, in many instances, have developed anxieties because they feel that their specialist brothers wish to "fence them in."

The specialists have many anxieties among themselves, manifested by "iron curtains" which establish who may enter a chest, who may do a neck dissection, who may give a caudal anesthetic, or who may wire a jaw.

The trustee finds himself in a strange world that does not behave like his bank, his factory, or his brokerage house. He runs a business at the hospital in which medical care is dispensed by individuals on a personal service basis and is in no way subject to the personal wishes of the trustee. All this leads to anxiety.

The administrator, often caught between the board and the staff, keeps his antacid bottle filled and handy and hopes that some day he may understand it all.

In this anxious atmosphere many dedicated people do a superb job in caring for the sick, but no one seems to be attacking the problem which robs us all of complete job satisfaction and enjoyment in our work.

Of the three groups of victims of anxiety—the governing board, the medical staff, and the administration—only one, the physicians, has been truly trained in the proclivities of the mind. Surely medicine must lead the way to a better understanding, a greater confidence, and a more cooperative spirit. At least half the members of every medical staff are capable of diagnosing the problems and suggesting a solution, but nowhere is the statement more applicable that "What is everybody's responsibility is nobody's responsibility."

Here again we see the need for a well-adjusted, well-qualified, interested chief of staff in whom the members of the medical profession can place their confidence. We need a man without bias who appreciates the need for speed and the value of conference-table courtesy and who can clearly see the positive values in other people.

SUMMARY

The title of this chapter may appear inapt because no attempt has been made to develop a table of organization to identify the generals, majors, captains, and lieutenants. Much has been said elsewhere about such tables of organization and about bylaws. This is the time for something new, and I recommend that the essential ingredient for bringing about organization of the medical staff is a chief of staff who meets established standards. Organization will develop from his leadership. Without him, the finest set of bylaws will remain a paper document without flesh and blood and a soul.

BIBLIOGRAPHY

1. Report on Physician-Hospital Relations, June, 1964, Council on Medical Service, Committee on Medical Facilities of the American Medical Association, Chicago, 1964.

2. Crosby, E. L.: Issues in Voluntarism As the National Health Council Views Them, Paper presented to National Voluntary Health Conference of the American Medical Association, Chicago, September 17–18, 1964.

3. Bond, F. A. et al.: Preparation for Business Leadership, University of Michigan Bureau of Business Research, Ann Arbor, Michigan, 1964.

4. Rourke, A. J. J.: The Internal Medical Audit, Requisites and Principles, *Hospital Prog.*, 41:72–73 (Nov.) 1960.

2

Medical Staff Bylaws, Rules, and Regulations

By Robert R. Cadmus, M.D.

Robert R. Cadmus is president of the New Jersey College of Medicine and Dentistry. Prior to accepting this position in 1966, he was chairman and professor in the department of hospital administration of the University of North Carolina School of Medicine. He received the M.D. degree and his postgraduate training at Columbia University. For a number of years, Dr. Cadmus has actively engaged in hospital research, especially in the areas of improving hospital-physician relations and exploring a university's responsibility to community hospitals.

Many years ago in jolly old England and up the rugged fjords of Scandinavia, the people of the villages and the hinterlands—in the *byrs* or *bys* as they were then called—were burdened by disputes over farm boundaries, the trespass of cattle, and other minor personal conflicts which constantly pop up whenever people live close enough to one another to impinge upon each other's lives and property. Courts of law were few and not generally available for such petty matters. Certain local rules began to be laid down within these little *bys*, and it was natural that these codes of conduct became known as bylaws. (Bylaws are also discussed in Chap. 1.) As the years passed, this term took on a new and more modern meaning and came to refer to those subsidiary laws or regulations made by a public or private corporation or association for the regulation of its own local or internal affairs, for its dealing with others, and for the government of its members. This is not an unreasonable corruption or extension of the original meaning.

Medical staff bylaws have added a new dimension to the standard definition, the concept of public protection—placing restrictions on the members of the association not for the member's protection, but for the public's protection. It is this aspect of bylaws which attracts most attention, and it is around this concept that problems, misunderstandings, and difficulty in writing bylaws occur. Generally, there are few fireworks over whether the jobs of secretary and treasurer should be combined or separated or whether the meetings should be held on Tuesday evenings or Thursday noons. But a sonic boom can be created by the provisions of bylaws which involve the limitation of privileges, the election versus appointment of chiefs of service, emergency room coverage, completion of medical records, and required attendance at meetings. These are features which are included not to aggrandize physicians nor to stimulate a strong fraternal allegiance; rather, they are wholly incorporated to protect the patient whom the physician has already sworn to serve faithfully when he took the Hippocratic Oath.

It is little wonder, then, that many physicians in private practice rather sincerely ask, "Why are bylaws so important?" They are not required for office practice; they are not necessary to obtain medical licensure; they are not even mentioned as a part of medical education. Why have bylaws? The answer is simple. The medical staff of a hospital is a group of individuals, and as groups we live in a society governed by laws, not in an anarchy. There can be no group and no organized activity of life, particularly in a democracy, without rules—rules which describe the who, what, why, when, where, and how the game is to be played. When the game is on and everything is going according to Hoyle, there is no need for well informed players to flash the rule book. One needs the rule book only when some rascal fails to play by the rules and an argument ensues.

Obviously, one cannot make the rules after the game has started. The rules must be made before the game starts, and they must be mutually understood and accepted prior to the opening whistle. This is why before each major league baseball game the umpires review with the team captains and managers not only the general rules of the game but also the ground rules of the particular ball park in which they are playing. Medical staff bylaws are nothing more than the rules of the game as it is played by physicians in hospitals.

For the same reasons, medical staff bylaws should be not only available but familiar to each physician before he starts his practice within the hospital, and they should be reviewed again at every change of the bylaws or change of his status. Bylaws should be prepared and completely understood before problems arise with the physician who is unqualified, unethical, uncooperative, or even rarely alcoholic, drug addicted, or psychotic. During times of tranquility, one can talk rationally about the qualifications for membership, but it is immeasurably more difficult to talk about a specific delinquent physician with whom one may be emotionally involved. Therefore, as in baseball, the rules must be made before the game starts. After an infraction has occurred, neither the players nor the courts will permit rules to be made retroactively—to enforce a rule, yes; but to make a rule, no.

"Each physician *is subject* to the bylaws of the Medical Staff and *must* conduct his professional activities according to the standards, rules, and regulations adopted by it." Too strict? Dictatorial? This quotation is from a statement on medical staff organization adopted by the House of Delegates of the American Medical Association. The leadership of both the American Medical Association and the American Hospital Association recognizes that the operation of a hospital in the future will require much greater cooperation between physicians and hospital administrators than has ever been witnessed in the past. It is recognized that the civilized way of accomplishing this objective is through well-written medical staff bylaws, rules, and regulations.

Legal Nature of Bylaws

The creation of medical staff bylaws is in some respects the gateway to a terrifying legal jungle because these bylaws take on formal legal standing. They are accepted by the courts, and legal decisions are made in accordance with their provisions. The interpretation of law, even of hospital bylaws, may be difficult, and at times legal decisions are influenced more by the interpretation of words, or more often by the lack of words, than by the larger issues of right and wrong. There is not a more apt example than in hospital bylaws of the legal dictum, "Where the law is uncertain, there is no law."

That medical staff bylaws have formal legal implications is illustrated by two opposing cases. The first shows why one needs bylaws; the second shows that one must abide by the bylaws he has written.

In *Green v. the City of St. Petersburg, Florida,*[2] the bylaws denied full surgical privileges to any surgeon who was not first proved competent by being supervised in 20 cases. A physician who was refused full surgical privileges on his original application by virtue of this bylaw provision sued the institution. The courts sustained the hospital, saying that the bylaws were not discriminatory and were reasonable to establish and uphold high standards of medical care. Without that provision in the bylaws, any physician without surgical competency could have demanded and received full surgical privileges. As indicated earlier, the bylaws were interpreted by the courts not as a protection to the surgeon but rather as a protection to the patient.

In the second case, *Jacobs v. Martin*[2] in New Jersey, the bylaws of the hospital had no provisions covering the qualifications for surgery, but they did have provisions for the presentation of charges and a hearing before staff privileges could be suspended. When a surgeon was abruptly notified that his surgical privileges were being withdrawn, he sued the institution and won, not because the court judged that he was a competent surgeon or that it was proper for an incompetent surgeon to practice but rather because a hearing was not held and the hospital thus failed to follow its own rules. The court said that, "absence of compliance with their own rules and regulations renders invalid the disciplinary action of the medical staff."

How Bylaws Are Created

How are bylaws created, and how may they receive a major revision? Perhaps it is carrying coals to Newcastle to discuss this, but with the advent of Medicare many hospitals have become involved in the serious process of revising bylaws for the first time and a few hospitals will be writing new ones. Whose responsibility is it to create bylaws—the administrator, the trustees, the hospital attorney, the medical staff?

The governing board has the final responsibility to insure the creation of adequate medical staff bylaws, and they have the power to reject or to formally adopt and accept them. But this does not mean that they should write them. To avoid any justified claims of interference, it is proper for the physicians themselves to prepare the rules under which they will work. An ad hoc bylaws committee from members of the medical staff should be appointed by the chief of staff, and it is wise for the administrator to be an ex officio member. A permanent on-going committee is usually not necessary if the bylaws have a formal amendment mechanism. When changes are recommended or when the status quo has existed for as long as five years, it may then be time for another ad hoc committee to review and recommend amendments. It is common knowledge that both medical practice and hospital operation are dynamic functions; as these change, so should the bylaws. New emergency room patterns emerge; recovery rooms or intensive care units are added; further departmentalization occurs with the addition of a pediatrician or a psychiatrist; a utilization committee is organized in response to Medicare; or some other internal change is made—all of these should be reflected in the bylaws.

There are many models or sample bylaws to follow, but a warning is in order. In the *Hospital Law Manual* [2] there is a whole section entitled "Litigation Involving Bylaws and Rules Similar to Provisions of Model Documents." Copying polished bylaws does not protect a hospital from possible trouble, but this should not deter one from consulting models. The one offered by the Joint Commission on Accreditation of Hospitals [3] is the proper starting point. Although the American Medical Association is a member of the Joint Commission, it urges physicians to refer also to the *General Principles of Medical Staff Organization*. [1]

The creation of bylaws follows a series of sequential steps. The first is the preparation of a recommended set by the Bylaws Committee. This draft is taken to the medical staff for further review and possible amendment. Eventually a revised draft is adopted by the full membership.

The staff recommendations are then forwarded to the governing board; they consider them and formally adopt them if they concur. If the governing board finds objections to the suggested bylaws, the problems should be ironed out in a joint conference of appropriate representatives of the staff and the board. The revised draft should then be reviewed and approved by the full medical staff membership before it is resubmitted to the board. The governing board should notify the medical staff of the eventual adoption of the bylaws, and the signatures of the appropriate medical staff and governing board officers should be affixed to the document.

Finally, to give the bylaws full legal standing they must be incorporated within the hospital corporation's own bylaws; in lieu of this, a reference must be made in that document that the medical staff bylaws are considered a part of the institution's bylaws. At this point, they become the law of the institution and are enforceable by the courts.

A significant and often overlooked final procedure is for all physicians, including those present and those who join at a later date, to sign a statement indicating that they have read, understand, and are willing to abide by the bylaws.

What is the difference between bylaws and rules and regulations? Actually, they serve the same general purpose and both have equal legal standing. The model bylaws suggested by the Joint Commission include the rules and regulations as an article within the bylaws themselves. According to legal opinion, bylaws should state the basic principles—the source of authority, the general organization, and the overall conduct of the group. Accordingly, they are technically somewhat less subject to amendment. Rules and regulations, on the other hand, outline the mechanics and the details by which the goals of performance are carried out; they are more easily and more frequently amended to meet changing needs and conditions. The hospital attorney should settle the form, and the medical staff should settle the contents.

Essentials of Bylaws

What are the essentials of good bylaws and well-written rules and regulations? Obviously, one should study the model prepared by the Joint Commission on Accreditation of Hospitals. There should be an opening statement giving the source of authority, the name of the organization and the essential definitions. The following outline gives the fundamental provisions which should be embodied in every set of staff bylaws:

A. A statement of purpose
    1. To insure quality of care
    2. To handle medical-administrative matters
    3. To maintain staff self-government
    4. To maintain educational standards
B. A statement concerning membership
    1. Qualifications—medical licensure in state
    2. Ethical conduct
    3. Terms of appointment
    4. Procedure of appointment and withdrawal of appointment
    5. Appeal procedure
    6. Temporary appointments
C. A descriptive outline of the medical staff organization
    1. Categories of membership: honorary, consulting, active, associate, courtesy
    2. Listing and description of clinical departments
    3. Listing and description of officers
D. A statement concerning medical staff functions (these functions must be accomplished, although not necessarily by a committee or by separate committees)
    1. Executive
    2. Credentials
    3. Joint conference
    4. Accreditation
    5. Surveillance of quality of patient care
        a. Records
        b. Medical records, tissue and audit reviews
        c. Utilization
        d. Infections
        e. Pharmacy and therapeutic services
    6. Others as indicated
E. A statement concerning delineation of privileges
F. A statement concerning meetings
    1. Annual
    2. Regular—staff and departmental
    3. Special
    4. Attendance records
    5. Rules of order
    6. Agenda
G. Rules and regulations incorporating at least:

1. A provision for keeping accurate and complete medical records
2. A provision that tissue removed at operation be sent to the laboratory
3. A provision for routine examination of all patients upon admission and the recording of preoperative diagnosis prior to operation
4. A ruling permitting surgical procedures only on the consent of the patient or his legal representative except in true emergencies
5. A provision for compulsory consultation in special cases
6. A regulation insisting that physician's orders be in writing and signed

H. A provision for amendments
I. A statement indicating adoption

If dentists are to be granted membership, the bylaws should be entitled "Bylaws of the Medical and Dental Staff," and specific reference should be given to their qualifications, privileges, and responsibilities. Every dental patient should have a general history and physical examination by a physician in addition to the dental history and local physical examination. General medical support, if needed, should be provided by a physician.

Whether the rules and regulations are separate or an article within the bylaws, the model of the Joint Commission on Accreditation of Hospitals suggests some 30 separate items, only a few of which were mentioned in the outline as fundamental. Actually, all are worthy of adoption but need not be enumerated here.

How tight, how stringent, how detailed should these bylaws be? There is no better definition of this delicate point of balance than that made by the chairman of a women's auxiliary as she presented a major rewrite of the auxiliary bylaws to the membership. She said: "Bylaws should be like a well-fitting girdle—strong and specific enough to give support where it is needed and large enough to cover the subject adequately, but loose enough to permit reasonable movement and comfortable enough to avoid any temptation to discard it."

Problem Areas

How well do the bylaws and rules and regulations in community hospitals conform to these standards? The Department of Hospital Administration of the University of North Carolina School of Medicine has the opportunity to review a large number of hospitals and their bylaws. From this experience, as may be expected, the findings varied from terrible to superb. If the bylaws fail, it is in one of two respects: poor bylaws, or poorly enforced bylaws. Here are some of the more common problems we have found:

1. There was a lack of bylaws or an inability to find them. When

hospital administrators are asked for a copy of their medical staff bylaws, several have some excuse such as, "They are around here someplace, but I can't lay my hands on them at the moment." They may gracefully blame the situation on a new secretary.

2. The creation of bylaws by administrators with only tacit medical staff participation is another problem. This breach of routine usually occurs for one of two reasons: rarely, the administrator may be trying to control the staff for some ulterior reason; more commonly, the medical staff is inactive and abrogates its responsibility. The responsibility to control the quality of medical care and to maintain self-government must be accepted by the medical staff. Proper bylaws offer the one democratic mechanism by which they can and must exert their responsibility.

3. Unimaginative copying of model bylaws is another common fault. This practice may lead to stupid and ludicrous situations as shown in the following true examples (Figs. 2-1 and 2-2). These and the other illustrations are actual photographs of the documents found in community hospitals. It is obvious that the bylaws shown here were thoughtlessly copied, inadequately prepared, and perfunctorily approved. But do not laugh—they may be your own. Can you imagine the dilemma these bylaws would create for hospital and physician alike in trying to convince a court of law of the hospital's high integrity and the due care it exercises over its everyday operation?

4. The delineation of the qualifications for membership is another major problem. (See Chap. 7 for discussion of the legal aspects of qualifications for staff membership.) Almost every copy of bylaws that we review includes such qualifications as graduation from an AMA approved medical school, membership in the county medical society, an internship requirement, and often board certification. One fully recognizes the intent of these provisions, but in the case of *Greisman v. Newcomb Hospital* [2] the courts have said that bylaws requiring graduation from an AMA approved medical school and membership in the county medical society are invalid. Relying on an earlier *Falcone* [2] case, the court said that a hospital has no claim to immunity from judicial supervision or control where it possesses a virtual monopoly on hospital services in its geographic area. This means that one cannot throw up

21. The hospital shall admit patients suffering from all types of disease except the following (specify diseases not treated). Patients may be treated only by physicians who have submitted proper credentials and have been duly appointed to membership on the medical staff.

11. The hospital shall admit patients suffering from all types of diseases except the following: (Specify diseases not treated). Patients may be treated only by physicians who have submitted proper credentials and have been duly appointed to membership on the medical staff.

Fig. 2–1

PROGRAM COMMITTEE: The Program Committee shall consist of three members of the
Medical Staff, and it shall be responsible for the preparation of
all programs for regular staff meetings in accordance with these
By-Laws, as specified in Article _____, Section _____.
If the hospital has a Pathologist, he shall be Chairman of the
Committee.

Fig. 2–2

legal barriers against admission other than medical licensure even in private hospitals, and particularly if it is a one-hospital community. Public and private hospitals have been treated differently in the sight of the law in the past, but the margin of difference is being steadily and rapidly narrowed. The legal interpretation of hospital bylaws will likely be made through public-oriented glasses.

It is for these many reasons that the model bylaws of the Joint Commission on Accreditation of Hospitals are rather brief on this subject and merely require licensure within the state, not medical society membership, not board certification, nor any other possibly discriminatory provision. This is a reason for the staff to involve the hospital attorney in the preparation and review of any new or revised bylaws. There is little profit is polishing up the wording of an illegal provision.

5. The procedure of appointment is a common problem. Most bylaws contain in some detail the mechanism of appointment through application, through the credentials committee, through the medical staff, and ultimately through the governing board. But when one tries to match compliance with the bylaws, it often cannot be done. The applications themselves may be incomplete if not lacking. Often there is no record of appointment either on the application or in the minutes of the medical staff or of the board of trustees. There is no doubt that some action has been taken, but such actions cannot be traced on paper.

In contrast to such easy appointment, there are examples of such extreme rigidity of appointment that there are no staff physicians under the age of 50 years and no appointments since World War II. These hospital staffs are "closed corporations" in which there is an uncrackable monopoly except for two things: the public is learning to bypass hospitals with restricted medical staffs in favor of those which offer a more talented and qualified group, and the courts are acting.

A recent issue of *Medical Economics*[4] carried an article entitled, "When a Hospital Staff Is Closed." This is a shocking story of how bylaws are used to "protect the public" who, in fact, created the facilities in order to provide quality medical care for themselves, not to donate a sheltered workshop to a self-limited group of physicians. In this case, the bylaws required an applicant to practice in the community for two years before he could apply for staff membership in the only hospital in the community. The chief of staff had the power to make exceptions, which he did to snuff out competition. This example may be extreme, but it illustrates the discrimination and self-interest in which some staffs indulge. The courts are very clear in requiring that appointments be made on objective criteria and not on provisions which in any way can be considered arbitrary, capricious, or discriminatory.

6. The delineation of privileges is another concern of many staffs. This is one of the most difficult parts of bylaws, and it is an area in which the Joint Commission on Accreditation of Hospitals is much concerned. The model bylaws try to help to determine privileges by suggesting such words as "training, experience, and competency," but these are broad terms and are difficult to define and administer. Quite properly, the Joint Commission leaves this matter to the local medical staff; but because of the lack of more specific standards, there is much drifting on the sea of confusion.

When bylaws do delineate privileges, they usually concern surgery, obstetrics, and gynecology, apparently to protect the public from mismanagement at the hands of an unskilled surgeon or obstetrician. There is generally no protection for a patient with a complicated metabolic problem from mismanagement at the hands of an unskilled general practitioner or internist.

To solve the dilemma of privileges, some medical staffs evade the issue by granting full privileges to every physician. Unless otherwise specified, this would apparently include organ transplants in a rural 50-bed hospital. There are men in small hospitals who at times do not hesitate to do relatively major surgery. Open chest surgery and artificial

ARTICLE VIII

CLASSIFICATION OF CERTAIN SPECIAL PRIVILEGES

Section 1. Surgery

   Major surgery is defined as all other procedures not listed under minor surgery. Privileges for Tonsillectomy and Adenoidectomy shall be granted separately from minor surgery.

   Minor surgery is limited to the following procedures:

Incision
Drainage of furuncle, steatoma or small subcutaneous abscess
Drainage of onychium or paronychium with or without complete or partial avulsion,
   of nail
Excision
Biopsy of Skin
Local excision of cicatrix, inflammation, congenital or benign neoplasm, or
   nevae
Suture
Primary Suture of accidental wounds
Minor skin grafting (Such as pinch graft)

MUSCLES

Incision
Drainage of abscess, hematoma ^-

NOTE: Listing of procedures continues for 3 pages under 22 anatomical
         sub-headings.

Fig. 2–3

```
        Physicians residing and practicing in the community as of
September 11, 1961, and who were members of the Medical Staff of
the hospital on that date shall be privileged to continue the type
of practice which has been their custom.
        No one shall be permitted to perform tonsillectomies unless
he meets one of the following requirements:  (1)  Completion of
at least two (2) years residency training in diseases of the ear,
nose, and throat;  (2)  Participation in fifty (50) tonsillectomies
during the past 12 months prior to his first application for such
privileges, with an accepted surgeon, twenty-five (25) of which
he has performed himself.
```

Fig. 2–4

kidney dialysis are currently being done in one 50-bed hospital that is located very close to a major referral center.

Other staffs have gone to the other extreme and list each procedure included in minor and major surgery. In Fig. 2-3 one sees the listing of minor surgery, leaving everything else to be considered major. This apparently means that if a physician has major privileges, he can do neurosurgery, open chest surgery, orthopedic surgery, plastic surgery, and organ transplants. I believe a court would so interpret these bylaws.

One hospital, in outlining its tonsillectomy provision, rather stringently demands 50 cases in the year before a physician can even receive privileges (Fig. 2-4). This bylaw provision almost forces unnecessary surgery.

There is no secret formula for delineation of privileges, but it is a task that must be done, and it must be done by the staff and not by the trustees or the administrator. It is not too difficult for a chief of a well organized surgical service to delineate privileges for his staff members. It becomes more difficult, however, for a staff of general practitioners to define surgical privileges for the surgeon, and most difficult for one surgeon to determine the privileges of his arriving competitor. To write medical criteria frustrates the best.

Some staffs have approached the delineation of privileges from the negative rather than the positive side and have declared that full surgical privileges in that hospital does not include open chest surgery, neurological surgery, major reconstructive surgery, or other types of surgery for which the hospital is inadequately equipped or staffed. This technique actually has a lot to offer.

7. The withdrawal of privileges is an even greater problem, especially in the pathetic case of a productive surgeon who has begun to show senile changes (Fig. 2-5). A question regarding this problem was asked by a reader of *Medical Economics*.[5] The answer given did not consider education, boards, or even an evaluation of surgical competency; it merely referred to the bylaws. One cannot help wondering, "Did he at a more tender age vote for that bylaw provision?" or "Did he really think he was an exception?"

8. The section on officers is an area where frequent problems arise because it stipulates too brief a period of tenure. To be effective, officers should hold office long enough to learn it, long enough to live with their decisions, and long enough so that they cannot procrastinate and refer the tough problems to the man who will take over in a few months. A good tenure of office would be three to five years.

In this same section one may see the word "elected" but with no mention of the method of nomination or the quorum necessary. Although it is not written in the bylaws, in practice one sees these positions of leadership rotated on the basis of alphabet, social popularity, or some other unmeritorious selection. There are other outlets for real or pseudo honor, and these jobs should be real working assignments held by administratively capable physicians.

9. The sections under committees are usually well written, but again compliance is often poor. One finds either inadequate minutes or no minutes at all. The committee chairman sometimes refuses to sign the minutes of the medical records committee or the tissue committee for fear of legal involvement. The provisions of Medicare and now of the Joint Commission on Accreditation of Hospitals require that every hospital have an active utilization review mechanism. This is an innovation not yet written into most bylaws, and it will force most hospitals to review their bylaws, perhaps for the first time in many years. No committee or function should be created without official recognition in the bylaws.

Physicians serving on record or medical audit committees should act like physicians not like clerks. They should ask for information, evaluate it, and make recommendations. They should not pore over records checking for signatures, looking for compliance or lack of compliance with bylaws, nor perform other tasks which are clerical in nature. Good committee function can be interesting and productive—poor committee work, dull and wasteful.

Practice
MANAGEMENT Q&A

How an elderly M.D. can regain full privileges

Question: The younger men who control the votes on my hospital's medical staff executive committee passed a resolution that prevents men over age 65 from operating. How good are my chances if I sue to get my privileges back? . . . *Answer:* Not very good. If the staff acted in accord with its bylaws, chances are that it's on legally solid ground. If, after reviewing the bylaws, you feel you have a case, consider turning the matter over to your attorney.

Fig. 2–5

20. Recognizing that the hospital's chief source of income is from its paying
     patients and that it is essential for the hospital to be in sound financial
     position, the Members of the Medical Staff will make every effort to see
     that their patients pay the hospital bill and agree that the hospital has
     first priority in the collection of accounts. They further understand and
     agree that if their ratio of non-paying to paying patients averages 15%
     higher than the mean average of the total Medical Staff, that this will
     constitute grounds for dismissal.

Fig. 2–6

10. Medical records is another subject in which there are usually fairly good bylaws but poor compliance. At times, the bylaw provisions for the time limits or deadline for completion of medical records are impossible to follow, so no one tries. We have recommended that deadlines be made less strict and more realistic.

The questions are repeatedly asked: "How does one get compliance with these rules?" and "What about the desirability of a clause concerning the suspension of privileges for failure to write records?" The courts have upheld, as in the case of *Memorial Hospital v. Pratt*[2] in Wyoming, that suspension from the medical staff for failure to keep records is not arbitrary but rather it is protection for the public and is therefore enforceable, provided, of course, that regulations requiring such records are in the bylaws. Whenever one must consider withdrawing privileges for failure to complete records, the situation has so deteriorated that one has a rather deep-seated hospital-physician or physician-physician problem. The problem should be put back where it belongs—on the medical staff—but not before one can be assured that the bylaws are reasonable and that the medical records committee is organized properly and operating effectively.

11. The oddment of irrelevant items which improperly creep into bylaws is the final problem to be mentioned in this listing of bylaws irregularities. Figure 2-6 shows an example of unfair, unworkable, and probably unconstitutional economic restrictions which have no place in bylaws. Requirements for such things as disaster or emergency room assignments are reasonable, but not so are such restrictive covenants as economic control, building fund assessments, race, or national origin.

Need for Physician Understanding

The biggest problem concerning bylaws, rules, and regulations is not the mechanics of writing and evaluating bylaws but that of convincing practicing physicians that the creation of bylaws and the compliance with them serve the best interest not only of their patients but also of themselves.

Requirements for bylaws are not created by Chicago or Washington, nor are they the sinister creations of boards and administrators. They are the end products of the best thinking of dedicated physicians at the local level. They are the rules that physicians feel are necessary to guarantee freedom for themselves and quality care for their patients. They give the physician legal protection and simultaneously force him to live by his own rules. If he accepts the concept that there is need for us to be our brother's keeper, that freedom is not absolute but limited, that what is good for the goose is good for the gander, and that the whole purpose of medicine is to provide the finest possible patient care, then he should have no conflict in accepting the concept of bylaws.

But this is not only the author's idea. As was said at the beginning, it is the idea of the American Medical Association, the American Hospital Association, and the courts. In a recent issue of the *Journal of the American Medical Association*,[6] the president of the Federation of State Medical Boards of the United States, writing on the subject "What Should the Profession Do About the Incompetent Physician?" said: "The local hospital staff is the logical body to control the incompetent physician." He did not say the county medical society, the licensing authorities, the AMA, or the Supreme Court, although all of these might appear on the chain of appeal.

The courts have been even more clear, particularly in the recent *Darling v. Charleston Community Memorial Hospital** decision, now sustained by the U.S. Supreme Court. It supports the contention that such standards as hospital accreditation, state licensing laws, and adequate hospital bylaws serve as useful evidence in evaluating the quality of care which a hospital must provide. This means that one cannot avoid having bylaws; that they must be adequate and up-to-date; and that they must be objectively enforced. Anything less is not enough.

Members of medical staffs and hospital administrators share not only in the preparation and enforcement of bylaws but also in the greater responsibility of educating members of the medical staff to accept bylaws willingly to keep things under control.

BIBLIOGRAPHY

1. General Principles of Medical Staff Organization, as Adopted by the House of Delegates, December, 1964, *JAMA*, 193:627 (Aug. 16) 1965.

2. Litigation Involving Bylaws and Rules Similar to Provisions of Model Documents, Sect. 3, Medical Staff, "Hospital Law Manual," vol. II, Health Law Center, University of Pittsburgh, Pennsylvania, 1959.

3. Model Medical Staff Bylaws, Rules and Regulations (under revision in accordance with *Bull. Joint Commission Accreditation Hospitals*, No. 40 (Dec.) 1965), Joint Commission on Accreditation of Hospitals, Chicago, 1964.

* *Darling v. Charleston Community Memorial Hospital*, 211 N.E. 2d253 (1965).

4. Heimlich, H. J.: When a Hospital Staff Is Closed, *Med. Econ.*, 42:82–94 (Sept. 20) 1965.

5. Practice Management Q & A, *Med. Econ.*, 43:157 (Jan. 10) 1966.

6. Derbyshire, R. C.: What Should the Profession Do About the Incompetent Physician? *JAMA* 194:1287–1290 (Dec. 20) 1965.

3

The Chief of Staff—The Hospital's Man or the Staff's Man?

By Kenneth J. Williams, M.D.

Kenneth J. Williams is the medical director of Saint John Hospital in Detroit. He was a high-rigger in logging camps in British Columbia for several years before entering the University of Manitoba Medical School from whence he received the M.D. degree. After eight years of private practice in British Columbia, he entered Yale University and earned the M.P.H. degree in Hospital Administration in 1959. He was medical director of St. Joseph's Hospital in Hamilton, Ontario, for five years, during which period he was a surveyor and field representative for the Canadian Council on Hospital Accreditation and consultant medical director to three other hospitals. He is a Fellow of the American College of Physicians and a member of the American College of Hospital Administrators. He is also consultant medical director to the Hospitals of the Sisters of St. Joseph of Nazareth, Nazareth, Michigan.

The Guide Issue of *Hospitals*, *JAHA*, August 1, 1965, gives the following data on Saint John Hospital: Beds, 292; Admissions, 15,606; Census, 282; Bassinets, 80; Births, 4,798; Newborn census, 58; Total expenses, $5,182,000; Payroll, $3,140,000; Personnel, 735. (*Ed. Note: Since this issue of* Hospitals, *Saint John Hospital has opened up a 200-bed addition, bringing the total bed capacity to 500.*)

There is considerable but unnecessary misunderstanding and confusion in the minds of many physicians as to just whose man the chief of staff is. Several physicians active in medical staff affairs were asked, "In your opinion, who does the chief of staff represent?" The answers reflect a wide divergence of opinion: "He is the patient's man;" He is not anybody's man;" He is the same as the president of the staff;" "He is everybody's man;" "He is the hospital's man;" "He is the staff's man and has to protect the staff from the administration;" and so on.

Examination of some basic principles may give a clearer answer to this question.

THE SOURCE OF AUTHORITY OF THE HOSPITAL

A hospital is a social institution. It is for patients. Society imposes demands upon its institutions as it does upon its citizens. Society demands that the many and varied interests of its members be safeguarded when they are admitted to hospitals. To this end, society has vested the control and management of the hospital in the hands of a board of trustees. This is the keystone of our voluntary hospital system, and it is not merely a theoretical concept. It has long been accepted and advanced by hospitals and the medical profession alike. It is clearly stated by the American Medical Association: "The governing authority, by whatever name called (e.g., board of trustees) is legally and morally responsible for the conduct of the hospital as an institution." [1] This principle has been well endorsed and substantiated by statutory and common law.

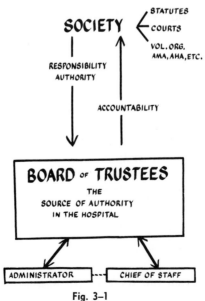

Fig. 3–1

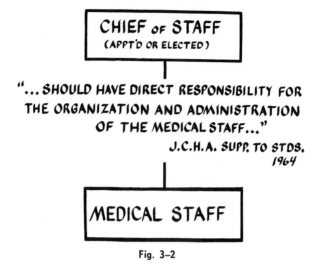

Fig. 3–2

Any authority vested in hospital officials, medical or non-medical, must initially stem from the board of trustees. Accountability must flow in reverse, for these officials must answer to the central source of authority for the effective discharge of their responsibilities and for the proper exercise of the authority delegated to them. (See Fig. 3-1.)

AUTHORITY AND ACCOUNTABILITY OF THE CHIEF OF STAFF

The chief of staff is also an official of the hospital. He should, as the Joint Commission on Accreditation of Hospitals recommends, "have direct responsibility for the organization and administration of the medical staff. . . ." [2] (See Fig. 3-2.) In delegating this responsibility and the commensurate authority the board of trustees does not and cannot abdicate or abrogate its final responsibility for the effective functioning of the medical staff organization. *The chief of staff is therefore accountable to the board, not to the medical staff.* He is the hospital's man, the trustee's man—the man the governing authority of the hospital has placed in charge of the most important single department of the hospital, by virtue of the hospital corporation's bylaws and the medical staff's bylaws.

This does not mean that the chief of staff may function in a totally autocratic fashion. On the contrary, the astute chief of staff is attuned to the desires of the general staff and takes these into consideration in all decisions and actions. He works closely with the medical staff to make sure that its voice is heard through the staff organization, and he maintains close liaison with the hospital administrator. It by no means infers that the chief of staff is a "yes man" to the board or administrator or that he cannot disagree with them. However, when a divergence of philosophy or of objective arises between the trustees and the medical staff, the chief of staff is the trustee's man and not the staff's man.

There are several important aspects of medical staff organization which commonly give rise to misunderstanding, conflict, and ensuing breakdown of medical staff leadership.

CHIEF OF STAFF AND PRESIDENT OF STAFF

The first of these areas concerns the potential misunderstanding of the distinct and separate roles of the chief of staff and the president of the staff.

It is essential to distinguish between the chief of staff and president of the staff because they are frequently regarded as one and the same, and the terms may be erroneously used interchangeably. The Joint Commission on Accreditation of Hospitals recognizes the importance of these two officers when it states that they ". . . are the key personnel in the proper organization and functioning of the staff in the hospital." The duties, responsibilities, and functions of the chief of staff are clearly set forth in the explanatory *Supplement to the Standards of the JCAH* (Joint Commission on Accreditation of Hospitals).[2] Yet we know that in many hospitals these two key positions are combined into one office with the incumbent carrying one or the other title. There are distinct advantages to be gained by keeping the two offices separate.

First let us consider *the medical staff organization in which the two offices are combined.* The chief of staff directs and administers the medical staff organization through his cabinet, the executive committee,

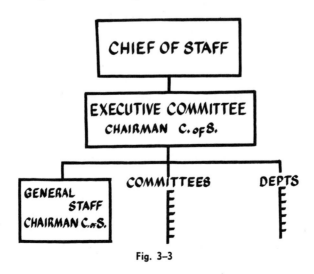

Fig. 3–3

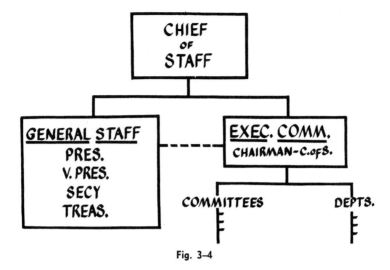

Fig. 3-4

of which he is the chairman. His primary efforts must be directed toward structuring a coordinated and durable cabinet which willingly accepts responsibility for the professional practices of the medical staff.

The department chiefs, whether appointed by the board of trustees or elected by the staff, are members of the executive committee and are answerable to it and to the chief of staff. The staff committees are appointed by the chief of staff in consultation with the executive committee, and they report directly to that body.

When the two positions are combined, the chief of staff usually chairs the general staff meetings. This may work well in some hospitals, but at times the chief of staff may be forced into a tenuous position by having to chair both the executive committee and general staff sessions. The individual staff member who is concerned over the protection of his rights may ask, "If the chief of staff is the hospital's man, then who is my spokesman?" (See Fig. 3-3.)

In the medical staff organization providing for both offices the staff member is assured who his representative is. At the same time, the chief of staff's load is lightened, and the entire organization is strengthened. In addition to the president of the staff there should be a vice-president, a secretary, and a treasurer, all of whom should sit on the executive committee. (See Fig. 3-4.)

The Functions of the President of the Staff

Let us consider the functions of the president of the staff, bearing in mind that as the JCAH points out, it is the chief of staff ". . . who has direct responsibility for the organization and administration of the medical staff." [2] The president of the staff does not have authority vested in him by the board of trustees; as we have seen, that authority is vested in the office of chief of staff. The president's responsibility is to the general staff. He is answerable to them—they elected him—and his function is primarily that of representing them. He is the official voice of the staff in executive committee deliberations and he must be a member of that committee. He must also represent the staff in deliberations with the board of trustees and must therefore be a member of the joint conference committee.

The president's forum is the general staff meeting which he chairs. He must encourage the staff to express itself, and he must convey the staff's feelings to the executive committee and to the board of trustees by way of the joint conference committee. He must be prepared to take a firm stand in support of the staff's position. So that he may be conversant with all aspects of the staff organization, he should be an ex officio member of all committees. He has an obligation to report back to the general staff on all policy matters discussed by the executive committee and the joint conference committee.

The president of the staff should not be a one-year honorary position simply signifying "reward for good service." For continuity, he should hold office for at least a two-year period. He and the other three officers should be elected by a free vote of the general staff and not by means of a nominating committee appointed by the executive committee. The election of the president of the staff should be planned and conducted on the same deliberate basis as are county medical society elections. It should not be by a last minute, late-at-night show of hands.

Perhaps one of the reasons the separate office of president of the staff has not been used by many staffs is that the JCAH has not clearly delineated the relationship of the president to the chief of staff. Under the heading of "President of the Staff—Chief of Staff," the *Supplement to the Standards* emphasizes the importance of these two offices when it states that they ". . . are the key personnel involved in the proper organization and functioning of the staff in the hospital." [2] Yet in the following paragraph it states that in many hospitals the two offices are combined, and in the ensuing discussion the two offices are treated as one under the title of the chief of staff. Similarly, the *Model Medical Staff Bylaws, Rules and Regulations* of the JCAH does not clearly distinguish between the two positions. It suggests that the president should appoint all committees other than the executive committee,[3] whereas the *Explanatory Supplement to the Standards* states that the chief of staff should appoint all committees other than the executive committee.[2] Unhappily, there is much confusion in terminology and concept.

Election or Appointment of the Chief of Staff

In the foregoing sections, much has been said and inferred about the functions of the chief of staff. A situation which may preclude the staff from fully appreciating the fact that the chief of staff is answerable to the board and not to them exists in hospitals where the chief of staff is elected by the staff. It is not difficult to understand why they feel that because they elect their chief he should be their man and should be answerable to them. The chief of staff himself may be confused. He may feel beholden to the electorate, and it may be difficult for him to see exactly whose man he is. Filling this important office by election unnecessarily clouds the question of the direction of responsibility. But whether the chief of staff is elected by the staff or selected by the board, the fact remains that he must discharge the responsibilities and exercise the authority delegated to him by the board of trustees, and he is answerable to them and to them alone.

SELF-GOVERNING MEDICAL STAFF

Another aspect of medical staff organization which can confuse the issue of whose man the chief of staff is relates to the various interpretations which may be placed upon the term, "a self-governing medical staff." To many physicians this means that the staff is autonomous; they believe that the medical staff is the sole authority on which type of medical staff organization is to prevail, and they believe that the chief of staff and the chiefs of services are answerable to them. It is understandable how the term "self-governing" gives rise to such beliefs. But this ignores the fundamental fact that the board of trustees has total responsibility for the conduct of the institution, and it must be the final authority to approve or reject the form of medical staff government. As Arthur F. Southwick points out, there is "no such thing as a completely 'self-governing' medical staff for the reason that the governing board will always be ultimately responsible for the medical standards of the hospital." [4] (See Chap. 7.)

But the medical staff is self-governing to the extent that it is given the responsibility for the establishment and maintenance of professional standards and for supervising the professional practices of its members. To assure that these responsibilities are properly exercised by the staff, the board of trustees must see that the office of chief of staff is vested with the proper authority through the medical staff bylaws, and the incumbent must answer directly to them.

Admittedly, there is a danger of becoming inflexible in attempting to demarcate categorically just who belongs to whom. In the hospital setting, where so much depends upon group activity and the acceptance of the team concept, this danger is of greater significance. It is imperative that all of us—board of trustees, administration, and medical staff—have a clear understanding of whose man the chief of staff is. An appreciation of this relationship can bring about improved group activity and a furtherance of the team concept and can do much toward eliminating the separatism and removing the "gauze curtain" which unfortunately exists all too often between medical staffs and trustees.

BIBLIOGRAPHY

1. General Principles of Medical Staff Organization, American Medical Association, Chicago, 1964.

2. *Explanatory Supplement to the Standards for Hospital Accreditation*, p. 16, Joint Commission on Accreditation of Hospitals, Chicago, 1964.

3. Model Medical Staff Bylaws, Rules and Regulations, p. 9, Joint Commission on Accreditation of Hospitals, Chicago, 1964.

4. Southwick, A. F.: The Legal Aspects of Medical Staff Function, *Hospital Prog.*, 46:84–91 (Jan.) 1965.

4

The Functions of the Chief of Staff

By William W. Jack, M.D.

William W. Jack is an obstetrician and gynecologist in Grand Rapids, Michigan. He received the M.D. degree from the University of Michigan and his specialty training at the Lying-In Hospital of the University of Chicago and at the University of Colorado School of Medicine. He is a diplomate of the American Board of Obstetrics and Gynecology, a Fellow of the American College of Surgeons, and a Fellow of the American College of Obstetricians and Gynecologists. He has been chairman of the Committee on Maternal Health of the Michigan State Medical Society since 1961. Dr. Jack was chief of staff at Blodgett Memorial Hospital in Grand Rapids, Michigan, from 1962 to 1964, and he has served on many staff committees.

This decade continues to produce vast changes in the whole fabric of medicine. New drugs, new techniques, new capabilities are an almost daily occurrence, and "miracle drug" and "breakthrough" are terms which are nearly jaded from overuse.

Beneath this spectacular display of progress lie other changes of equal importance. The increased interest of the general public in our profession is an example. Medicine has ceased to be mysterious to our patients as the reading and viewing public has become conversant with such esoteric terms as the hyperbaric chamber and cardio-version techniques. Moreover, the courts no longer fear to tread on medical ground, and lack of complete success in the care of a patient may sometimes seem to be equated with negligence. Finally, government and politics exercise an ever increasing influence. Health has now been written into the Bill of Rights.

This change, this accelerated evolution, has produced grave stresses and strains in many quarters. It has become necessary to reappraise many traditional concepts, to discard, to modify, to seek new answers to old and new problems.

THE HOSPITAL IS A SINGLE ORGANIZATION

The place of hospitals in medicine and the place of physicians within the hospital represent two related areas which require new thinking, new appraisal, and new understanding. The hospital has become the "center" of medicine within a community. The public, the courts, and the government are beginning to regard the hospital as a single organization, an indivisible unit. Yet there is still widespread misunderstanding in our profession with many still holding that a hospital is two organizations: one for the physicians who take care of patients; the other, quite unrelated, to provide facilities and personnel necessary for the doctor to take care of these patients. This concept of fragmentation must be discarded. A new understanding of the relationship between physicians and hospitals must be developed. Physicians must acknowledge that their responsibility extends beyond one patient to include all patients, to include the hospital; they must admit, however reluctantly, that the hospital is no longer just a "doctor's workshop." The one-to-one, doctor-patient relationship is sacred and inviolate only so long as the one doctor provides good care for the one patient.

The administration and the governing board must acknowledge, however reluctantly, that their responsibility extends beyond raising money, hiring help, paying bills, and building new facilities. Should the care provided by one doctor for his one patient be less than the accepted standard, the hospital has the moral and legal responsibility to take whatever steps are necessary to improve that care.

This concern over fragmentation was one of the common threads that ran through several papers at the Colorado meetings. (ED. NOTE: *Chiefs of Staff Conference, October 22–24, 1964, Denver, Colorado; Hospital Medical Staff Conference, October 11–13, 1965, and Conference on Medical Education in the Hospital, October 14–16, 1965, Estes Park, Colorado.*) Keith Taylor, director of the course in Hospital Administration at the University of California, made this statement: "Coordination depends upon clear communication, upon the understanding of hospital problems by members of the staff and of medical problems by board and administration." [1]

The executive director of the Catholic Hospital Association, Father John Flanagan, put it this way:

> I am appalled at the growing chasm of misunderstanding that is dividing health care in the United States. Good physicians feel that

they have no voice in making policies which affect their activities in the hospital. Many are completely uninformed about routine management policies and have not understood the relationships between good management and good patient care . . . Too many good physicians become frustrated; feel they are kept in ignorance of hospital policies and lapse into a sort of cold war of cynical indifference—a fatalistic coexistence with "city hall." [2]

This is harsh judgment against both administration and medical staff. It does not suggest that either is without sin or that either is totally sinning. It does suggest that a "gauze curtain" [3] seems to have fallen between two professions that must work together to achieve the common goal of ever better care of sick people.

The medical staff is a working participant in the daily operation of the hospital.[4] If I were to draw a diagram of this concept, it would be an equilateral triangle with one side marked Administration, one side marked Medical Staff, and one side marked Nursing. Surrounding this triangle is a circle I would mark Governing Board. None of the three sides of the triangle should try to function independent of the other two, or of the policies and authority of the governing board.

THE CHIEF OF STAFF IS THE LEADER OF THE STAFF

Where does the chief of staff fit into this picture? He is the leader of the staff and the voice of the staff. It makes little difference what he might be called, how he attained his position, how long he serves, or whether or not he receives a salary. The important consideration is that he leads and that the staff acknowledges his leadership. He must realize that he is the chief of the entire staff. Special interests within his own department or personal crusades must not conflict with his leadership of the whole staff. However, this leadership needs definition.

LIAISON WITH ADMINISTRATION AND BOARD

Probably the most important phases of leadership lie in his association with the administration and with the board. The chief is a liaison person who must transmit, and interpret if necessary, the thinking and collective judgment of the staff to the administration and to the board and, conversely, of the administration and the board back to the staff.

Liaison with Administration

Let us examine his relationship with administration. Ideally, this is the easy, trusted association of two good friends. Beyond this, I urge that a regularly scheduled meeting be set up between the chief and the administrator. The interval at which a meeting is held is probably less important than that it is held. In my own instance, we met for an hour once a week if each of us was available. On alternate weeks the director of nursing was included. Many problems of administration are problems for nursing and for the staff. Similarly, many problems of nursing are problems for administration and for the staff, and many problems of the staff are problems for administration and for nursing. The opportunity for the three most interested and responsible persons to meet regularly and to discuss problems freely and frankly is the very heart of effective liaison. Without these meetings the chief of staff cannot know what is going on, and the voice of the staff is silent.

An alternative is to hold meetings only when there are problems that demand attention. This is "government by crisis," and it provides an unsatisfactory type of leadership.

When the chief of staff takes office, he is strictly an amateur in the complex profession of hospital administration. We learned nothing about it in medical school, and until recently there has been little in the literature that was helpful. The chief must therefore learn from the available trained professionals. Administrators can speak our language much better than we can speak theirs. The chief must learn from the administrator, and the weekly meetings serve this educational function well.

Liaison with Board

The relationship between the chief of staff and the governing board may exist at three levels: no contact at all, contact through the joint conference committee, or membership on the board. The first alternative is to be deplored. The technique of the joint conference committee may work well and may permit a relationship that is as pleasant as it is profitable. The agenda of the meetings should include any and all hospital problems, and frankness and honesty should characterize the discussions. These meetings, too, should be held regularly to avoid "government by crisis." It is as important for the board to understand the problems of the administration and the staff.

Membership of physicians on the governing board is now widely accepted; and I feel this is as it should be, but only if it is the chief of staff who is the member. Since he is the leader of the staff, only he should speak for the staff.

APPOINTMENT OF COMMITTEES

Committee work is the backbone of staff administration. The chief of staff must exercise his leadership in their selection, and committee appointments should actually precede the chief's inauguration so that these people are ready to serve when the chief takes office. These appointments may represent the chief's first major decisions. Service on committees has been described as the "tithe" doctors must pay for membership on a staff.[5] This is not a bad way of looking at it.

Basically, we have too many physicians on too many committees. Too many committees are appointed because of tradition or because of extramural pressure; too many committees exist without clearly defined aims and purposes; too many committees have too little to do to maintain the interest of the members; too many committees suffer from lack of communication with the chief of staff and the executive committee. The net result is frustration, exasperation, loss of interest, and loss of the contribution the committee should be making to the staff and to the hospital. A bad committee may be worse than no committee at all.

With each committee appointment, the chief should ask himself three questions. First: "Am I appointing this committee because it performs a useful function within this hospital?" Second: "Will the chairman and the members know and understand the task for which I am appointing them?" And third: "Do I, as the chief of staff, know and understand the task for which I am appointing them?" The answers are self-evident. There is another question: "Have I appointed committees whose aims and purposes overlap or are related, and would it not be better to name one committee with wider responsibility than to name two or three with too little to do to justify their existence?" Few gardens can profit as much from periodic weeding, pruning, and transplanting as the garden we call our committee structure.

STAFF DISCIPLINE

Leadership involves discipline and the enforcement of the staff bylaws. Disciplining one's associates is never easy. There are two varieties of discipline: the first is the kind that is written into the bylaws, such as suspension of privileges for delinquent records or for failure to attend meetings. These should be so clearly written and so well known and understood by the staff that the chief need play no part in their enforcement.

The second, more serious variety involves alleged breaches of personal or professional conduct. The appropriate punishment fitting these crimes may range from reprimand to dismissal from the staff. Any serious action must be predicated upon full access to the facts, full discussion with the staff executive committee, the full knowledge of the administrator and the board, and complete compliance with staff bylaws. It is dangerous for a chief of staff to attempt to sail alone between the Scylla and Charybdis of breach of contract, libel and slander, or conspiracy. He should have the administrator holding his left hand, the hospital attorney holding his right, and the president of the board hovering overhead as a guardian angel. Each hospital should carry sufficient liability insurance for its chief, for all the staff officers, for department and division chairmen, and for committee men to protect them in the event of legal action incurred in the performance of their staff duties.

STANDARDS OF PATIENT CARE

Another area of leadership by the chief of staff lies in maintaining standards of patient care. Although ultimate legal responsibility for patient care lies with the governing board, these men who are not physicians obviously cannot take an active role. Accordingly, they give a mandate to the staff. That the staff fulfills the responsibility inherent in this mandate is a proper concern to the chief of staff. The chief is supported by the chairmen of the clinical departments and divisions. Most specific questions can be referred to these physicians because they constitute immediate and urgent matters for the departmental or division chairmen. The chief's responsibility is not thus removed, nor is the necessity for an answer from him removed; rather he delegates the investigation and corrective action to the appropriate chairman.

Quality Control

There is other help in promoting high standards of patient care which has many names but which is often known as "quality control." This concept has two faces. The more notorious one is the witch hunt, the seeking out of those members of the staff with poor practice habits or even the downright scoundrel. A good chief, and certainly a good department chairman, usually needs no help in identifying these individuals.

The other face of quality control is far more important. By systematic analysis of current patient care we may assure ourselves that each patient is getting the best care possible. An additional factor, now as never before, is that the public in general, and governing boards in particular, are requiring proof of the effectiveness of our mandate.

CONTINUING EDUCATION

Several factors taken together make it necessary for the chief to assume the leadership for continuing medical education within his hospital. First, the body of medical knowledge is burgeoning so rapidly that the physician who stops learning today is out of date tomorrow.

Second, in most metropolitan areas, the county medical society is no longer the traditional "medical home" for today's physicians.

Third, because of the extent of specialization, a physician who may be reasonably current within his own province finds it difficult to be even modestly abreast with the mainstream of medicine.

If these premises are true, and I believe they are, our hospital must assume the role of a latter-day alma mater.

Hospitals with House Staff

For the hospital with a house staff, the concept of including the active staff in the existing educational program is almost as easy as moving the conferences to a larger room—almost. These teaching hospitals already have a basic science course, a clinico-pathological conference, a tumor conference, general staff meetings, and department and division meetings. In addition to an existing program, the staff also has the annual stimulation of new interns and residents. In seeking approval for training programs, the staff asks for the responsibility of teaching. One other point is worth making. We can teach them the art, we can teach them the science, and we can teach them by continuing to learn ourselves. The habits of continuing education that we demonstrate will stay with them all their professional lives.

Hospitals Without House Staff

For the hospital without a house staff the concept of continuing education within the hospital may be revolutionary, but it can be done. Fundamentally it depends upon a properly qualified, properly motivated, and properly led professional staff. Our hospital has become our nourishing mother. It will do its job well or poorly depending largely upon the leadership provided by the chief of staff.

INTANGIBLES OF LEADERSHIP

Leadership is an intangible thing. It is honor, the highest honor a staff can confer upon one of its members. It is a state of mind. It is a conscious updating and modifying of staff plans and policies. It is bringing to fruition the planning that was begun in years past. Leadership is an excursion into the future. No chief can be content to deal only with the moment, only with the present. Regardless of the years required to attain a goal, leadership involves beginning the project now.

SUMMARY

The chief of staff is the keystone in the structure of better relationships and better understanding within the hospital. He is the leader in tearing away the "gauze curtain" and closing the chasm of misunderstanding. But he cannot do this alone; he must have the support of his staff. He must have wise and faithful lieutenants on his executive committee, and he must have effective staff committees. The staff owes him this support for the time and effort that he must spend in his position. He must have the support of administration and the board; he must have their understanding, their counsel, their advice.

Yet why should he lead? Why should we regard the hospital as a unit? Why are better relationships and understanding so desirable? Why do we seek coordination, cooperation, communication? Why must our goals be the same, and why must we reach for them together? The answer to these questions is the same—for better patient care. Collectively our best is better than any of us can achieve alone.

BIBLIOGRAPHY

1. Taylor, K. O.: What Does the Hospital Owe the Doctor? *Hospital Prog.*, 46:65–68 (Jan.) 1965.

2. Flanagan, J. J., SJ: Implications for Hospitals, *Hospital Prog.*, 46:125–127 (Jan.) 1965.

3. Williams, K. J.: Your Medical Staff—a Potential for Hospital P.R., *Canadian Hospital*, 39:52–55 (Sept.) 1962.

4. Jack, W. W.: Duties of the Chief of Staff, *Hospital Prog.*, 46:77–81 (Jan.) 1965.

5. Patients, Surgeons, and Hospitals, American College of Surgeons. (In press.)

5

The Functions of the Medical Director

I. THE VIEWPOINT OF THE CHIEF OF STAFF

By James B. Osbaldeston, M.D.

James B. Osbaldeston received the M.D. degree from the University of Toronto and practices general medicine in Hamilton, Ontario, where he is an active member of the medical staff of St. Joseph's Hospital. In addition to being chief of staff, he has served as president of the staff and as chairman of many staff committees, including the executive committee, the credentials committee, the medical audit committee, and the education committee. He is a part-time field staff representative for the Canadian Council on Hospital Accreditation.

The Guide Issue of *Hospitals, JAHA,* August 1, 1965, gives the following data for St. Joseph's Hospital in Hamilton: Beds, 765; Admissions, 24,538; Census, 566; Bassinets, 125; Births, 3,-984; Newborn census, 72; Total expenses, $8,-108,098; Personnel, 1,686. The population of Hamilton, Ontario in the 1961 census was 273,991.

(ED. NOTE: *The two sections of this chapter present different viewpoints, that of a chief of staff in a hospital that employs a medical director, Dr. Osbaldeston, and that of a physician who has served as medical director in several hospitals, Dr. Williams.*)

In the search for better methods to improve patient care, the position of hospital medical director has evolved, and it promises to exert a dominant influence. The position is pivotal in the relationship between administration and the medical staff. The medical director is the administrative officer who is vitally concerned with all medical staff affairs and who is oriented to the staff's needs. He supervises medical staff organizational activities and directs the review and analysis of patient care.

The appointment of a medical director alters the organizational pattern because he assumes many of the traditional functions and responsibilities of the chief of staff. In some hospitals, the office of chief of staff has been discontinued in favor of that of the medical director. In those hospitals that retain the office, the chief of staff serves primarily as the chairman of the executive committee.

In administrative relationships, the medical director is appointed by the board of trustees, and he is responsible to them through the hospital administrator. The director's work is more effective if he has direct administrative supervision over certain departments such as radiology, laboratories, pharmacy, and medical records.

Qualifications. This sensitive position requires a mature physician who is trained and experienced in medical administration and who is held in high esteem for his integrity. On occasion he may be called on to meet difficult situations with resolute action. A background of medical practice is important to this new career in medicine because it forms a basis for the medical director's understanding of the everyday affairs of the physician and the physician's patients.

Authority. All members of the medical staff are under the jurisdiction of the medical director, whose authority and responsibility stem directly from the board of trustees. To illustrate, consider a surgeon who ignores the protests of the chief of surgery and attempts a procedure beyond his competence and outside of his delineated privileges. In support of the chief of the service and the bylaws, the medical director suspends the offender until the executive committee can meet. Repercussions will likely follow; and without proper authority the medical director, as well as the chief of the service, would be lost, and the medical staff bylaws would become meaningless. With the unchallenged authority of the medical director, the offending surgeon is corrected, and others will be less likely to test the rules in future.

The authority of the medical director is not so much a personal possession as a means of authority for the medical staff organization. Although an authoritarian approach may occasionally be required, the director more often operates from an educational position, acting as a catalyst to effect change when it is required.

Function, Objectives, and Philosophy. There are two major reasons why a hospital should have a medical director: First, the physician who has been trained in the many phases of hospital organization and operation is better equipped to assume the management of the professional activities of the hospital. The second reason is the matter of available time. A physician committed to a medical practice simply cannot meet all of the demands of a senior medical staff office as effectively as a full-time medical director. Sometimes a medical director is engaged to solve a staff problem or to correct a poor pattern of operation; but a well organized, efficient hospital receives even greater dividends from the appointment of a medical director because his role as a corrective agent is only a minor part of his overall function as a builder.

Medical Staff Organization. A major concern of the director is to build a sound medical staff organization with a strong executive committee that acts in accord with the responsibility and authority delegated to it. To insure a durable organization, the resources and knowledge of the medical director must be used by the executive committee to write bylaws that define terms of reference and methods of procedure for the medical staff. A well-intentioned executive committee without proper guidance may get into serious difficulties in dealing with problems such as medical incompetence, not because they misjudge the physician's incompetence but because their method of managing the problem is wrong. It is not to be concluded that the medical director is a "hatchet man;" this would not only impair his own effectiveness but would also weaken the executive committee by their abdication of responsibility. The executive committee must examine, evaluate, and make recommendations to the board of trustees in such problems. The medical director's expert knowledge is invaluable in guiding their efforts in accord with a proper and fair method which has been predetermined and described in the bylaws. In all matters, the executive committee must function as the "cabinet of the medical staff" with the medical director acting as its expert advisor.

Selection and Development of Staff Officers. In many respects, the medical director is a management executive who must search out promising physicians and assist in their development for appointment to office in the medical staff organization. The appointment of a physician to a senior staff office should culminate a planned program of development that provides the appointee with experience and responsibility. Physician participation in all aspects of hospital operation is increasing, making it more important than ever that the best prepared individuals be selected and trained for office.

Supervision of Patient Care. Supervision of patient care requires an awareness of the everyday care rendered in the hospital and an assessment by competent physicians of the quality of that care. Department chiefs supervise the care in their own departments and report to the medical director, who is responsible for the supervision on a hospital-wide basis. When a problem relating to the quality of care is identified, the medical director presents the facts to the executive committee; they must evaluate the situation and recommend appropriate action, carrying it to the board of trustees if indicated.

Evaluation of Patient Care. The medical director provides leadership in the review and analysis of patient care. Department heads and departmental quality control committees review their own care, working with the director whose expert knowledge dictates the most effective methods of review. It is not uncommon for tissue committees, for example, to spend many hours in a superficial review of all surgical tissues when a review in depth of those from single disease entities would yield more useful information. Ineffective evaluation of care is a triple waste—it does not get the intended job done, it wastes the valuable time of physicians, and it causes committee members to lose interest. With the director's knowledge of medical audit, the quality control committees replace mere mechanical checking of patient charts with more exciting methods that involve the exercise of professional judgment.

The Commission on Professional and Hospital Activities, in their PAS-MAP programs, provides an invaluable tool to assist the evaluation of care, and its potential is staggering. However, the value of the program is proportional to one's ability and willingness to utilize it.

Coordination. The complexity of hospital organization may give rise to poorly coordinated activity among medical staff officers, committees, and members. This is commonly caused by ineffective communication. Committee action may be largely lost unless it is reported to the staff members. The physicians who serve on committees lose interest and initiative unless their recommendations are implemented and the results are made known to them.

Coordination, to the medical director, means the establishment and maintenance of channels of communication. As secretary of the executive committee, the medical director records and circulates the minutes of the meetings, lists the names of those responsible for actions directed by the committee, and places items requiring follow-up on the agenda of the next meeting. The medical director also channels hospital communications relative to the medical staff to all concerned. A medical director's newsletter is an excellent method of communicating scattered but nevertheless important items to the medical staff.

Education. The increased scope of education in the hospital necessitates better planning. There is a great opportunity in the area of continuing medical education which falls naturally to a medical director. He may delegate this work to a director of medical education, especially in larger institutions.

Physician Relationship. By stressing the function of the medical director in the organized medical staff, it is not implied that his role is small in relation to the individual staff physician. The director must be sensitive and understanding in dealing with individuals. On occasion he may oppose physicians, but he should covet their trust, and he should become the indispensable partner of the medical staff. Trust and confidence will bring staff physicians to the medical director to seek his counsel on many subjects.

SUMMARY

There is no argument that an effectively organized medical staff, assuming its role in the supervision and evaluation of patient care, can bring great improvement in the quality of care. But there is often some question as to how well organization, supervision, and evaluation can be achieved. The motivation of medical staffs is not in doubt but rather the time available and the specialized knowledge necessary to effectively conduct the affairs of even a moderate-sized hospital.

The creation of the position of medical director introduces a concept that has a powerful impact on hospitals, their medical staffs, and ultimately on every patient. Creation of this position stems from the need for a trained physician, employed on a full-time basis, to be responsible for the management of professional activities of the hospital. For the medical staff, the appointment of a medical director does not mean reduced participation in hospital affairs but rather a more meaningful and a more effective role in the hospital organization.

II. WHY A MEDICAL DIRECTOR?

By Kenneth J. Williams, M.D.

Kenneth J. Williams is the medical director of Saint John Hospital in Detroit. He was a high-rigger in logging camps in British Columbia for several years before entering the University of Manitoba Medical School from whence he received the M.D. degree. After eight years of private practice in British Columbia, he entered Yale University and earned the M.P.H. degree in Hospital Administration in 1959. He was medical director of St. Joseph's Hospital in Hamilton, Ontario, for five years, during which period he was a surveyor and field representative for the Canadian Council on Hospital Accreditation and consultant medical director to three other hospitals. He is a Fellow of the American College of Physicians and a member of the American College of Hospital Administrators. He is also consultant medical director to the Hospitals of the Sisters of St. Joseph of Nazareth, Nazareth, Michigan.

The Guide Issue of *Hospitals, JAHA,* August 1, 1965, gives the following data on Saint John Hospital: Beds, 292; Admissions, 15,606; Census, 282; Bassinets, 80; Births, 4,798; Newborn census, 58; Total expenses, $5,182,000; Payroll, $3,140,000; Personnel, 735. (*Ed. Note: Since this issue of* Hospitals, *Saint John Hospital has opened up a 200-bed addition, bringing the total bed capacity to 500.)*

(ED. NOTE: *This section is reprinted by permission of* Hospitals, JAHA, *39:74–84 (Nov. 16) 1965. This is a paper presented at the 1965 annual meeting of the American Hospital Association in San Francisco, August 30 to September 2, 1965. Dr. Williams also presented this material in a seminar at the Hospital Medical Staff Conference in Estes Park, Colorado, October 11 to 13, 1965.*

In contradistinction to the director of medical education—the person primarily concerned with the establishment, maintenance, and improvement of intern and residency training programs in the hospital—the medical director is the physician member of the administrative team who has been given the responsibility for directing all the activities of the entire medical staff.

At first glance, the phrases "all the activities" and the "entire medical staff" might conjure up visions that the medical director is a fearsome individual with unusual powers to be used for the subjugation of the practicing physician and the elimination of his clinical freedoms. This is obviously not the way the medical director—or any person in any organization for that matter—directs the medical staff, although one can expect a certain amount of this reaction when the medical director is superimposed on a long-established, traditional organization.

The relationship of the medical director to the administrator and to the governing board is usually shown in the table of organization in one of two ways. The first concept predicates that the medical director is a member of the administrative team and reports to the chief executive officer of the hospital. He is the administrator's chief assistant and is in charge of the most important area of activity in the hospital. Because of this and because his authority stems initially from the governing board,

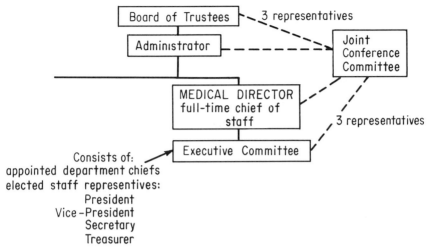

Fig. 5–1. One concept of the relationship of the medical director to others in the administrative team.

he should accompany the administrator to board meetings to report on medical staff activities. His presence there is as an assistant to the chief executive officer (Fig. 5-1).

The second concept entails a certain dichotomy of authority and responsibility within the internal organization of the hospital. Here the medical director answers directly to the governing board authority. Proponents of this arrangement maintain that inasmuch as the hospital governing board's prime responsibility to the public is for the maintenance of high professional standards it should therefore appoint an individual to organize and administer the medical staff organization and be answerable directly to the board. This is shown in Figure 5-2.

Whether the medical director reports to the board directly or through the administrator, there must be a close working relationship between the medical director and the administrator. Regardless of the way his relationship to the board is delineated, successful function and attainment of objectives are contingent upon the existence of mutual respect, trust, and understanding between the governing board, administrator, and medical director.

When the medical director is a member of the administrative team and reports to the administrator, he, in addition to being responsible for medical staff organization and activity, may be assigned such paramedical departments as the pharmacy, medical record department, medical library, and out-patient department. He may also be designated as the administrative officer in charge of laboratories and radiology, and be responsible for the working out of contractual arrangements for these professional departments. The extent to which he becomes involved

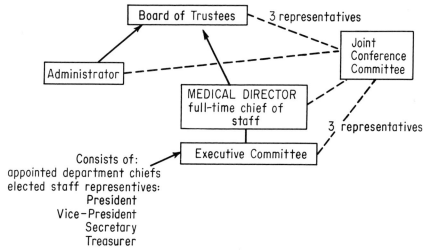

Fig. 5–2. A second concept of the relationship of the medical director showing a dichotomy of authority and responsibility.

in areas distinct from the medical staff organization depends upon several factors, such as the size of the staff, whether or not the chief executive officer is an M.D., whether there are full-time chiefs, the effectiveness and efficiency with which medical staff functions are carried out, the existence of medical school affiliation, and the extent to which house staff training programs have been developed.

Usually, the medical director in most community general hospitals will be involved in directing and guiding the establishment of sound medical staff organization and in assisting the medical staff in adequately fulfilling its numerous functions. In short, he assumes the duties and responsibilities of the traditional chief of staff position.

TRADITIONAL POSITION

Understandably, the idea of the disappearance of the traditional chief of staff position does not set well with some staffs or even with some administrators who may regard a medical director as a threat to their own security. Let us examine this thesis for a moment.

If medical care is the most important component of patient care, it follows that the chief of staff holds, next to the administrator, the most important position in the hospital organization below the governing board level. Does it not then follow that this person should have other qualifications besides several years of clinical experience? Should he not have some training in administration, be knowledgeable concerning overall hospital operation, be present and active in administrative conferences, and be informed on medical staff organization? Should he not be an expert on medical staff bylaws, rules and regulations, and be thoroughly conversant with the use of medical audit techniques in continuing medical education programs? Should he not also be physically present in the hospital to enforce the rules and regulations and to fulfill all the other functions spelled out for him in the *Supplement to the Standards* of the JCAH?

All the nonmedical aspects of the hospital organization are being examined and modern methods and techniques of management applied to job descriptions, employee performance ratings, uniform accounting, cost analysis, and work simplification programs. Courses have been established in human relations and management techniques for practically every person holding a supervisory position in the hospital, except for the one person who has charge of the most important single area of activity in the entire hospital operation: the chief of staff.

BASICALLY UNCHANGED

The medical staff organization and chief of staff role remain basically the same as when they were introduced to the hospital organization chart some 40 years ago. Yet the individual physician and the medical staff as a whole continue to exert an ever greater influence on practically all aspects of hospital operation. Quality, quantity, and cost of medical care in the hospital setting today are inseparably bound together. We cannot ignore the increasing demands to use improved methods for the review, analysis, and evaluation of clinical practice.

Although the chief of staff position has worked well in the past, this role must be reevaluated in the light of changing times. Should not the manager of the most important department in the hospital have continuity of office, training in management leadership techniques, as well as clinical experience, so that he can pursue all the administrative details for which he is responsible and be free of economic worries?

The heat that is sometimes engendered by the suggestion the chief of staff could be replaced by a full-time medical director is largely due to the fact that the role of the chief of staff is not fully comprehended. All too frequently one encounters the firm belief that the chief of staff is the medical staff's man, whereas in actual fact he is the hospital's man. The board of trustees have literally been given a trust by the public —by the patients for whom they must accept responsibility. This trust, under our voluntary hospital system, requires that the trustees have total accountability for all that goes on within the hospital. This includes being responsible for the establishment, maintenance, and improvement of professional standards. To this end they appoint, or cause to be appointed, a physician to whom they delegate the responsibility and commensurate authority. His delegated responsibility and authority stems from the board of trustees, not from the medical staff.

The mistaken concept that the chief of staff is the medical staff's man is the more prevalent in those hospitals where the chief of staff is elected and where he fills both the office of chief *and* the office of president. The basis for conflict here should be readily apparent. Once it is fully appreciated that the chief of staff is the hospital's (the board of trustees') man, much of the confusion is cleared away and there is a better understanding of the medical director's role.

The fact that a full-time medical director is present to assume the responsibilities of the traditional chief of staff does not prevent the medical staff from governing itself. He does not preside over the general staff meetings; that is the function of the elected president. He does not preside over the executive committee; that is the function of the chairman of the executive committee who has been appointed by them with the approval of the board of trustees. The medical director serves as the secretary of the executive committee, as the resource person and catalyst, as a guide, and at times as a conscience of the executive committee.

FORMAL LIAISON

The presence of a full-time medical director does not preclude formal liaison of the staff with the board of trustees through the joint conference committee or by physicians serving as board members. Such formal liaison is essential (Figs. 5-1 and 5-2). The medical director achieves his objectives—which are the same as those of the staff and board—by close cooperation with the staff and by gaining their respect and trust. He cannot work by the authoritarian approach alone. His personal actions and the guidance he gives to the staff must bear scrutiny by both the staff and trustees. Hence, formal meetings of liaison are imperative.

In considering the composition of the joint conference committee when the staff is organized and administered by a medical director—i.e., a full time chief of staff—it should be borne in mind that the medical director, although he may at times have to take a stand along with the staff, he is nonetheless the trustees' man. It is recommended that the joint conference committee consist of the president and two other members of the governing board, the elected president of the medical staff and two other members (from the executive committee), the administrator and the medical director.

The presence of a full-time medical director does not restrict the clinical freedoms of physicians. He does not interject himself between patient and doctor. Instead, he develops strong departmental chiefs and a strong and durable executive committee which makes the clinical value judgments on individuals and which discharges the collective responsibility of the staff.

The presence of a full-time medical director does not preclude the staff or executive committee from placing—and to quote from the Joint Commission on Accreditation of Hospitals—the "heavy emphasis on group participation in evaluating clinical practice." On the contrary, his experience in clinical practice, his knowledge of medical audit methodology and data retrieval techniques, and the fact that he has the time to devote to these educational programs permit him to provide a wealth of data to the extent that there can be an even greater degree of group participation.

The growing interest of trustees, administrators, and medical staffs in the role of the medical director suggests that the most important area of hospital operation should have a full-time, trained person in charge.

6

Control of Quality of Medical Care

By Karl S. Klicka, M.D.

Karl S. Klicka, president of the Appalachian Regional Hospitals, has a distinguished record in hospital administration and planning. The organization he directs is a non-profit, non-sectarian corporation operating a system of ten community hospitals in Kentucky, Virginia, and West Virginia. These hospitals have 1,021 beds and serve 25 counties. The ten hospitals employ 1,800 people. Dr. Klicka received the M.D. degree from Western Reserve University and the Master's degree in Hospital Administration from the University of Chicago. His hospital experience began as the assistant director of the Grasslands Hospital in Valhalla, New York, and continued after three and one-half years as a medical corps officer in World War II. He was director of Woman's Hospital in New York, then director of St. Barnabas Hospital in Minneapolis, and later director of Presbyterian Hospital in Chicago, where he supervised an expansion program and a merger between Presbyterian and St. Luke's (Episcopal) Hospitals. Before Dr. Klicka assumed his present position, he served for nearly five years as executive director of the Metropolitan Hospital Planning Council of Chicago. He worked with the officials and physicians of 145 hospitals in developing new hospitals and renovating and expanding existing hospitals for a seven-county area inhabited by almost 7 million people. Dr. Klicka was appointed Executive Director of the Peoples Community Hospital Authority, Wayne, Michigan, on September 12, 1966.

The word "control" in the title of this chapter is rather forceful, but there is no doubt regarding its meaning. Control connotes responsibility and authority. It implies the right to insist that certain rules of conduct be obeyed and the right to penalize those who do not obey. Control also means power, and it is achieved in various ways. It may be bestowed by election by those who wish to be governed. It may be established by legal process. It may be given as an appointment by a person in a higher position of authority. But always it is handed to a person or persons presumed to have the wisdom and leadership for properly exercising control.

Control is not necessarily permanent. The person elected or appointed to a position of control retains this position so long as he satisfactorily serves those who chose him.

People react differently to control. Some seek it because they like power. Some reject it because they prefer to be led. Some abhor it because they fear it will affect their freedom. Some support it because they feel it will assure stability.

GOVERNMENT CONTROL

The American Medical Association, in opposing federal legislation for payment of hospital care to aged persons receiving social security benefits, fought from the platform of fear of control. The position of American medicine was always crystal clear. The doctors' argument was merely that this action by the federal government was another step toward control of the practice of medicine. I think, however, it is more of a leap than a step. Whether there will be other steps, I think, depends upon us doctors, and I shall have more to say on this subject later. Meanwhile, we might reflect on the fact that members of the medical profession helped to draft the new government program; and our fellow physicians will play an important role in the top-level administration of it.

Certainly, our elected representatives in organized medicine have demonstrated their reaction to fear of control. These physicians fought against the amendment of the Social Security Act even though many of them knew that it offered a way of paying for the hospital care of patients who found it difficult or impossible to do so themselves. Most physicians who have carefully considered this problem know that financing the care of the aged and the care of the sick poor—whether they be aged, middle-aged, or young—has been an increasingly serious problem in this country for many years.

Unfortunately, conventional methods of financing have not solved this problem in our hospitals, whether they are publicly owned or voluntary non-profit hospitals. Blue Cross and Blue Shield have been unable to do it. The amendment to the Social Security Act gives reasonably good indications that a greater portion of this problem can be solved. But despite this, organized medicine opposed the program primarily because of fear that in the administration of the program, control by the federal government would emerge in a much larger form than had ever existed before.

Like it or not, the proposed amendment has passed and exists as Public Law 89-95. There is no question in my mind that the government now will exercise greater control than heretofore. It remains to be seen, however, whether this control will be harmful or beneficial, for it may be either. But the point that should be emphasized is that this control need not increase substantially or increase in a way that will handicap us as physicians, unless this becomes necessary. By necessary I mean that government personnel who have been put into a position of control will be guided by the electors of this nation. These electors will direct them to increase or decrease their control over the practice of medicine on the basis of how satisfied or dissatisfied the average citizen is with the quality and quantity of medical care available to him in hospitals and doctors' offices.

A doctor fears control because to him it means regimentation, restrictions, and the imposition of rules and regulations that may infringe on his freedom to practice his profession as he feels he properly should. It is understandable, therefore, why doctors react as they do to new controls that may affect their method of practice.

I purposely say "new controls," for many controls already exist that doctors have learned to live with. We can cite as examples the public health controls that regulate the conduct of physicians as they practice in communities. Generally speaking, physicians accept the controls laid down by the city, county, and state health departments as being in the public interest. Doctors have also come to accept the controls imposed by community hospital planning agencies, but with the proviso that such planning be kept on a voluntary basis. This field is undergoing rapid changes; however, unless community hospital planning can demonstrate that it will work successfully on a voluntary basis, we may very well see legislation passed to make it compulsory. Already in New York State a new law has brought a certain amount of regulation into community hospital planning.

QUALITY OF MEDICAL CARE IN HOSPITALS

We are specifically interested in control as it applies to the quality of medical care and the manner in which quality is controlled in hospitals. We will focus our attention on the role of the chief of staff as the delegate of hospital trustees in controlling the quality of medical care.

The Role of Trustees

Since the 1920's the control of the quality of medical care has been recognized as a function of hospital trustees, and the courts of law have clearly held that this is their responsibility. Some physicians, nevertheless, still question the right of trustees to control the quality of medical care in hospitals. Because of this persistent questioning, the issue will be explored at some depth.

It seems proper to begin with the basic assumption that things which are in the public interest should be controlled by public representatives. At this point in our civilization there can be no question regarding the public's interest in health. The public looks at good health as a right in the same way that it looks at proper housing, food, education, and a good life regardless of race, color, or creed. We as physicians are fortunate to have training which enables us to restore good health to the sick and to prevent poor health by seeing that certain safeguards are established. Also, we have reached a point where the establishment of many protective health measures is now largely a matter of law. This is the field of public health.

In the area of the specific practice of medicine, there are no laws prescribing the manner in which we should treat sick people, and our profession understandably wishes to prevent the establishment of such legal controls. The public, however, wants to be assured that when they are sick and place their lives in the hands of physicians, the process of curing will be done as quickly, effectively, and inexpensively as possible. This, then, is our challenge. The public is very interested in this process and manifests its interest by voraciously reading articles on this subject in the popular magazines and newspapers. The headlines acknowledge the publishers' recognition of the public's interest.

Although physicians like to believe that they are now voluntarily submitting to a maximum number of controls, it is apparent that some outside dissatisfaction does exist. As an example, in the amended Social Security Act (Medicare) the establishment of utilization committees in the medical staff organization is a basic requirement that a hospital must meet before it can participate in the benefits of this legislation. The utilization committee, as you know, checks on whether a patient is being retained in the hospital longer than is necessary or whether he should have been admitted to the hospital at all. By this we see that the federal government is already looking into whether quality care is being provided as inexpensively as possible.

Although we like to believe that physicians do subject themselves voluntarily to control by their colleagues as they practice together in hospitals, actually there are large voids in the systems currently used.

Surgeons know that the tissue committee helps to control surgery in a hospital. The internists, pediatricians, and all of the non-surgical specialists know that a technique similar to the tissue committee approach to quality control has not yet been developed for their specialties. The closest approach to it is the PAS and the MAP systems.* Although these are being adopted by an increasing number of hospitals, there are still many hospitals which do not use these systems properly. An adequate system, however, is essential to the proper control of medical practice by physicians, and hospital trustees look to their medical staffs to develop and to administer the system.

Trustees are bankers, industrialists, merchants, lawyers, housewives, engineers, and tradesmen. They are not doctors and therefore cannot directly control the quality of care in their hospitals, even though they are all aware that legally, by statute, trustees are held responsible for the quality of care practiced in their hospitals. They must insist, therefore, that the system used by doctors in controlling the practice of medical care be practical and effective.

Trustees do what they can to help. They work with the hospital administrators to provide facilities that are conducive to the practice of good medicine. They should also provide proper financing so that adequately paid personnel are available to carry out the orders of the staff physicians. In other words, the trustees working with administrators should do everything they can to provide the proper environment for the practice of medicine.

The Role of the Medical Staff

How does a medical staff assure the trustees that every physician on the staff is practicing as competently as a physician should be expected to practice within the framework of today's knowledge? Medical staffs have bylaws setting forth rules and regulations that each physician is supposed to follow. This is important, and the Joint Commission on Accreditation of Hospitals examines these bylaws quite critically to see whether they establish proper safeguards for patients who come to the hospitals for care. The Joint Commission surveyors are the first to acknowledge, however, that it is difficult for them to measure the extent to which physicians follow these bylaws. It is difficult also for the surveyors to determine how well the chiefs of the various departments and the chief of staff of the hospital carry out the role that the trustees expect them to play in controlling the quality of care.

Being a chief of staff is not easy and takes courage. There are many

* The Professional Activity Study (PAS) and the Medical Audit Program (MAP) of the Commission on Professional and Hospital Activities, Ann Arbor, Michigan.

situations in which the solution of a problem is hard and may even lead to the break of a longstanding friendship with another physician.

A problem of this nature came up recently in one of our hospitals in the mountains. The chief of staff and his chief of the surgical service telephoned me to report this situation:

> A physician on the staff was treating a 14-year-old girl for a displaced fracture of the lower leg. The radiologist twice had reported a poor position of the fracture to the child's physician. The chief of the surgical service concurred with the radiologist that the child would have an improperly functioning leg unless the fracture were manipulated and properly set. The chief had told the child's physician that the patient should either be transferred to an orthopedic surgeon or placed in the care of a general surgeon. The physician was not impressed by the opinion and went so far as to say he would resign from the staff if the chief of service interfered in the treatment. It was at this point that I was called. In the course of our conversation I was told that the young girl's parents were not available for consultation. The surgeon did not feel it wise to confront the young patient with the fact that in his judgment she was not receiving adequate care. I thanked them for calling me and for taking the course of action they had followed. I urged the chief of surgery to assume the responsibility for the care of the child and to transfer her to his service. At the time of this writing the doctor involved has not resigned from the staff, and it seems unlikely that he will do so.

The example illustrates how the chief of staff, the chief of service, and the hospital administrator can work together as teammates in controlling the quality of care in a hospital. The chief of staff had been alerted to the potentially dangerous situation in the hospital by the chairman of the department of surgery. After the chief of staff and chairman of the department had evaluated the problem, they made a recommendation. By accepting their recommendation, I assured them of my support in the event of further complications regarding the physician involved.

The physician, taking umbrage, could have done more than resign. He could have taken the issue to the board of trustees. In anticipation of such developments, the administrator and the chief of staff should be in agreement regarding any action that interrupts a course of treatment being pursued by a doctor on the staff. Should an issue be made about it, they then can stand together in explaining why they acted to protect the patient's interest.

We can recognize that each time a patient's interest is protected the interests of the trustees and the hospital are protected. When a patient sues a hospital on the basis of alleged malpractice by a member of the medical staff, the trustees must show that they have taken every reasonable precaution in the appointment of physicians and in the administration of the rules and regulations governing the practice of medicine in the hospital. And, I need not point out that the trustees, the chief of staff, and the department heads, in taking all necessary precautions, are protecting the interests of the physician.

The Chief of Staff and the Department Chiefs

Let us consider further the manner in which the chief of staff works with department chiefs in exercising control.

The chief of staff looks to his lieutenants—the chiefs of the services—to control the quality of medical care in their individual departments. In larger hospitals, department chiefs delegate the control of quality to physicians holding subordinate positions. These subordinates, in turn, control junior physicians lower in the order. This order of responsibility might be expressed in a little jingle: "Fleas have little fleas upon their backs to bite them, and these little fleas have littler fleas and so ad infinitum." Each physician must bear the bite of his section chief or department chairman who in turn is responsible to the chief of staff for the proper performance of physicians in his department. The top man, the chief of staff, is responsible to the board of trustees who represent the public interest.

In summary, *whether we like it or not, someone must exercise control in our hospitals to assure that the quality of care is at the highest possible level.* By statute this control is given to trustees who are responsible to the public served by the hospital. Trustees exercise this control by delegation of responsibility to the medical staff which is organized so that each physician is supervised by a physician senior to him. The typical medical staff organization thus provides stability and assurances that the watchful eye of one physician upon another is always present. The extent to which this eye is alert definitely determines the manner in which medicine is practiced in that hospital.

Departmental Meetings

An effective device for implementing control is the appraisal process that takes place in departmental meetings. Here, case reviews permit the free exchange of ideas between physicians regarding patient care. When these meetings are held frequently so that the cases are fresh on everyone's mind and when doctors feel free to express their opinion of the adequacy or inadequacy of the patients' management, the process of quality control becomes relatively easy to administer. It is in these meetings that control develops, and this pattern, in my opinion, is basic and absolutely necessary. Participation by every physician in the process of control is assured. It is an effective mechanism for checking the performance of the most senior physician as well as the most junior, because in this forum everybody stands equal in his opportunity to praise or criticize the work of others.

We come then to the realization that for all practical purposes the medical staff controls its own destiny. Hospital trustees rely upon medical staffs for the self-discipline that goes hand-in-hand with self-government. So long as physicians conscientiously conduct their affairs to the satisfaction of the hospital trustees, the physicians will control themselves.

When the system of control does not function to the satisfaction of the hospital trustees and hence to the satisfaction of the general public, an alternate method of control will be found. When hospital control has changed hands in other nations, the direction has almost always been toward increased government control. This is the alternative we face in the United States if we cannot perform satisfactorily within our present system.

THE NEED FOR CONTROLS

It would seem that the need for control of the quality of medicine in our hospitals and the efficacy of the system devised to meet that need are so apparent and simple in logic that they should not warrant exposition in detail. Unfortunately, human frailties—call them excessive pride, overconfidence, or shortsightedness—tend sometimes to obscure the truth. Edmund Burke once said, "Society cannot exist unless a controlling power upon will and appetite is placed somewhere." All of us are aware of *the necessity for controls in every facet of our society*. If traffic jams up at a busy intersection, we summon a policeman to control it. If a saloon threatens to encroach on a respectable subdivision, we pass a zoning ordinance. When contamination of streams becomes a public menace, we enact a law to control pollution. The medical profession itself has successfully fought for the enactment of many, many laws controlling human conduct in order to protect the health of society.

In every case, a need had to precede the imposition of a control. The need for vesting in hospital trustees the authority to control the quality of medicine practiced in their hospitals is well established, despite the occasional dissenter. Let us not forget that we doctors first asked that lay trustees assume this responsibility—it was the American College of Surgeons which emphasized this need as it developed its hospital accreditation program in the 1920's.

As we fear the spectre of federal government control of the practice of medicine, we might find guidance in Plato's warning: *"The punishment suffered by the wise who refuse to take part in government is to live under the government of bad men.*" The doctors, because of their acknowledged wisdom in a special field, are entrusted with full control of the methods of practicing medicine. So long as they discharge that responsibility wisely and participate vigorously and conscientiously in the governing of their profession, they will not create a need for governmental control. I am confident that the medical profession will never allow that need to arise.

7

Legal Aspects of Medical Staff Function

By Arthur F. Southwick, Jr.

Arthur F. Southwick is professor of business law
in the Graduate School of Business Administration at the University of Michigan. He received
the B.A. degree from the College of Wooster,
Ohio, and the M.B.A. and LL.B. degrees from
the University of Michigan. He is widely known
for his writings in the field of hospital law.

THE HOSPITAL AS A CORPORATE INSTITUTION

The primary purpose of a non-profit, community hospital is to provide patient care of the highest possible quality. The whole trend of
social, economic, and legal events supports this assertion. As will be
noted in detail subsequently, significant and influential court decisions
have asserted, in effect, that a community hospital is directly responsible to the patient for providing competent medical care. Accordingly,
failure on the part of the hospital to control adequately medical staff
appointments and privileges, to "supervise" the attending physician, to
require the attending physician to seek consultation in problem cases,
and to remove him from a case in extreme situations may result in legal
liability. Patient care, medical education, research, programs relating
to home care, and preventive medicine are in no sense separate, nonre-
lated purposes or functions of a hospital. Rather, all aspects of the institution's work should be interrelated and integrated toward the single
goal of providing the best possible medical care.

A hospital, therefore, does not consist of two organizations or institutions—business and medical. Rather, it is a single organization. It is
imperative that all who serve the hospital recognize this concept. Accordingly, smooth and harmonious co-ordination between business administration and medical administration must be achieved to carry out the
purpose of the hospital. The organizational structure of the medical

65

staff, lines of communication, areas of responsibility, and the site of ultimate authority must be well established, respected, and utilized.

Legally, as well as ethically, the board of trustees of the hospital is ultimately responsible for standards of patient care. Hence, the medical staff is "subservient" to the board of trustees in the sense that the board is ultimately responsible for staff appointments, reappointments, privileges, the rights and responsibilities provided for in medical staff bylaws, all changes or amendments to the bylaws, and discipline of medical staff members.

This is as it should be because it is perfectly evident in today's environment that both the public and the medical profession view the community hospital as an institution where medical care is provided and not simply as a place where an unorganized group of private practitioners care individually for their patients. The public's increasing use of the hospital's emergency room is only one manifestation of the view that a hospital provides medical care. Another manifestation is the fact that outpatient services and home care programs are expanding rapidly. The advent of Medicare will, of course, accelerate these developments. From the view of the physician, his practice is more and more hospital oriented. Specialization of medical practice leads inevitably to the need for consultations, team work, and practice in groups. Arrangements for the payment of a salary by the hospital to one or more key staff physicians are bound to grow in importance and significance. The result of all this— the changing expectations of the public and the changing patterns of medical practice—is that the institutionalization of medical care is rapidly accelerating. Again, this is as it should be as available evidence indicates that there is a direct relationship between the institutional orientation of medical practice and the quality of care.* In the main, legal and ethical doctrines do not stand in the way of or inhibit these developments.

The Corporate Practice of Medicine

To be sure, from a legal point of view, the hospital cannot be formally licensed to practice medicine. Most non-profit hospitals are corporations, and lawyers are familiar with the fundamental common law rule that corporations cannot practice medicine. Under the medical practice acts of the various states, a hospital, as an organization, cannot qualify for a license to practice. In only a few states, however, do the statutes say specifically that hospitals cannot practice medicine. Even these do not specifically prohibit a non-profit institution from practicing. The result is that the rule of law banning the corporate practice of medicine is judicial in origin in most states, implied from the medical practice acts.

* Milton I. Roemer, Growth of Salaried Physicians, *Hospital Prog.* Vol. 45, No. 9, pp. 79–83, 104 (Sept.) 1964.

Therefore, such generalized legal doctrines as the corporate practice rule are significant and relevant only to particular questions in individual cases in particular jurisdictions.

Salaried Hospital Physicians. One such particular question is whether or not a non-profit hospital may employ a licensed physician on salary and bill patients for a fee. In only a very few states has this question been authoritatively answered in the negative by statutory or judicial law.* In fact, the corporate practice rule as announced by past judicial decisions originated in the context of profit-oriented business and in an age of medical quackery and commercialization. It can be forcefully argued that it should have no application to a non-profit hospital attempting to attain and maintain high standards of professional excellence.

In some states the Attorney General has issued opinions to the effect that a charitable hospital should not enter a salaried arrangement with a licensed doctor. However, such opinions do not constitute law. The Ohio court recently impliedly approved a salaried employment contract between a non-profit hospital and a medical specialist, contrary to previously announced opinions of the Attorney General.† In the light of the current state of the law as a whole across the country relative to the corporate practice rule as applied to charitable institutions, it is fair to conclude that legal doctrines do not present significant barriers to the assertion that a hospital's purpose is to provide patient care. To put the matter another way, the law of most jurisdictions, generally, does not require that the hospital as an institution confine its role to simply the providing of facilities for medical practice. A hospital is a single, vibrant institution with a purpose and not merely physical space and equipment.

Furthermore, the ethical standards of the American Medical Association do not prohibit salaried arrangements between a hospital, or other institution, and a staff doctor so long as the professional work of the physician does not result in a commercial profit to a third party and so long as there is no lay interference in the exercise of clinical judgment by the physician. A salary, per se, is not inconsistent with professional, clinical freedom. The report on Physician-Hospital Relations by the Committee on Medical Facilities, Council on Medical Service, adopted by the American Medical Association's House of Delegates at the 1964 San

---

* Litigation on this issue in the State of Iowa is noted and reported in 166 J.A.M.A. 374 (1958) and 160 J.A.M.A. 58 (1956). But, significantly, there is a distinct absence of appellate court decisions ruling specifically that a non-profit hospital may not employ a licensed physician on salary. Employment of a physician on salary by a profit corporation is more likely to be condemned. Actually, the cororate practice rule is based, historically, in most states upon premises applicable only to profit-making enterprise.

† *Lundberg v. Bay View Hospital,* 191 N.E. 2d 821 (Ohio 1963). The relevant (and inconsistent) Attorney General Opinions are #1751 (1952) and #3197 (1962).

Francisco Convention, stresses the fact that the medical staff of a hospital has responsibility for the quality of medical care in the institution and recommends that the staff be considered an integral part of the institution's administrative team.*

Standards of Professional Care

In establishing and maintaining an institution's standards of professional care, the board of trustees must, of course, regularly turn to the medical staff and its committees for advice and recommendation regarding staff appointments, reduction or restriction of privileges, and rules and regulations relative to professional and nonprofessional conduct of staff members. Indeed, failure to do so might well be a breach of legal duty by the board for the reason that in the performance of its responsibilities the board is expected to formulate policy and make specific decisions consistent with recommendations from competent professional sources. In seeking advice and recommendation, however, the board is not limited to the hospital's own medical staff. On occasion, the governing body may deem it wise to seek counsel from professional sources outside the institution. In summary, then, the fundamental role of the medical staff is to provide the hospital's governing body with advice and recommendation relating to all aspects of the institution's professional work. The staff occupies this role as a result of authority voluntarily delegated by the board of trustees.

ORGANIZATION AND BYLAWS OF THE MEDICAL STAFF

To fulfill adequately its role of advising and recommending with respect to the hospital's professional standards, the medical staff must be properly and efficiently organized. In general, a lawyer can assert his opinion that the fact of institutional medicine and the theme of joint lay and professional responsibility for the institution's standards of care require that the medical staff's executive committee be held directly accountable to the board of trustees for the quality of medical care. As pointed out by Kenneth J. Williams, M.D., the chief of staff and also the staff's executive committee are essentially the hospital's men and not the staff's. They should be selected and appointed by the board, not elected by the staff. The lay administrator of the hospital should be a member of the executive committee because he has a real concern with the hospital's professional standards. All medical staff committees having responsibility for matters relating to standards of care, especially

* "Physician-Hospital Relations," Vol. 190 *J.A.M.A.*, No. 1, October 5, 1964, pp. 74–79.

for example the credentials, tissue, medical records, pharmacy, research, and utilization committees, should be directly accountable to the executive committee. Similarly, the chiefs of the various services should be accountable to the executive committee after selection and appointment by the hospital's governing body. All of this means, of course, that individual staff physicians must take the time from personal, private interests to serve medical staff functions.

The medical staff bylaws establish the pattern of staff organization and fix rules for the internal management of staff. They should be made an actual part of the hospital's own bylaws. Ideally, as a lawyer, I would prefer just one set of bylaws for the institution—one document pertaining to both the corporation's business affairs and professional affairs. But I see no harm and probably, in fact, some psychological benefit in having two documents—the hospital bylaws and the medical staff bylaws—as long as the latter are legally incorporated into the former so that medical bylaws are part of the hospital bylaws and thereby binding upon the board of trustees. The legal mechanics for making the provisions of medical staff bylaws binding on the governing body may differ from state to state. In general, it can be said that the board of trustees must be bound by corporate action before medical staff bylaws are effective to grant rights to a member of the staff and establish responsibilities. Certainly, as a matter of justice and fairness staff physicians should be given protection from arbitrary and capricious action terminating or restricting staff privileges.

As a legal matter, the provisions of medical staff bylaws not made a part of the hospital's own bylaws are meaningless and do not operate to grant legal rights to a staff physician. Accordingly, staff physicians sometimes think they have certain rights relative to staff appointments and privileges when, in fact, they do not. To illustrate, the staff bylaws of a private, voluntary hospital provided that in pending cases of dismissal from the medical staff the physician was entitled to a statement of the charges against him and a hearing before the staff executive committee. In fact, the board dismissed a staff doctor without furnishing a statement of the charges and a hearing. The Iowa court held that the staff bylaws were not effective to create a right to a hearing.* It is a principle of American law, generally, that a member of the medical staff of a non-profit, private, voluntary hospital facing dismissal or suspension has no legal right to a statement of charges or to a hearing unless such procedures are provided for in the hospital bylaws.

Even where the medical staff bylaws have been "approved" by the hospital's governing body, the provisions of the staff bylaws may not

* *Natale v. Sisters of Mercy of Council Bluffs,* 243 Iowa 582, 52 N.W. 2d 701 (1952).

create legal rights in some states. For example, if the staff bylaws provide for a hearing but the hospital's own bylaws do not, some states have held that a hearing need not be provided in action removing a doctor from the hospital's staff.* Clearly, in such situations, the hospital's own bylaws should detail the procedures to be followed relative to staff appointments, renewals of appointments, suspension, and dismissal. In other states, however, approval of staff bylaws by the governing body will be sufficient to bind the hospital. In sum, one way or another staff bylaws should be made a part of the hospital bylaws.

Amendments. The medical staff bylaws should determine the procedure for amendment. If they have been properly incorporated into the hospital bylaws, the board and the medical staff are both legally bound by the procedure agreed upon. Again, this affords some protection to members of the medical staff against arbitrary and capricious action by the board in regard to medical staff privileges.

MEDICAL STAFF APPOINTMENTS AND PRIVILEGES

Generally, it is clear from what has already been said that the law of the United States does not give a licensed physician any absolute legal right automatically to attain or retain medical staff membership or privileges. Certainly, the state licensure laws are not a satisfactory vehicle for establishing and controlling professional standards. For one thing, these statutes specify only minimal qualifications for admission to the practice of medicine; furthermore, the disciplinary powers of the state licensure board are often quite limited. Licensing laws furnish no continuing control over an individual's professional competence.†

Legal Distinctions Between Public and Private Hospitals

In briefly reviewing the law pertaining to medical staff appointments and privileges it is necessary to draw a distinction between the public, or governmental, hospital and the private, voluntary hospital. As a general rule, the governing body of a *public or governmental hospital* must not act arbitrarily, capriciously, or unreasonably when granting,

* *Weary v. Baylor University Hospital,* 360 S.W. 2d 895 (1962).
Wolf v. LaCrosse Lutheran Hospital Assn., 181 Wis. 33 (1923).
Manczur v. Southside Hospital, 183 N.Y.S. 2d 960 (1959). Apparently a contrary position is taken in *Joseph v. Passaic Hospital Assn.,* 26 N.J. 557 (1958). Further, Pennsylvania law is clearly to the contrary. If medical staff bylaws provide for a hearing and if they have been approved by the hospital, the provisions are binding. *Berberian v. Lancaster Osteopathic Hospital Assn.,* 149 A. 2d 456 (Pa 1959).
† For a recent discussion of staff privileges see James E. Ludlam, Medical Staff Privileges: Legal Snares for the Hospital, *J. Am. Hospital Assoc.,* Vol. 38, Part I, p. 38, August 1, 1964.

withholding, or restricting medical staff privileges.* The case law indicates that a governmental hospital should have well stated rules regarding staff appointments and also rather precise and fair procedures pertaining to enforcement of the rules. The courts will inquire into the reasonableness of any given rule at issue in a staff appointment or privilege controversy and will also investigate the procedure followed by the hospital's governing body in applying the rule. In other words, a physician may succeed in court in attacking the rule as unreasonable; or, even if the rule is reasonable, he may be entitled to the procedural rights of notice and a hearing. State statutes may play an important role in the decision of specific cases, especially in California.

For example, it is unreasonable for a governmental hospital to require that staff physicians be members of the local medical society,† to require that an applicant be eligible for membership in the medical society, to decree that a physician who practices "contract medicine" is ineligible for staff membership,‡ or to rule that the board must be satisfied that patients will be given the best possible care before an individual is extended staff privileges.§ A recent California case held that a district hospital could not require its staff doctors to carry malpractice insurance as such a rule results in an unjustified delegation of authority to determine staff privileges to organizations outside the hospital.¶

On the other hand, a governmental hospital may have rules which state recognized professional criteria as a condition for staff membership. To illustrate, rules regarding the maintenance and completion of medical records and rules relative to professional qualifications as a prerequisite for defined privileges will be upheld by the courts. Surgical and specialty privileges may be restricted as long as the rules are reasonable, definite, certain, and objective.** A city hospital may have a closed staff in the radiology department as long as there are adequate reasons for such actions.††

In the majority of states, at present, the governing body of a public

---

* *Bronansh v. City of Parkersburg*, 32 Law Week 2692 (W. Va. 1964).
There are many other cases to the same effect.
† *Hamilton County Hospital v. Andrews*, 227 Ind. 217, 84 N.E. 2d 469 (1949).
Ware v. Benedict, 99 Ark. 604, 280 S.W. 2d 234 (1955).
‡ *Group Health Co-operative v. King County Medical Society*, 39 Wash. 2d 586 (1951).
§ *Wyatt v. Tahoe Forest Hospital District*, 174 Cal. App. 2d 709 (1959).
Rule too vague and hence invites arbitrary action.
¶ *Rosner v. Hospital District*, 36 Cal. Rep. 332 (1964).
** *Hamilton County Hospital v. Andrews*, 227 Ind. 217 (1949).
Jacobs v. Martin, 20 N.J. Super 531 (1952).
Green v. City of Petersburg, 154 Fla. 399 (1944).
Selden v. City of Sterling, 316 Ill. App. 455 (1942).
Memorial Hospital v. Pratt, 72 Wyo. 120 (1953).
†† *Benell v. City of Virginia*, 258 Minn. 559 (1960).

hospital can deny staff privileges to licensed osteopathic physicians and to members of other schools of the healing arts. But a court may reach a contrary result based upon its interpretation of local statutes or simply upon public policy.*

An applicant for staff privileges in a public hospital should be given a hearing, and, similarly, a hearing should be held whenever a present member of the staff is not re-appointed or whenever surgical privileges are restricted. In California, the governing body's decision must be based upon current information and facts and not upon past misconduct of the doctor.† "Temperamental unsuitability" not related to professional qualifications or competence is an invalid basis for deciding whether or not one should be granted hospital privileges in a district hospital in California.‡

But, in summary, it is perfectly clear that the public or governmental hospital may, in general, have and enforce rules controlling medical staff privileges so long as those rules bear a reasonable provable relationship to patient care and the hospital's professional standards.§ Procedures for enforcement of the rules must be fair and provide adequate opportunity for the staff member or applicant to be heard. During recent years the fundamental trend of the law generally has been to enlarge the powers of the public hospital's governing body relative to control of the institution's medical standards. Hence, the freedom of the licensed physician to practice where and how he wishes has been correspondingly reduced.

The law relative to medical staff privileges at the *private or voluntary hospitals* is largely a matter of judicial decision on a state to state basis. However, state statutes dealing with particular issues are beginning to appear and are having an impact. Moreover, Federal Constitutional Law has become significant. Both of these developments, together with state court decisions in some jurisdictions quite aside from statutory or constitutional law, have the effect of reducing the area of freedom previously enjoyed by the voluntary hospital's governing body in appointing staff physicians. Correspondingly, the physician's ability to gain staff privileges has been enhanced. The result is that the fundamental trend of the law pertaining to privileges in the private hospital may be in the opposite direction from the trend of the law pertaining to the public or governmental hospital.

* For example, see *Stribling v. Jolley*, 253 S.W. 2d 519 (Missouri 1952).
† *Wyatt* case, supra.
‡ *Rosner v. Eden Township Hospital District*, 25 Cal. Rptr. 551 (1962).
§ *North Broward Hospital District v. Mizell*, 148 So. 2d 1 (Florida 1962). Governmental hospital may determine and enforce rules for staff standards more restrictive than the rules of state licensure board. Specifically, proof that the frequency of a physician's erroneous diagnoses was excessive is an adequate basis for suspension of surgical privileges. *Mizell v. North Broward Hospital District*, 175 So. 2d 583 (Florida App. Court 1965).

Historically and traditionally the board of trustees of a voluntary hospital has not been under a legal compulsion to have reasonable rules pertaining to medical staff appointments, re-appointments, and surgical privileges. In other words, medical staff membership has been strictly a privilege and not a right. The courts have generally said that a voluntary hospital can, in effect, be arbitrary in its decision making process by giving to the governing body an almost unlimited and absolute discretion when granting or withholding appointments to the medical staff. However, if the hospital's bylaws contain provisions for a hearing, or other procedural safeguards, whenever privileges are withdrawn or restricted, the board of trustees is under a legal compulsion to follow the dictates of its own voluntarily adopted procedural rules.* The basis for this traditional posture of the courts is simply that a voluntary hospital is a private organization and, hence, may adopt whatever rules it wishes to control staff appointments and privileges.

This traditional attitude has been recently reaffirmed by courts in the District of Columbia, West Virginia, and Kansas. In *Shulman v. Washington Hospital Center*, 222 F. Supp. 59 (D.C. 1963) it was held that the governing body of a private hospital may deny reappointment to a staff doctor, providing only that bylaw requirements relative to procedural safeguards are followed. Similarly, the West Virginia court has held that a voluntary hospital, even though it receives money from the Hill-Burton program and certain tax revenues from state and county government, retains its status as a private corporation; the governing body in its discretion may exclude an individual from the medical staff without giving a reason for its action.† In the *Sams* case the physician was apparently denied staff privileges as a consequence of his participation in a closed panel group practice, although such was never formally stated as a reason for his exclusion. The Kansas Supreme Court has held that the board of trustees did not abuse its discretion in relying solely upon the recommendations of the medical staff's credentials and executive committees in rejecting an application from a surgeon for admission to the medical staff.‡

However, an important 1963 New Jersey case departed from the traditional judicial attitude and may take its place in history as the basis for a new trend—a new philosophy—relative to medical staff appointments in a private, non-profit hospital. In *Greisman v. Newcomb Hospital*, the court invalidated the bylaws of a voluntary hospital which required all staff physicians to be graduates of a medical school approved by the

* *Levin v. Sinai Hospital*, 186 Md. 174, 46 A 2d 298 (1946).
West Coast Hospital v. Hoare, 64 So. 2d 293 (Florida 1953).
Shulman v. Washington Hospital Center, 222 F. Supp. 59 (D.C. 1963).
† *Sams v. Ohio Valley General Hospital Association*, 140 S.E. 2d 457 (1965).
‡ *Foote v. Community Hospital of Beloit*, 405 P. 2d 423 (1965).

American Medical Association and members of the county medical society.* Specifically, the court held that the governing body of the hospital must at least consider the application of an osteopathic physician for staff privileges. The case followed *Falcone v. Middlesex County Medical Society* which had determined that the defendant's denial of medical society membership to a licensed osteopathic physician was in violation of the state's public policy.† Such denial was said to be an arbitrary and unreasonable exercise of power over the practice of medicine. Consistent with the declaration of public policy in *Falcone,* the court in *Greisman* said that a voluntary hospital is vested with a public interest and should not be treated strictly as a private organization, at least when it is the sole hospital in the immediate geographical area. In short, the discretionary powers of a non-profit hospital's board of trustees are "deeply imbued in public aspects and are rightly viewed, for policy reasons, as fiduciary powers to be exercised reasonably and for the public good."

Arizona has already adopted the reasoning of the *Falcone* case by ruling that a local medical society cannot arbitrarily deny membership if there is a relationship between society membership and hospital staff privileges.‡ In effect, then, these courts are saying that a medical society is not a private social club. Accordingly, in Arizona and New Jersey, at least, hospital bylaws arbitrarily excluding fully licensed physicians from staff privileges on the basis that they have not attended a medical school for at least four years or on the basis that they are ineligible for membership in the local medical society are likely invalid as contrary to public policy. All of this, of course, is consistent with the merger of the osteopathic and medical professions in California and the possible merger in other states.§

Consistent with the new trend in enhancing a physician's ability to gain staff privileges in a private, non-profit hospital, certain local statutes which restrict the discretionary powers of the hospital's board of trustees are making an appearance. For example, in Louisiana a statute prohibits a voluntary hospital from denying medical staff membership solely because of participation in group practice or lack of membership in a specialty body or professional society.¶ A similar statute relating to

---

* 40 N.J. 389, 192 A. 2d 817 (1963).

† 34 N.J. 582, 170 A. 2d 791 (1961).

‡ *Blende v. Maricopa County Medical Society,* 393 P. 2d 926 (1964).

§ A recent Missouri case is relevant and should be compared. On the basis that a Missouri statute requires that a degree obtained by a doctor be awarded by an institution actually attended by the doctor, the court approved the action of the licensing board in refusing to recognize an osteopathic physician as an M.D. The doctor had obtained the M.D. by simply registering with a California medical school. *Mitchem v. Perry,* 390 S.W. 2d 605 (1965).

¶ La. Rev. Stat. Ann., Paragraph 37:1301 (1964).

group practice and non-profit health insurance plans is in effect in New York.*

State law relating to *unlawful restraints of trade* can be used as a legal theory, or vehicle, to attack a voluntary hospital's arbitrary denial of medical staff privileges.† In the future this theory could be an increasingly popular allegation by physicians who have been denied appointments. But, fortunately, a recent California decision has held that an exclusive privilege contract for the operation of a private hospital's radiology department does not violate the restraint of trade laws as long as such a contract is entered into to assure high quality care and is in the best interests of both the public and the hospital's medical staff.‡

There is, of course, further evidence that the courts and legislatures are inclined to restrict the "private" character of a voluntary hospital and treat it as a quasi-public institution with positive duties to the public. Even prior to the Civil Rights Act of 1964, which prohibits discrimination based on race, the Federal Courts had decided that a private hospital receiving Hill-Burton funds could not discriminate on the basis of race or creed when making medical staff appointments or in admitting patients. To do so was said to be "state action" denying equal protection of the laws and hence in conflict with the 14th Amendment to the Federal Constitution.§ Moreover, quite aside from the Hill-Burton program, a voluntary hospital could not discriminate on racial factors in circumstances where a governmental unit had appointed the members of the original governing board, where certain local taxes were appropriated to the hospital's use, and where the deed to the hospital's land provided that title would revert to the county if hospital use should cease.¶

The climate of our times and the moral of legal trends are rather clear. *A voluntary hospital is never truly private in character and outreach.* It is perfectly evident that social and economic factors shape law and policy; the result is that the non-profit hospital must consider itself to be a public or quasi-public institution. *With respect to hospital medical staff appointments and privileges, the sole, overall guideline for policy must be, simply, quality of medical care.* Hospital bylaws controlling privileges must be precise, concise, and reasonably related to professional excellence. Ideally, each new applicant for appointment should be extended the opportunity for a hearing focusing upon his professional qualifications and proven ability. Certainly, a staff physician who is

---

* N.Y. Session Laws, c. 770, Par. 2 (1963).

† For example, *Willis v. Santa Anna Community Hospital Assoc.*, 20 Cal. Rep. 466 (1962).

‡ *Blank v. Palo Alto-Stanford Hospital Center*, 234 Cal. App. 2d 442, 44 Cal. Rep. 572 (1965).

§ *Simkins v. Cone Memorial Hospital*, 323 F. 2d 959 (1963).

¶ *Eaton v. Grubbs*, 32 U.S. Law Week 2523 (1964).

not to be re-appointed or whose privileges are to be restricted should be given a hearing before the appropriate medical staff committee which then makes recommendations to the board of trustees. Accordingly, an active and responsible credentials committee is a necessity for every community hospital. By the same token regular, objective review of the reports from the tissue committee will furnish evidence of competence, or incompetence, and thereby support the governing board's action in individual cases.

The law relating to medical staff privileges is interested in protecting the welfare of the public and in promoting fairness and justice for the individual physician. Conflicting interests must be balanced. Certainly, the law should fully sanction bonafide efforts to establish and maintain professional standards.* It is always wise for hospital management—lay and medical staff working jointly together—to anticipate trends and implement appropriate policy rather than waiting for specific legal compulsion in individual cases. Legal trends relative to professional standards and the vital interest of lay administration in these matters will now be examined.

THE VITAL INTEREST OF HOSPITAL ADMINISTRATION IN PROFESSIONAL STANDARDS

As previously emphasized, the matter of joint co-operation and responsibility between lay hospital administration and medical staff for the quality of medical care is a matter of utmost importance. There is ample evidence, in general, medical politics notwithstanding, that the medical profession is ready to co-operate more closely with lay administrators and the hospital's governing body in hospital management. In turn, the lay administration must be prepared to assume a more active role in the joint effort to control quality. Legal trends as expressed in judicial decisions make this imperative. The courts, to an ever increasing extent, are pin-pointing the vital interest of lay administration in professional standards.

For one thing *the courts are expanding, or even changing, the historical, traditional statements of the law relating to professional liability.*

* In *Levin v. Doctors Hospital,* 233 F. Supp. 953 (1964) the court upheld the bylaw of a proprietary hospital refusing podiatrists the right to admit patients and write orders for their care and resticting them to patient care only under the supervision of a medical staff member. Undoubtedly, the decision would apply to a voluntary hospital. Significantly, the court commented favorably upon standards promulgated by the Joint Commission on Accreditation of Hospitals. But a higher court has now ruled that the hospital's motion for summary judgment should not have been granted. There must be a trial on the merits of the plaintiff's claims that the bylaw provision was the result of a conspiracy between the Joint Commission and the hospital in violation of antitrust laws. *Levin v. Joint Commission* 354 F. 2d 515 (1965).

Traditionally, the standard of care legally required of a physician in diagnosing and treating illness has been defined by reference to the knowledge possessed and the standards exercised by other like physicians of the same school of medicine practicing in the same or similar communities. In any particular situation, the performance of an individual doctor has been measured against the performance of his colleagues similarly trained, qualified, and situated.

But, significantly, the "same or similar community" is no longer a local, geographical area. This is a natural development in our era of technological advance, mass communication, and widespread dissemination of knowledge. In effect, judicial decision is demanding that the "best" methods be adopted and accepted by all. The courts are likely to test the validity of standards existing in a particular area of geographical region against those which prevail in a distant region. The result is that there is a decided tendency to refrain from giving special protection to doctors practicing in rural or semi-rural communities. Similarly, it is no longer a valid defense to a professional liability claim that malpractice is not proved as long as nobody else performs the omission complained of or as long as everybody else in the more or less local "community" follows standards utilized by the defendant.

These observations apply with equal force to claims against both an individual physician and/or a hospital. *The performance of staff at the local community hospital is likely to be measured against standards prevailing at much larger metropolitan medical centers.*

To illustrate, in *Favalora v. Aetna* a radiologist was said to be liable in damages for failing to review the patient's history when she fainted and fell while standing on the footboard of an X-ray table even though it was not customary in the local community for radiologists to check the medical history of their patients. A review would have revealed the patient's history of fainting spells, and, further, there was evidence to the effect that medical school faculties and teaching hospitals recommend that radiologists should follow such precautions.* Further, the failure to count surgical instruments could not be excused on the ground that no other nearby, similar hospital counted instruments.† *In short, the fact that everybody in similar circumstances is negligent does not justify the defendant's conduct.‡*

* 144 So. 2d 544 (Louisiana 1962).

† *Leonard v. Watsonville Community Hospital,* 47 Cal. 2d 509 (1956).

‡ See also, *Kolesar v. United States,* 198 F. Supp. 517 (1961) where the court held physicians to higher standards of care than the community was willing to tolerate.

A most significant decision to the same effect is *Darling v. Charleston Community Hospital,* 211 N.E. 2d 253 (1965), where it was said that a hospital could not defend itself on the basis that it conformed to the practices and procedures of other similar community hospitals. The *Darling* case is discussed in detail subsequently.

Furthermore, new standards of care are being created every day in this age of scientific and technological advance. As is to be expected, these *new standards are quickly reflected in the law by both judicial decision and statute.* An example is the very recent, widespread adoption of statutes requiring hospitals to test for PKU in new-born infants. In states not yet having a statute, the courts could easily hold that failure to conduct the test creates legal liability. Both physicians and lay hospital administrators must be ever alert to advancing, changing standards of care.*

As new and improved standards of patient care are established, is it the task of the medical staff or the task of lay administration to initiate changes in a particular hospital? Actually, it must be the task of both, managing the institution in concert. The standards of professional care in the hospital are the legitimate business of every responsible person in the hospital. As has been previously emphasized, the governing body of the hospital is ultimately, legally responsible for standards of care. The lay administrator's vital interest must not be interpreted as "interference" in the clinical practice of medicine. When things go wrong in the hospital, both the institution and the attending physician are sued. It serves no real purpose for the hospital to blame the doctor and the doctor to blame the hospital, or its lay administration, or its nursing staff. *All possible defendants are likely to be joined in a lawsuit.* Accordingly, mutual efforts by lay administration and medical administration must be regularly carried out to assure control of such matters as surgical privileges for individual physicians, sponge counts, instrument counts, patient identification, medication errors, and surgical consent procedures. It is now legally well established that members of the hospital's board of trustees and lay administrators are entitled—indeed, responsible to the hospital corporation—for knowing what is going on professionally within the hospital. Specifically, a member of the board has the right to inspect patient medical records for the bonafide purpose of investigating alleged improper, non-consensual experimentation on patients. In other words, a board member has a legal duty to protect the hospital corporation, and the possibility of corporate liability gives him the right to learn the truth relative to the professional standards and activities of the medical staff.†

The vital legal interdependence between lay hospital administration and the medical staff is dramatically illustrated by an Illinois Supreme Court decision just announced. The result of this case, entitled *Darling v. Charleston Community Hospital,* in effect makes the hospital directly

---

* The legal implications of scientific advance are thoroughly explored by Oleck, New Medicolegal Standards of Care and Skill, *Cleveland Marshall Law Review,* Vol. II, No. 3, p. 443, September, 1962.
  † *Hyman v. Jewish Chronic Disease Hospital,* 258 N.Y. 2d 397 (1965).

responsible to the patient for providing competent medical care, although it is not the first decision to show a trend in this direction.*

In *Darling* the plaintiff's leg was broken during a football game, and he was taken to the emergency room of the community, voluntary hospital. A general practitioner on emergency call examined the patient and set the fractures with the assistance of hospital personnel. The leg was enclosed in a plaster cast. From the outset the patient complained of severe pain, and the attending nurses noticed and recorded swelling in the toes. The toes became dark, cold, and insensitive. After a few days the physician split the cast, and an infected laceration of the leg was noted. Everyone caring for the patient noticed a strong odor in the patient's room. For the following ten days the hospital nurses frequently informed the attending physician of the patient's continuing complaints of pain, and the doctor prescribed a number of pain relieving medications. At this point the patient was removed to a St. Louis hospital. He was placed under the care of a specialist who found that the leg contained a large amount of dead tissue resulting from circulatory impairment caused by swelling and hemorrhaging while the leg was enclosed in the cast. Ultimately, after several surgical attempts to save the leg, amputation was necessary.

Suit was brought against both the attending physician and the hospital. An out-of-court settlement was quickly concluded with the doctor, and the case proceeded to trial against the hospital. Allegations against the institution included claims that the hospital was negligent in allowing this particular doctor to engage in orthopedic practice when he was not qualified to carry such responsibility, that the institution had not reviewed the physician's qualifications following issuance of his license to practice medicine nearly three decades ago, that the hospital had failed to review the reports of the tissue committee for the purpose of determining the qualifications of all members of the staff, and that the tissue committee had failed to meet regularly to review surgical procedures being undertaken within the hospital. Also, significantly, the plaintiff alleged that the lay administrator of the hospital knew from the nurses' daily reports and other sources that this case was a "problem" and that nobody had taken steps to enforce the medical staff bylaws which required consultations with specialists in such cases. In sum, the plaintiff maintained that the nurses were at fault for failing to impress upon the administrator the seriousness of the case, and/or that the administrator was to blame for failing to involve the medical staff, and/or that the

* *Darling v. Charleston Community Memorial Hospital*, 211 N.E. 2d 253 (1965). The appellate court decision in this litigation is reported in 200 N.E. 2d 149 (1964). An application for rehearing was denied by the Supreme Court of Illinois on November 18, 1965.

staff itself was negligent in not supervising the physician and requiring consultation as provided for in the medical staff bylaws.

In support of his allegations that the hospital had failed to perform its duties to the patient, the plaintiff relied upon the standards of the Joint Commission on Accreditation of Hospitals and the standards of the Illinois Department of Health as expressed in regulations pertaining to the licensure of hospitals. Both, in essence, recite that the governing body of the hospital is ultimately responsible for patient care and the professional standards of the institution. In addition, the plaintiff called attention to the then applicable ethical standards of the American College of Hospital Administrators which stated, in effect, that an administrator's reluctance to interfere in a physician's handling of the case should never be permitted to jeopardize the patient's welfare. In summary, then, the plaintiff argued that licensing, accreditation, and ethical standards, as well as bylaw provisions, make quite clear the hospital's duties to the patient and that violation of these responsibilities creates legal liability.

The case proceeded to a jury trial, and the trial court permitted the jury to determine whether the hospital had violated its duties to the patient. The court's affirmation of the jury's verdict for the plaintiff means, in effect, that the law has sanctioned a literal application of standards promulgated by both public regulatory bodies, i.e., state hospital licensure boards, and private bodies, i.e., the Joint Commission on Accreditation of Hospitals.

Actually, the jury's verdict in this litigation against the hospital should not be surprising. The jury was not sympathetic with the hospital's contentions that it operated the same as other nearby community hospitals, that a corporation cannot practice medicine, and that a hospital is unable ever to forbid or command a physician's act in the practice of his profession. By its verdict, the jury has, in effect, said that a hospital is considerably more than a place which furnishes physical facilities for the practice of medicine by an unorganized group of practitioners. Lay people often do not understand the sometimes subtle distinction between "hospital services" and "medical services." Further, it is only natural in this age that lay people from the community at large believe that a hospital should be required to adhere literally to licensing and accreditation standards and follow provisions in medical staff bylaws. At the trial it was conceded by witnesses for the hospital that it was the governing body's responsibility to delineate medical staff privileges and that the chief of staff had not been active in this situation, in which it was widely known throughout the hospital that the attending doctor was having difficulty with the case. Moreover, it was conceded that nobody had specifically asked the chief of staff to consult with the attending physician or arrange for a consultation.

Neither should it be surprising that the Supreme Court of Illinois has now permitted the jury's verdict to stand. To be sure the decision greatly broadens a hospital's legal responsibility for the quality of professional care, but the courts have been moving in this direction for a significant period of time. In *Seneris v. Haas* the California court held a hospital liable for the malpractice of an anesthesiologist who was on regular on-call duty for the hospital, although the doctor billed the patient independently for his fee.* Three years later, in 1958, California said that a hospital was responsible to a maternity patient of whom the nurses knew of dangerous bleeding due to the physician's failure to suture properly, and they failed to notify hospital administration of the situation.† In sum, *on one legal theory or another, the courts have been saying for some period of time that a hospital is responsible to the patient for knowing what is going on professionally within its walls.*

In the *Darling* litigation the Supreme Court relied heavily upon a quotation from a 1957 New York case.‡ In that year the court said:

> The conception that the hospital does not undertake to treat the patient, does not undertake to act through its doctors and nurses, but undertakes instead simply to procure them to act upon their own responsibility, no longer reflects the fact. Present-day hospitals, as their manner of operation plainly demonstrates, do far more than furnish facilities for treatment. They regularly employ on a salary basis a large staff of physicians, nurses and interns, as well as administrative and manual workers, and they charge patients for medical care and treatment, collecting for such services, if necessary, by legal action. Certainly, the person who avails himself of hospital facilities expects that the hospital will attempt to cure him, not that its nurses or other employees will act on their own responsibility.§

To this the Illinois court added its own comment: "The standards for hospital accreditation, the state licensing regulations and the defendant's bylaws demonstrate that the medical profession and other responsible authorities regard it as both desirable and feasible that a hospital assume certain responsibilities for the care of the patient."

Specifically, the court said that the jury's verdict was supportable on either the basis that the hospital failed to have an adequately trained nursing staff capable of recognizing the patient's serious condition and of bringing the matter to the attention of administration and the medical staff so that adequate consultation could have been secured *or* on the basis that the hospital had negligently failed to require the attending doctor to consult with specialists.

What genuine implications, legally and practically, does the *Darling*

* 45 Cal. 2d 811, 291 P. 2d 915 (1955).
† *Goff v. Doctors Hospital,* 166 Cal. App. 2d 376, 333 P. 2d 29 (1958).
‡ *Bing v. Thunig,* 2 N.Y. 2d 656, 143 N.E. 2d 3 (1957).
§ Ibid, 143 N.E. 2d 8.

decision have? The case continues and expands upon a legal trend long in the making. It recognizes the realities of our age that the hospital is a community institution which furnishes medical care. It will have a very significant effect upon the management of many community hospitals because it demands that fragmentation within the walls of the institution be minimized. In other words, the historical separation between lay hospital administration, on one hand, and the clinical practice of medicine, on the other, is clearly deemphasized, if not abolished.

But lay administrators and physicians must not be emotional about these implications. The decision does not mean that the lay administrator is bound to embark upon the clinical practice of medicine nor that the chief of staff must make daily patient rounds in order to assure that all is going well. Still, the court's opinion and result of the case are likely to raise these seemingly difficult questions in the minds of administrators, nurses, and medical staff. When is the lay administrator or chief of staff justified in "interfering" or "intervening" in an attending physician's handling of a particular case? When do nurses report to the administrator —or the chief—that a staff physician is encountering difficulties in the treatment of a patient? Must lay administration minutely control the doctor's clinical practice?

The answer to the last question is clearly in the negative. Only a physician can exercise clinical judgment. But it does not follow that lay administrators, or nurses, are incapable of exercising sturdy common sense relative to "interference" or "intervention." When, in particular situations and in particular cases, there is knowledge of trouble or knowledge of incompetence, responsibility demands that lines of communication within the institution be open and functioning in the interest of patient welfare. The interest of all within the hospital, lay and medical, is the same—specifically, high quality of care.

Accordingly, the *Darling* opinion emphasizes the *need for active, continuing programs to establish, maintain, and enforce professional standards.* Such programs must be conceived and implemented by the mutual efforts of administration and medical staff. Responsible medical staff committee work is indispensable. Review of quality standards and enforcement of rules providing for consultations must, by necessity, be accomplished by the medical staff. Every hospital needs an energetic and responsible chief of staff and departmental heads whose judgment commands respect. *It is the administrator's task to be certain that his hospital has a well established and functioning procedure for quality reviews and for consultation.* This, then, does not mean that the lay administrator is called upon to practice medicine because he is not the one actually conducting reviews of clinical practice or doing a consultation. Rather, he, together with the chief of staff, is only making certain that an organized medical staff is performing its delegated responsibility.

In other words, it is the administrator's task to make certain that doctors are continually working and talking together in implementing programs designed to assure professional excellence.

All of this is simply a recognition that a hospital is a single institution which brings together a host of people of varying training, skills, and attitudes, all striving together to realize the rightful expectations of the public relative to quality health care.

8

Achieving an Effective Staff

By Floyd C. Mann, Ph.D.

Floyd C. Mann is professor of psychology at the University of Michigan. He is the director of the Center for Research on the Utilization of Scientific Knowledge (CRUSK) of the Institute for Social Research of the University of Michigan. He was formerly a study director and then program director of the Institute's Survey Research Center.

Dr. Mann has long had an interest in the problems of achieving organizational effectiveness in the hospital medical staff and in applying research findings which have been found to distinguish effective from less effective organizations.

(ED. NOTE: *An earlier version of the first part of this paper was published in* Hospital Progress, January, 1965. *The ideas in this paper were reviewed and extended in three discussion seminars in the University of Colorado Postgraduate Conference for the Hospital Medical Staff in October, 1965. Much of the work on this paper was made possible by a contract with the Health Communications Branch, Division of Community Health Service, Public Health Service.*)

In the last two decades a great deal of quantitative research has been undertaken in complex organizations to learn what distinguishes the more effective from the less effective organizational units. Studies have been done in all types of organizations: industrial and business firms, governmental agencies, voluntary associations, and hospitals. From this research[1,3,9] a pattern of findings is emerging that allows behavioral scientists to make predictions to units—such as medical staffs—which have not yet been studied intensively.

Medical staffs, like hospitals, undoubtedly differ markedly in their effectivess. While there are virtually no carefully designed, systematic studies of how the more effective medical staffs differ from the less effective ones, it is reasonably safe to predict some of the factors which would distinguish such units. High on such a list would be (1) the type of organization—the way the medical staff is organized and actually functions; (2) the type of leadership given the staff—the way the chief of staff and related associates handle the supervisory and administrative aspects of their role; and (3) the type of problem-solving procedures used within the staff—the way the key officers and the members of the medical staff identify and work toward the solution of problems their staff and hospital faces. In this paper we will draw on this growing, general body of scientific knowledge about how effective units differ from ineffective units and relate it to the practical experiences of men like Dr. Kenneth Williams, who has been actively engaged in improving the functioning of medical staffs. Our objective will be to identify some of the principal organizational and motivational forces that contribute to developing an effective medical staff.

THE ORGANIZATIONAL FORM OF THE EFFECTIVE UNIT

Organizational research has indicated that the more effective organizations are made up of relatively small work groups, or organizational families, that work together in a particular way toward the attainment of the total objectives of an organization. The individuals within the organization do not function as discrete entities but as members of a team working to meet the objectives of each subunit. The subobjectives and activities of each unit are, of course, a part of the total structure of objectives of the organization. Each of these teams is interlocked with other teams through the activities of the persons in the coordinative or supervisory roles—roles in the medical staff, such as chief of staff, department head, or chairman.

In the hospital one important task with which the chief of staff must concern himself is the development of an overlapping group form of organization. The chief of staff and his department heads need to be shaped into a cohesive organizational family working on the solution of the problems of the medical staff as a whole. Each member of this group in turn needs to develop the members of his own departmental staff into one or more equally effective problem-solving units to meet the problems for which the department is responsible. Whether the members of these groups are elected by their colleagues or appointed by the chief of staff does not matter as much as whether they recognize the multiple representational and coordinative obligations of their roles. Each department head, for example, must be able to represent the problems faced by

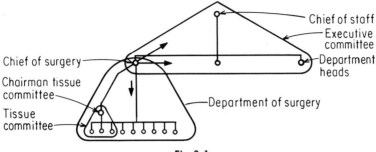

Chief of staff

Executive committee

Chief of surgery

Department heads

Chairman tissue committee

Tissue committee

Department of surgery

Fig. 8–1

his group to the next higher echelon group, to other groups on the same level, and to represent the problems faced by the higher echelon group to those in his own group. It is through these interlinking roles that the work with the medical staff is coordinated and interrelated. This co-ordination is essential for it has been found that the more effective hospitals differ from less effective hospitals in just such processes of coordination.[2]

The general model of this overlapping group form of organization we are describing here can be depicted graphically in Fig. 8-1. Arrows show the three-way interlinking function.

Research in all types of complex organizations has indicated *the importance of occupants of the key leadership roles establishing a group pattern of operation rather than a man-to-man pattern.* Occupants of key interlinking roles who work with others as single individuals do not build organizational work units which tap the full intellectual or problem-solving potential of the men in their group. They do not obtain the full motivational and commitment potential of others. Nor do they create the situation in which the full potential of the group for controlling the behavior of an individual member can be brought to bear. Figure 8-2 shows the man-to-man pattern on the left, the group pattern of organization on the right.

Organizational teams function best when all of the members of each unit, not just the key man, know what the objective is, what the obstacles

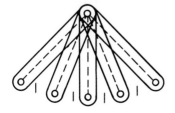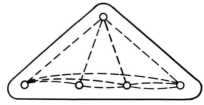

Fig. 8–2

are, and are able to pool their ideas and experiences to find ways past the obstacles to the objective. Research has shown again and again[6] that participation in group problem-solving gives an individual:

A greater opportunity to contribute his ideas
A fuller understanding of all the facets of the problem being worked on
A clearer definition of the objective
A sense of responsibility for the success of the decision

Equally important to the establishment of an overlapping group form of organization is the establishment of general goals, purposes, and specific objectives of each group. Much of this is often done in hospitals in bylaws or preambles to bylaws. Groups need to have the goals spelled out so that each member knows exactly what the group is trying to accomplish. Clarity in the statement of goals is essential because the executive committee of the medical staff needs to be able to remind itself at times that the interests of the patient are primary, not secondary, to those of the physician. Specific objectives need to be set by the member of a group and concentrated on for a particular time, then other objectives can be set and worked toward for a time.

Along with the definition of goals and the creation of organizational teams, *workable bylaws and rules and regulations need to be developed and kept up to date.* The hospital, and the medical staff in particular, needs to have this formal organizational side of its house in order. Relationships among departments and committees must be spelled out and reporting processes specified in terms of time and manner. The recommendation that the records, tissue, and audit committees report once a month in writing to the executive committee of the medical staff is only a minimal requirement of the Joint Commission on Accreditation of Hospitals.

THE SKILLS OF THE EFFECTIVE LEADER

Type of leadership is another factor that consistently distinguishes the more effective from the less effective organizational unit. There are several facets of the role of the leader that we need to understand before we note how effective leaders differ from ineffective leaders.

The key position of the role of the leader in interlocking organizational units in a complex social system like a hospital or a medical staff within a hospital was visually evident in Fig. 8-1. Research has shown that such roles as chief of staff, department head, chairman, and supervisor have a great deal in common with one another.[7] We have already noted how they serve as "structural coordinative linking pins," linking together different work units within a system. Equally important to this structural, sociological function of the role is its "motivational link pin" function, for it is through this aspect of the role of the leader that organizational objectives are finally related to individual member needs and goals.

The raison d'être of every organization is to accomplish some objective. The physical and mental capacities and energies of men are among the principal means and resources through which the objectives of organizations can be attained. But men—the potential members of an organization—also have their own goals which they want to attain through working in the organization. The interests of the individual members of the organization and the goals which they are trying to attain may or may not be the same as, or compatible with, those of the organization. One of the basic problems of organizations is how to reconcile, coordinate, or integrate member needs and goals with organizational requirements and objectives. This social psychological aspect of the role of the leader in the complex organization is of key importance; it is here that the leader must deal with the *motivational* problem of relating man and system.

This brief description of the role of the leader suggests two of the three classes of skills that an effective leader has: (1) administrative or organizational skill; (2) human relations skill; and (3) technical skill. *Administrative skill* refers to the ability of the leader to think and act in terms of the total system within which he operates in terms of the organization as a system of people and physical objects with its own image, structure, and process that functions as a continuing complex problem-solving arrangement to attain particular objectives. *Human relations skill* refers to the ability of the leader to use pertinent knowledge and methods of working with people and through people. It includes an understanding of general principles of human behavior, particularly those that involve the regulation of interpersonal relations and human motivation. *Technical skill* refers to the ability to use pertinent knowledge, methods, techniques, and equipment necessary for the performance of specific tasks and activities and to the ability to direct such performance. The three kinds of skills concern organization, people, and tasks, respectively. We might think of these three skills as dimensions and show them diagrammatically in Fig. 8-3.

This approach to thinking about the leadership role evolved from studies of leadership in a wide variety of organizations. Our quantitative research has shown us that different combinations of these three classes of skills are required for different levels of jobs in the same organization and at different times in the life of an organization.

What is the meaning of this to our understanding of how to achieve a more effective medical staff? Let us think a bit first about what mixture of skills chiefs of staff should have and then what mixture of skills department heads should have. Remember that since no studies of medi-

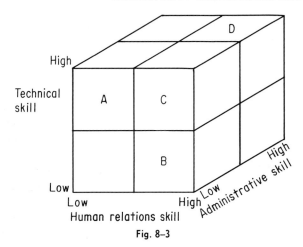

Fig. 8–3

cal staffs employing this framework have been done as yet we are actually only generating hypotheses using what the findings of research with other key groups in complex organizations would suggest.

The Chief of Staff

For the chief of staff role, it is safe to predict that all three dimensions are important and that the chiefs of the more effective staffs score high on all three dimensions of skills. (The chiefs in cell D of Fig. 8-3 probably have more effective medical staffs than chiefs in any of the other cells.) Another way of saying this is that it is not enough for a chief of staff to have only medical or technical skills, nor is it enough that he know how to work with other doctors to relate organizational and individual doctor's goals. Even the combination of medical and human relations skills is not enough in the hospital that has any complexity.

The Department Head

For the department head role, medical or the technical skills and the human relations skills are the most essential, with administrative skills useful but not as necessary as in the case of the chief of staff. Research has shown administrative or organizational skills to be important only in the highest levels of an organization unless the organization is very young and is just getting organized.

PROBLEM-SOLVING PROCEDURES WITHIN THE EFFECTIVE UNIT

Groups vary markedly in their capacity to solve problems. Medical staffs must vary as much as other groups in this respect. What are some of the research findings here?[4] Groups that are evaluated as more effective than other groups in doing their job are more likely to be groups where:

The members feel free to discuss the problems they have about their work openly with their department head and their associates.

The members feel that those higher in the organization ask them for their opinions and ideas about how to handle problems that arise.

The members feel that those over them in an organization are easy to go to and talk to.

Both members and the leader feel they have a great deal of influence in the decision-making process.

There is a great degree of mutual respect, trust, and confidence among the members of the group and between the members and the leader of each unit.[5,8]

Group Function

The more effective groups are consistently different from the less effective units in two respects: in the knowledge and ability their members have to perform both the functions necessary for orderly problem identification and solution, and in the functions necessary for the maintenance and development of the *group as a group*. The more effective group knows where it is both in terms of the problem-solving steps through which it is moving and in terms of whether it is building or reducing the group's ability to handle problems openly. It is *not enough for the leader and the members to understand the steps that are involved in high quality problem-solving*—steps such as the statement of the problem, clarification of the problem issues, identification of alternative solutions, testing of alternatives for both feasibility and motivational commitment by those who will have to execute the plan, selection of a plan of action, and the establishment of procedures for subsequent review of the decision. *The leader and at least a few of the group's members must also know how to improve the group's functioning as a group.* This involves eliciting the participation and ideas of those who do not contribute, expressing standards for the group to attempt to achieve in its functioning, applying such standards to the evaluation of the group's processes, and helping the group to handle the man who feels that his are the only ideas that are worthy (the dominator), or the only ideas that he is going to allow to be accepted (the blocker). Thus, both the group-task roles and the group-building and maintenance roles are recognized and become the concern of the group in the more effective staffs. *Particularly important is the group's ability and willingness to evaluate its own process.* This means agreeing to set aside a few minutes of each meeting to look at the way the group has been functioning—to critique the meeting, to discuss the effectiveness of the group's own processes of solving problems and working together.

Another key to effective problem solving is *well organized information about how a system is functioning*. Where is the system for which the group is responsible running well? Where are there problems that need attention? The people in key positions in business and industry have long recognized the importance of having careful research made of what is happening within their systems, but a great deal is also invested in organizing and summarizing these data. The auditing of all manner of things and functions is standard operating procedure. Data are summarized so that the incidence and magnitude of problems can be ascertained long before they snowball into properties that are hard to handle. The establishment of careful record keeping and the processes for reduction and summarization provide the basic body of information necessary to monitor and to change the functioning of a system. Feedback systems are an essential to effective problem solving. The decision-making processes are most likely to improve when the group can use objective data to assess a situation and decide what needs to be done in one period, implement their decision, and then use objective data from a subsequent time period to ascertain the effectiveness of their decision.

Knowledge of results has long been recognized as an important aid to learning. Careful and regular use of data collection and summarization procedures by committees within the medical staff, such as the medical audit, the tissue committee, the transfusion committee, provide the basis for better decision-making and for monitoring the effectiveness of how the various organizational units and committees are functioning.

SUMMARY

A recurrent underlying theme in this paper is that to achieve an effective medical staff it is necessary to create and maintain a more effectively functioning social organization within this sector of the hospital. In many hospitals, the skeleton of organization exists within the medical area. But such a bare outline or structure of an organization is not enough. There is a vast difference between an "organization" that is only an organization on paper with the names of men written in the boxes of the organizational chart who do not know or really perform their duties, and an organization in which the members know what they are trying to attain, have set their own goals and objectives for the system, understand and agree among themselves about how their respective roles interrelate, and work together in concert to attain the organization's objectives.

Common and shared expectations about each other's roles and about what is appropriate behavior is not attained by any simple process.

Common norms and values and similar frames of reference are built only through discussional processes. The persons in the key roles who understand what it means to develop "a sense of organization" in the people in a system must be continually on the lookout for opportunities to strengthen the members' conceptual and behavioral understanding of organization. As in other fields, the concepts alone are not enough. It is necessary to show the way these ideas about how to work together translate into the specific acts of working together every day. If this is seen as a continuing educational process—not something that is supposed to be done once for all time—the problems that occur because some individual or group did not think about the organizational implications of an act can be welcomed as providing an additional chance for further training in the processes of organization and effective self-government.

Lest we become too impatient in accomplishing the many things that have to be done to develop and maintain an effectively functioning medical staff, we should remember that much of this represents new knowledge and requires a high order of behavioral skills which we are only beginning to be able to conceptualize and train.

SELECTED EXCERPTS FROM TAPES OF THREE SEMINAR DISCUSSIONS OF THE PRECEDING MATERIAL WHICH ILLUSTRATES SOME ASPECTS OF GROUP PROCESS

FCM: Groups are usually quite good at identifying problems on which to work; they may or may not be good at working through to the solution of their problems. But the understanding of how to help a group develop its skills in problem solving is not readily understood. These are skills that may, however, be learned. They have to be learned intellectually and behaviorally, and usually there is a considerable gap between what we understand at the head level and what we are able to do behaviorally. We have to learn to look at both the *content* of the discussions and the *process*—the way the discussion is unfolding. Groups which can monitor their process can improve their effectiveness markedly.

Let us begin our work in this small group by forming a circle. This will help us work as a group should. Even these little physical arrangements make a difference. It is difficult to talk to the back of a person's head and even more difficult to influence him. It is also important to monitor factors that affect the physical comfort of a group, things like ventilation, heat, and the sun moving into people's eyes. How you arrange things helps the group in focusing its energies on the solution of the important problems.

[Each member of the group introduces himself and identifies his role in his hospital.]

FCM: Our topic here is "achieving an effective medical staff." But in all honesty, as far as I am concerned, it is "achieving an effective group." These ideas probably hold for a tissue committee, or for the chairman of the board with his trustees, or for the director of nursing with her nursing group. The process points out how group functions are relevant to all such groups.

What are the costs of *working man-to-man—one superior to one subordinate?* That approach often means five conversations if he has five subordinates. If the leader could get all the members of his group together, he could first share the information about the problem and then get the ideas of the five men. This would give him a wider range of ideas than if he worked on a man-to-man basis. There are many arguments for working as a group rather than man-to-man.

[A suggestion is offered by a member of the seminar that a chairman, before a meeting, phone the members and see what ought to be on the agenda and what the problems are. Then, when they come to the meeting, it is a combination of these man-to-man conversations.]

FCM: If you know you have a particularly delicate problem on the agenda, it is often useful to *explore the topic with individuals before the meeting.* This is not a case of building an agenda. The problem is clear; the question is how to handle it. The leader wants to know how different people see this before he tries to bring it out into the open. Someone asked if you would always bring everything out in a group the first thing. I would expect that we would agree that we would not. Why would you check with different people first before you try to pull them together in a meeting?

A member of the seminar: In my position I have to know what the group is thinking—what facets of the problem they are going to bring in. Many times these people give me ideas.

FCM: You make me feel a bit uncomfortable, because it sounds as if you might be telephoning all the members before the meeting to "case it out," so that you can manipulate a decision by knowing exactly what the tolerance of the group is for the decision you want.

Same member: I think it's wise to go to any committee with your homework done and your thoughts prepared instead of wasting five other men's time while you try to think about a problem that you should have thought about before coming. I believe leaders should contact their committee members and ask them to prepare their thoughts—write them out if necessary—so that it won't take five hours to do the work. We can then go through it in two hours.

FCM: You want good staff work in advance. That would be an index of good responsible leadership.

Same member: Yes, I think it is a waste of your committee's time if the committee members come unprepared to present their thoughts.

Another member of the seminar: I call my committee members because I want to get their opinions. I don't trust myself—I have only one mind. My committee is made up of seven or eight minds, and they're good minds. And they will give me fresh ideas so that by the time of the meeting they are thinking, and I have been refreshed by all these good ideas.

Another discussant: Communication should be not only between the group leader and his subordinates but also between subordinates and their peers and subordinates. If the agenda item should warrant this, I would expect them to go and talk with their subordinates so that they bring the ideas of their group to the committee meeting. But if it is a matter of policy—such as a change in the bylaws—and the subordinates have never been involved in this kind of a decision, I do not think they should waste the subordinates' time.

FCM: Did you ever have a meeting where you knew that there were some clear positions that one person is likely to take in opposition to another, but one of these is going to be so timid or such a poor group member that he won't bring his idea out? You want to check it out and be sure you understand that man's position. You know the man is not likely to face up to the responsibility of being a responsible member of that group. You may want to check his ideas in advance and know how he's really feeling. Then when the time comes in the group meeting, you can be sure to sharpen and draw the issue out. How does the leader find out where that man is if he does not do some advance work? The real question here is the way in which the leader uses this knowledge— the product of his advance work. If he uses it to manipulate, that is out. If he uses it to help the group to understand and to sharpen up its problems, that is probably all right. If the leader comes to the meeting with the feeling that he has learned all he can and done what staff action he can for the group, he is then able to give them ideas as to how different people see the situation if these differences are not getting expressed. Out of a good group discussion there will probably come a new solution, a new decision that is different from any held by members before the meeting. You can do a lot of staff action in advance if you do not use the information to manipulate—if you use it for the development of the group.

A seminar member: Certain situations face every chairman where he must guide the group; he must hold the reins, otherwise he is not an effective chairman. This, in effect, is manipulation. If the group considers a doctor's hospital privileges, a responsible chairman must think in terms of the hospital: "Is this man a menace to the public?" A chairman in this situation must lead his committee into thinking in terms of what is good medical practice.

FCM: What I seem to hear you saying is that *the leader may want to emphasize some of the goals the members hold in common.* There are times when certain things the group values must be stressed. At times the leader will want to re-emphasize these as a common set of norms under which we work together. Is that manipulation?

A seminar member: It is not manipulation for gain or personal evolvement, but it is guidance along a train of thought to achieve an end as quickly as possible, and as effectively as possible.

FCM: This gets around to the fact that *an effective group is able to handle conflict.* If you look through the problem-solving literature, you find that the better groups tackle differences more openly, and often head-on. The research literature also indicates that heterogeneity is what gives a group strength. So *in some way, you must bring out into the open the minority position.* All of our group problem-solving literature points out that *you can be solution-minded too early* and not work long enough at understanding and stating the problem. You can also be too docile as group members and not bring out and share the problems that you know are in the room. After all, it is your organization, it is your society and staff, and you are trying to govern it in a self-government way. Differences need to be valued and worked through, *if* the group has the strength to do it. That is the important variable.

It is not enough to identify the steps with which you must march logically to a decision. You must also look at the way in which you are doing it. What are you doing to the motivation of the members of the group to contribute ideas subsequently, to their willingness to carry out the decisions arrived at?

Do you feel that each time you manipulate, someone finds you out and calls your hand?

A member: They certainly do in my case!

FCM: Do the rest of you feel that when you see a man manipulating and running a pretty anti-democratic kind of show you let him know—you feed back this fact to him?

Members: It depends on who he is. Sometimes you say, well, he is certainly dogmatic and I do not agree with him, but he gets things done.

FCM: I have come to feel that I do not really know many professionals or scientists who know how to work in an organizational setting, to set up an effective arrangement for self-government. We are living in a society that believes it draws its strength from a democratic way of living. You, as doctors, are tied together into a voluntary association which should be self-governing.

Member: How do you deal with the guy who talks too much?

FCM: That is a good question. Let us talk about that. We have to learn how to handle such problems in a group.

Another member: Is that not the right of a leader?

FCM: That comment makes me feel uneasy because that suggests that everything has to be done by the leader. We have begun to develop into a group now; each of you is a member of this group, and I would hope that everyone here can see that all the responsibility for handling this meeting cannot reside in the leader's role. The leader has the responsibility to see that the work of the group is not reduced by the member who talks too much. But the leader has to help the group learn how to monitor its own processes and manage its own members. *Each person must learn to share the responsibility for the group's progress or lack of movement.* If a guy like that has to be handled and nobody else has the courage to do it, or if the intellectual understanding that it is the responsibility of the group as a whole to work on this is low, then the leader has to do it.

A member: Could he not make this one of the ground rules before the meeting?

FCM: Yes, has anybody tried ground rules? What would you do? You could set a timer on each speaker. What else could be done?

A member: I remind my committee members that if we do not get through the agenda we will have to have another meeting next Thursday because we must finish the agenda before the next board of directors' meeting.

FCM: That is a very potent threat. You are really saying, "Now, if you do not all get busy here, we will have to have another meeting, and you all know how we feel about another meeting." That is one way of handling it. What else have you found effective?

Another member: We use mimeographed newsletters. We can make announcements, and I have found that the locker room is a wonderful place to let off steam. Some men require this. And I also get some asides from the other members there. Another device we use is to assign tasks to smaller committees instead of bringing the problems up in a staff meeting of 175 physicians.

FCM: Let us return to our problem. How do you handle the man who wants to talk too much? You have an agenda, and here is this man who has a paragraph and a half on each one of the items about which he wants to make a speech. He may even be an instructed delegate, and he is sure he has got to be heard.

Seminar member: You can ask each member of the executive committee to forego discussion at the meeting and bring his thoughts in writing to the next meeting.

FCM: For the next five or ten minutes let us talk about the way in which we have been working so far this afternoon—not the content of the discussion but how we feel about how we have worked as a group. If we could develop this as a norm in our meetings of doctors, do you think that might help us alter our behavior as group members? Let us look at our own process as a group.

A member: We have had the ideas of three or four people here who have shared their ideas, but we have not heard from all the others. I think the more people we hear from, the more we will all benefit.

Another: I do not think a person has to say something if he is in agreement with what somebody else says, other than "I agree," or "I have nothing new to add."

Still another: Do we, as a group, know what we are doing?

FCM: We are now beginning to catch the idea. We have been looking at process. I stated the purpose at the beginning. I found I stated it three times this morning for one group, and they still did not understand it. You see, focusing occasionally on process—how we are working together as a group—is not part of the way we usually work; it is not a part of our experience.

In this brief hour or so, the *content* of our discussion is about how the more effective groups differ from the less effective groups. We also want to learn a little about how groups function by looking at the way our group here is functioning (the *process*). As we begin to learn to monitor our own process, we should see ways of handling the man who wants to dominate a meeting or draw out the person who is not contributing to the discussions. By occasionally stopping to talk about the process and progress of our own meeting, we can learn how to improve group meetings in general.

Members often have lots of ability to read what is going on in a meeting; but typically we do not share what we see and feel, so the group cannot improve its process. We just leave it up to the other person, and especially the leader—"That is his job, let us see if he can do it."

FCM: Do you ever find yourself in the *situation where members of a meeting are talking past one another and getting increasingly more angry at each other?* What do you do as a member or a leader?

[*Discussion:* Most responses seemed to indicate that they would tend to be quiet and listen, while the two in conflict would keep trying to hammer out their differences.]

FCM: A useful suggestion is for each person to refrain from making another comment until the other person's ideas and feelings have been clearly stated before putting another idea into the discussion. For example, if I were one of the verbal combatants, I would not be able to make another comment until I had demonstrated that I had listened so carefully to the other person's ideas (instead of trying to figure out how to slap him down again) that I could tell him to his satisfaction that I understood exactly what his points were. And I would have to state his position in such a way that he would know I understood the feeling with which he had said those ideas. I would have to be able to reflect both his facts and his feelings. Once I had done this, I would have the right to go ahead and try to tell him what it was that I was trying to say.

If I have done this well, the other person will recognize that I have had the courtesy to listen to him and have attempted to really understand all of his ideas and feelings. The other man is then obliged to listen to my position. I may even ask him to attempt to restate the ideas I consider important and significant to the argument. It is surprising how fast an agreement to discuss a problem in this manner will reduce the level of emotionality in the discussion. Often, before instigating a discussional role such as this, the parties are not sure what they are fighting about. Each party is sure the other man is not understanding him, so each gets more emotionally involved in making his point. Both stop listening.

If, during the discussion under these rules, you find the other person is operating under a totally unacceptable set of value assumptions— things that seem unethical or indefensible to you—then you have found something about which to fight. This is not a process for eliminating all conflict, only one to make sure we know what we are fighting about.

If either party finds there are value issues that the other is unaware of or indifferent to, then the discussion shifts to these to see what each sees as right, as consistent with the basic values for living and working together.

A careful definition of the way each party sees the situation often solves the problem. If we find basic differences, we at least know where the battle lines are drawn.

A member: Are these skills a leader should expect others to acquire? Is it proper to try to develop group members to do things like this?

FCM: In other words, what right do I have to train my colleagues in such skills for improving group process? Do we as leaders have this as an obligation? It is, of course, my feeling that we do.

BIBLIOGRAPHY

1. Cartwright, D., and Zander, A.: "Group Dynamics: Research and Theory," Harper & Row, Publishers, New York, 1960.

2. Georgopoulos, B. S., and Mann, F. C.: "The Community General Hospital," The Macmillan Company, New York, 1962.

3. Likert, R.: "New Patterns of Management," McGraw-Hill Book Company, New York, 1961.

4. Maier, N. R. F.: "Problem-Solving Discussions and Conferences," McGraw-Hill Book Company, New York, 1963.

5. Mann, F. C., and Baumgartel, H.: "Absences and Employee Attitudes in an Electric Company," Human Relations Series 1, Report 2, Survey Research Center, Institute for Social Research, Ann Arbor, Michigan, 1963.

6. Mann, F. C., and Neff, F. W.: "Managing Major Change in Organizations," The Foundation for Research on Human Behavior, Ann Arbor, Michigan, 1961.

7. Mann, F. C.: Toward an Understanding of the Leadership Role in Forman Organization, in R. Dubin, G. Homans, F. Mann, and D. Miller, "Leadership and Productivity," Chandler Publishing Company, San Francisco, 1965.

8. Mann, F. C., Indik, B., Vroom, V.: "The Productivity in Work Groups," Survey Research Center, Institute for Social Research, Ann Arbor, Michigan, 1963.

9. McGregor, D.: "The Human Side of Enterprise," McGraw-Hill Book Company, New York, 1960.

9

The Hospital Trustee and the Medical Staff

By Fred H. Zuck

Fred H. Zuck is the president of the board of trustees of the Good Samaritan Hospital of Sandusky, Ohio. He has held this position for the past 12 years, and he was a member of the board for many years before that. Mr. Zuck received the A.B. and LL.B. degrees from Western Reserve University. He is a member of the Ohio State Bar Association, and the Erie County, Ohio Bar Association. He is a well-known international industrialist.

Participation in the financial and industrial worlds and service as an officer of the board of trustees of a 170-bed hospital for many years permit me to make comparisons between what occurs in financial and industrial organizations and what occurs in the conduct of a hospital. The problems are parallel in many respects.

Despite the widespread belief that a hospital cannot be run like a business, experience has shown that it can be. In fact, if it is to succeed, it must be because *the hospital is a business—a big business.* To understand how big a business the community hospital is, compare the number of employees and the gross operating cost of your hospital with the cost of your city government or of your public school system, or of your average industrial plant. In our community of 32,000 people, the three hospitals employ approximately 700 people, with annual patient billing of over 4 million dollars. (See Table 9-1.) In the nation's 7,127 hospitals registered by the American Hospital Association, employment reached 1,887,000 in 1964; the combined payrolls were nearly 8 billion dollars; and the total expenses were in excess of 12 billion dollars. Yes, the operation of hospitals is big business, and it is going to get bigger because hospitals are becoming community centers.

By necessity and by law the responsibility for all affairs of a hospital

TABLE 9-1. Comparison of Hospital, School, and City Government Expenses in Sandusky, Ohio

	Operating Expenses in Thousands		Personnel	Beds	Admissions	Census	Births
	Total	Payroll					
Good Samaritan Hospital	1,300	680	198	169	4,448	90	465*
Providence Hospital	1,580	887	227	147	6,183	113	688*
Memorial Osteopathic Hospital	1,192	649	235	108	4,724	85	434
	4,072	2,216	660	424	15,355		1,587
Sandusky public schools	2,693	2,039	386				
City of Sandusky	2,675	1,472	287				
	5,368	3,511	673				

* Guide Issue, *Hospitals, JAHA* (Aug.) 1965.
NOTE: Figures given for beds, admissions, census, and births represent 1964 statistics.

is vested in the board of trustees. As there are no stockholders, *the board of trustees represents the public interest.* Membership on the medical staff is a privilege and can be obtained only by approval of the board of trustees, but treatment of the patients is exclusively in the hands of the medical staff. Staff membership can continue only so long as the physician complies with the staff bylaws, rules, and regulations controlling hospital conduct. These rules and regulations must be established or approved by the board of trustees. Unfortunately this has caused many physicians to feel that the board of trustees is intruding upon staff prerogatives and has resulted in suspicion and conflict where none should exist.

On the other hand, members of the governing board often are not sufficiently knowledgeable and are not personally willing to assume the necessary leadership.

Poor communication between administration and the medical staff is all too frequent. Safety of the patient and adequacy of patient care, which must be the first consideration of all parties, often become secondary to personal issues. Overall community planning of hospital facilities and proper utilization of both facilities and trained personnel, including physicians, are virtually impossible when such issues develop. The lack of planning and facility utilization would drive many hospitals into insolvency if they were in the competitive world of business. All of us are familiar with the unmanageable rise in the cost of hospital and medical care. Except for third party payments and government subsidies, few could function with the present financial requirements. The public, sensing this situation, has become articulate. The pressure is on, and we must revaluate our position and our policies.

In considering trustee-medical staff relationship, at least five basic points of common interest exist.

Location of the Hospital

Most hospitals are situated either in relatively small communities or in rural areas. This fact has an influence on the types of doctors attracted to the community as well as on the attitude of the community toward its doctors. The contact of these doctors with the constant changes in the science and practice of medicine is often limited to local professional society meetings and medical journals. The influence of the large teaching centers may be quite remote, and for the most part there is a lag in the application of new knowledge.

Increasingly over the past 10 or 15 years, the small town doctor has found himself in ideological conflict with the city specialist. This has created a situation which is often confusing and has resulted in "choosing up sides" in many communities. Add to this the rise of the osteopathic physician and the ever increasing awareness among trustees of their final accountability, and the stage has been set for serious problems.

The General Public and the Public Interest

During the development of this country, the medical doctor was often relatively unobtainable, and even today a similar situation exists in some communities. A quick look at the early days pinpoints the necessity of doctors in influencing community growth. The shortage of doctors led to the horse and buggy doctor. He was not a mere inhabitant of a community but was someone extraordinary. In community affairs it became common practice to attribute to him virtues and capabilities unrelated to medicine, which he did not always possess. Because of the close relationship between the doctor and his patient it is understandable how this situation developed. Its only significance at this time is its carryover effect. In those early days there were no hospitals as we know them today, and the relationship of the doctor to his patient and to the community was close. Today it is not always easy to find a doctor who will make house calls, and more and more the public looks to the hospital as a medical center.

It should be made clear that the right of a patient to be treated by a physician of his choice must be preserved and that no door be opened which would tend to interfere with the confidence of a patient in the physician of his choice. The president of a board of trustees must consider every public act or pronouncement as well as every internal position in board meetings from the point of view of its effect on the patient-physician relationship.

The environment in which the physician practices is changing, perhaps more rapidly than for any other profession. Today's complexities in the accomplishment of mutual objectives of hospital and physician can be resolved only by a sincere effort to bring about widespread public understanding of the soundness and cohesion of the system.

The Composition of the Medical Staff

Many factors influence the composition of a medical staff. Physicians have a choice of setting up practice on their own or entering into an arrangement with an established practice. In the case of the general practitioner, as well as the specialist, this constitutes a choice of association which is material in his future affiliations; if there is more than one hospital in the community, it will influence his future hospital relationships. If one hospital is sectarian and one is nonsectarian, this has an effect. If the community has osteopathic physicians and an osteopathic hospital, this presents a third major conflict within the community and its medical profession. Many of the established physicians are older in years and are well established in the community through personal associations as well as medical standing. Most of the younger physicians entering the community do not have these personal associations, but they are better trained academically. The catalyst for the interaction and reaction between young and old is the hospital. If for this reason alone, hospital staff privileges for all physicians are a must.

Thus, each physician sets his individual course within the profession, but to maintain public confidence, the profession must present a united front to the public in professional matters.

The Trustees—Their Motivation and Limitations

The trustees normally represent a cross-section of the community. The board is heterogeneous, but each trustee is a respected member of the community. The new member may rightly consider his election to the board as evidence of community recognition, but seldom does he have a true concept of the knowledge or responsibility which will be required of him, or the legal liability he has assumed. Each member is a competent individual in his own field but is completely unprepared for participation in the types of issues and decisions involved in the management of the hospital, his knowledge of the hospital usually being limited to personal contacts as a patient. Ordinarily he has no knowledge of the medical profession and its problems except those gained from the patient-doctor relationship. In short, he is unprepared for the moral and legal obligations he has assumed. *Trustee*, a periodical published monthly by the American Hospital Association, is doing an excellent job of educating trustees. An indoctrination manual or a training program for prospective board members should be a must.

The complexities of hospital management and the problems arising from the integration of lay management and physician medical care of the patient are not easy to understand, much less to solve.

The principal bridges between the lay and professional conduct of the hospital are the president of the board, the administrator and the joint conference committee. The president of the board must have the full confidence of the board and must be a knowledgeable and effective leader who gets things done. His job is not always pleasant, and he must be prepared to withstand criticism as he heads the board and safeguards the public trust given to him.

It has become desirable for the medical director and/or the chief of staff to be members of the board, but no other staff physicians should be included. Too often some members of the board will look to the physician member for the guidance in lay matters. This guidance must come from the president.

It is a function of the board of trustees to see that standards for medical care in the hospital are established, maintained, and improved. In framing the code of regulations of the board and the bylaws, rules and regulations of the staff, the recommendations of the Joint Commission on Accreditation of Hospitals are good benchmarks. The Joint Commission is a creation of the medical profession, and the majority of the members are physicians. Its standards serve as the most acceptable basis of establishing the minimum standards for the hospital. The information of the Joint Commission and its educational efforts have had a major influence in improving hospital care.

It is the responsibility of the board to preserve standards of medical care. Granting or withholding staff privileges is the ultimate method of enforcement. The medical staff alone, being the only competent body, should conduct its affairs and discipline its members in a fashion which obviates the necessity for any action by the board.

The Administrator

The administrator in most hospitals is a person selected by the board because he is known to them, or because he has business and administrative background, or because he is a professional who has been academically trained but perhaps has had little practicable business experience. In smaller communities, the selection of a professional administrator usually means importing one who has no local background.

Administration of the lay functions of the hospital is a highly specialized job. Not only must the administrator manage people and money, but he must carry out the board's policies, and, at the same time, maintain a sound relationship with the medical staff. By keeping in mind that two and one-half personnel are required for each patient and that 80 to 85 per cent of the income from patient billings is received from third party sources, one has a quick view of the broad scope of knowledge and skill required to manage the modern hospital. The hospital must maintain highly specialized service personnel and equipment. It must remain open 24 hours a day, 7 days a week. It must feed sick people with all the problems of poor appetites and special diets. It must maintain an emergency facility and see that it is properly staffed —an acute problem in many hospitals today. It must meet the ever increasing costs of operations. It must continuously modernize to meet the expanding requirements. These are some of the problems of a hospital administrator.

If the administrator demonstrates high competence in one hospital, he is in demand by larger hospitals, thus creating another serious problem of maintaining continuity of administration.

The administrator faces a difficult problem when a community is served by two or more hospitals. Usually the medical staffs are open, and there is considerable overlap. When this exists, the administrator is in the middle, and he is frequently under pressure by staff factions. Some staff members take the attitude that if they do not get what they want from one hospital, they will take their patients to another. This means that the staff rules and regulations are not always enforced. Rules on maintenance of proper records, for instance, can be written on the books but then ignored. Enforcement of the rules, even the insistence on adequate medical records, may mean the loss of patients and loss of income—problems for the administrator, and thus problems for the board. Failure of members of the medical staff to understand the legal and operational consequences, to themselves and to the hospital, of non-compliance with hospital policies can be a serious matter. It would appear that the attitudes of some physicians are largely based on fear —fear of being sued, fear of review of their medical judgments, fear of losing patients, fear of losing face. Of all professional people, the physician should know best that the elimination of fear can only be accomplished by knowledge. They should know that errors are certain to occur and *that professional responsibility, legal or moral, does not exceed the rule of reason in any given set of circumstances.* Somewhere in all of this complex structure an orderly process must emerge.

The medical profession must realize that most of the people who constitute our legislative bodies and our judicial systems are from small and rural communities and that the public interest will be crystallized into law through those legislative and judicial bodies. The major hospitals and teaching centers thus have a genuine responsibility to their small town confreres to extend their teaching efforts to the smaller communities. Success in these endeavors may have a major effect in shaping future laws and regulations.

The course which the hospital must take is fundamentally based upon the free enterprise system. For the hospital to survive the system must survive, and this means a system of checks and balances. Disregard of proper checks can result only in imbalance and an ultimate breakdown. Let us take a careful look at the facts:

First, *the medical staff is an essential part of the hospital structure* and its role is rendering patient care. In this field it is supreme, and it must accept total responsibility. The measure of its total responsibility is the safety of the patient.

Second, *the board of trustees is an essential part of the hospital structure,* and its role is the determination of hospital policy and the management of the physical facilities and financial structure. In its field it is supreme and must accept total responsibility. The measure of its total responsibility is the public interest.

How can the system of checks and balances be applied? In our American system, we vest the final authority in our judicial system. The law and the courts therefore fix the legal responsibility and adjudicate the ground rules. Both the statutory law and the courts are responsible to and ultimately reflect the public interest.

We come now to the crux of the problem. *What can we do to make the system work,* for none of us wants to accept what appears to be the only alternative—fully state-controlled medicine.

Foremost, we must recognize that every member of the medical staff and every member of the board of trustees is there because he wants to be there. He has accepted the obligation by his own choice. If we can keep this in mind, it will permit a more objective approach to the solution of the operational problems which arise. No longer is there a place in the hospital for the concept that a doctor is a rugged individualist and therefore above the checks which are imposed upon him. Nor is there a place for the medical staff to suspect that the lay board of trustees is dictating the manner in which they shall practice medicine. Every physician on the staff should be thoroughly oriented in the respective roles of the trustees and the medical staff. No longer is there a place for the member of the board of trustees who is unwilling to accept the legal and ethical responsibility to conduct the affairs of the hospital in the public interest. Members of the board holding contrary views should resign. The public interest means safety of the patient, adequate patient care at a reasonable cost, continuity of operations, and long-range planning.

Assuming that the medical staff and the board of trustees both accept their responsibilities, an operational structure will be developed with adequate communications between the president of the board, the medical director, and the administrator. This can be accomplished by a competent president of the board, a competent administrator, and a competent paid medical director. The president of the board usually will not be paid, for he serves as a volunteer. However, a voluntary medical chief cannot afford to take the time from his practice to carry the increasing burdens involved in the administration of the medical affairs of the hospital. The voluntary rotating chief of staff must be replaced by a long-term paid professional.

SUMMARY

Hospitals would be well advised to follow the organizational patterns which business has developed. This requires recognition of the necessity for a personnel structure competent to meet current needs and with sufficient depth of personnel to provide continuity. Because of the unusual character of hospital operations, this can be accomplished only by the board of trustees and the medical staff working together in common understanding.

10

What the Doctor Expects of the Hospital

By William W. Jack, M.D.

William W. Jack is an obstetrician and gynecologist in Grand Rapids, Michigan. He received
the M.D. degree from the University of Michigan and his specialty training at the Lying-In
Hospital of the University of Chicago and at
the University of Colorado School of Medicine.
He is a diplomate of the American Board of
Obstetrics and Gynecology, a Fellow of the
American College of Surgeons, and a Fellow of
the American College of Obstetricians and Gynecologists. He has been chairman of the Committee on Maternal Health of the Michigan State
Medical Society since 1961. Dr. Jack was chief
of staff at Blodgett Memorial Hospital in Grand
Rapids, Michigan, from 1962 to 1964, and he
has served on many staff committees.

The emergence of the hospital as the community medical center
began shortly after World War I when medicine outgrew the home and
the office. Through the years, the hospital has increased in importance
until its influence is now accepted throughout the community.

Three factors have contributed to this evolution. First, physicians
have developed new techniques, new tests, and new equipment that
are so complex and expensive that they can be used economically only by
a medical center and by many physicians for many patients. No longer
is the doctor's office the alpha and omega of diagnosis and treatment.
Second, the general public has continued to demand more and better
medical care. Third, the government has stimulated an intensified interest in medicine and the care of the sick.

Coincident with the increased importance of hospitals, a new profession has developed—the hospital administrator who is highly trained

and highly skilled in management. No longer can just "anyone run a hospital."

THE DICHOTOMY OF PHYSICIANS AND HOSPITALS

The result of these changes in many instances seems to be a dichotomy in patient care—physicians versus hospitals. Third-party payment plans have furthered this division: there is a Blue Cross plan for hospitals and a Blue Shield plan for doctors, and now Medicare legislation has produced a Plan A for hospitals and a Plan B for physicians.

These factors and many others have produced a divergence of the two most concerned parties, the physicians and hospitals. Deficiencies in coordination, communication, and interdependence have come about, and at times it seems there is lack of a common goal.

This fragmentation has been discussed elsewhere. (ED. NOTE: *Several of the contributors have referred to this concept of fragmentation.*) A plea is made for physicians and hospitals again to converge, and for physicians to spend the necessary time and effort to maintain the voice of the medical staff within the hospital.

SOME THINGS THE PHYSICIAN EXPECTS

The physician expects the hospital to be his "medical home." He expects that *membership on the staff will carry privilege as well as responsibility.* He expects the hospital to ask him to serve within the structure of the medical staff organization, and he does not expect this service to go unnoticed or unrewarded. Responsibility without privilege is as inexcusable as privilege without responsibility.

The physician expects an atmosphere in which *his opinions will be welcomed and even sought* with the common aim of providing ever better patient care.

He expects an atmosphere in which *each of his colleagues will provide quality medical care,* without the necessity of outside pressure and influence.

He expects an atmosphere in which *nursing care will be equally sincere and equally devoted* to providing quality care.

He expects *a physical plant that provides creature comforts for his patients.* He expects equipment and supplies for any and all procedures necessary for quality care.

The physician expects an atmosphere in which *continuing education for the physician, for the nurse, and for all hospital personnel* will be taken as a matter of course. He expects that the leadership in continuing education will be provided by the medical staff and that it will pervade all levels of hospital employees.

The physician expects an atmosphere in which there is a *continuing examination of the care provided,* where results are measured against today's standards. This self-examination must be extended to include comparisons of his hospital with other similar institutions. A hospital with no interest beyond its own walls, because of complacency or negligence, soon becomes second rate.

The physician expects an atmosphere in which *the governing board and the administration are familiar with medical problems* and are sympathetic toward solving them.

The physician expects *fiscal solvency* from administration.

He expects hospital care to be provided at a *cost to the patient consistent with the quality of the care given.* He expects a constant effort on the part of administration to hold down prices wherever possible. He expects to bear his share of the responsibility for this goal.

The physician expects his hospital to be *a focus of activity aimed toward attracting young people into the health fields.* This is a service that is at the same time selfish and altruistic.

The physician expects his hospital to create an atmosphere in which *his own desires toward research will find encouragement and support.*

SUMMARY

The physician expects the hospital to be *his* hospital. He expects membership on its staff to be an accolade. He expects his hospital to be the best in the community. He expects to help his colleagues and to be helped by them in providing the best medical care. He expects to be proud of his hospital and its place in the community, its physical plant, its equipment, its supplies, and its services. He expects to find professional stimulation to keep abreast with new developments. Within his hospital he expects to spend his professional life, happily, productively, and with the certain knowledge that his community is receiving medical care that meets the high standards not only of his own community but of the nation.

II

What the Hospital Expects of the Doctor

By Ronald D. Yaw

Ronald D. Yaw is the executive vice president of the Blodgett Memorial Hospital in Grand Rapids, Michigan, a post he has held for many years. He is the immediate past president of the American College of Hospital Administrators and a past president of the Michigan Hospital Association.

The Guide Issue of *Hospitals, JAHA,* August 1, 1965, gives the following data on Blodgett Memorial Hospital: Beds, 420; Admissions, 16,251; Census, 330; Bassinets, 66; Births, 2,475; Newborn census, 35; Total expenses, $5,721,000; Payroll, $3,597,000; Personnel, 988. There are two other general short-term hospitals in Grand Rapids, Butterworth Hospital with 467 beds and St. Mary's Hospital with 370 beds. The population of Grand Rapids in the 1960 census was 202,379.

What does the hospital expect of the doctor? For this discussion I consider the hospital to mean the total package—trustees, medical staff, administration, employees, patients, and supporters. And the term doctor means any member of that hospital's medical staff regardless of the presence or absence of any financial relationship with the hospital.

It is noteworthy that for all the years of my professional life, people have been giving talks on what some group expects of some other group, and I guess I have done my share. Medical record librarians, medical social workers, occupational therapists, and many more have heard what I expect of them, and perennially I have listened to talks on what is expected of administrators.

This concept of doctors and hospitals wondering what to expect of each other is a new one. Up until the past few years, we seemed to know by instinct, and it was no more necessary to ask this than it was to ask, "What do I expect of my brother?"

NEW THINGS IN THE HOSPITAL PICTURE

Clearly some things have entered the picture to make this subject worthy of discussion. Perhaps a look at these things and their impact will help us understand the current doctor-hospital problem and also provide some insight into what each may properly expect of the other.

I like Dr. Williams' term "gauze curtain" because in a modern hospital just about all of the gauze that is used is of the disposable variety.

The New Public—As a Citizen

The first new thing in the new concept of doctors' and hospitals' expectations of each other is the new public in its role as a citizen. This is the man who elects our congress. This is the man who, in the final analysis, decides what and where health facilities will be. It was not always so. A few men with the resources to dream and create their dreams out of their wealth were the decision makers. Today, to build, or expand, or improve a health institution without public understanding and acceptance is all but impossible. The new public looks upon health care as a right, not a largess to be dispensed. Hospitals are considered as utilities. The impersonal prepayment, from tax or payroll, is done more in the sense of paying a telephone bill than in the more emotional setting surrounding a recent illness or injury. Whether we like it or not, or whether we planned it this way or did not, *health care has become less personal both for the provider and the receiver.* This arm's length relationship with the public tends to be a source of frustration to us all, and in our confusion we blame each other. Doctors and hospitals feel that somehow the other is a major contributor to this not entirely understandable change in the patient public. Doctors are somewhat insulated from the public's changed attitude since theirs is still largely a personal one-to-one bedside relationship.

One thing, therefore, that hospitals should expect of their medical staff is that *the hospital will be defended by its doctors* when it needs defending. The doctor who is quick to agree with every petulant patient that "nurses aren't like they used to be," that "it wouldn't cost any more to stay at the Broadmoor," and that "they certainly are pushing the costs of medical care up"—this doctor remains on the staff and in good standing. But the nurse or technologist or admitting officer who vaguely implies that all doctors are not Oslers or Mayos has a hard and transitional life.

The New Public—As a Student

The second *new* thing is the new public in its role as a student. John Donne, poet and cleric of the 17th century, wrote, "I observe the physician with the same diligence as he, the diseased." The National Broadcasting Company has put Dr. Kildare on television twice weekly to meet the needs of our latter-day John Donnes. Today's physician, and hospital, exist in the spotlight of television, radio, *Reader's Digest, McCall's, Redbook, Life, Time,* and *Look.* The doctor who used to be considered some kind of nut if he did a rectal examination on an ulcer patient is now considered passé if he does not. A hospital has to be apologetic if it does not have a hyperbaric chamber or at least have one on order. The new public reads and watches its way into levels of pseudo-medical competence that were heretofore reserved for the products of more formal training. But this is not limited to clinical areas alone. Unions, government, and prepayment plans are all anxious to educate people about their health programs. As an example, I have been offered, exclusive of technical journals, through newspapers and the mail, a chance to get 17 booklets at little or no cost, all aimed at making me an expert on Medicare.

What has this to do with hospital-physician relationships? We all know the human weakness of assuming that competence in one field somehow produces competence in other fields. It is an easy jump for the semi-informed in some areas to assume the same knowledge in others. Through the eyes of the patient, the entire hospital structure is often seen as the man at the other end of the stethoscope. If the physician hurriedly gives partial information or misinformation, he creates misunderstanding and hours of needless work. Another thing a hospital has a right to expect, then, is that their *physicians should know hospital policies, procedures, and prices, or else know where to refer the patient for correct answers.* One cannot even estimate the number of man hours spent every day in American hospitals just responding to statements that start out, "Well, but my doctor told me. . . ."

The New Technology

A third new item is the new technology. Doctors have designed or inspired others to design hardware that is too big and too expensive to be anywhere other than in a central location. They have also taught or inspired others to teach highly specialized technicians, who are scarce and becoming scarcer, so they too must be centralized. The very existence of this hardware and the skilled minds to use it produces a steady change in hospital-physician relationships. So imperceptible and subtle is the change that it comes as a shock when finally noticed. A decade ago, a patient could receive a complete cardiac work-up in his internist's office. In 1966, such a work-up might involve a quarter of a million dollars worth of hardware weighing ten tons. What has this done to the relationships between internists and hospital? Between internists and radiologists in hospitals? Between internists and pathologists in hospitals?

Dr. George E. Miller, in an article entitled "Medical Education and the Rise of Hospitals," said: "It was not many years ago that most physicians used hospitals as a private workshop; a place to which they admitted their patients and in complete autonomy carried out the diagnostic and therapeutic activities . . . which seemed most appropriate." [1]

I think Dr. Miller was overly optimistic when he implied that this concept is a thing of the past, for in many hospitals physicians continue to feel that "the private workshop" is a good working description of physician-hospital relationships.

In the 1964 Stuart Crocker Lecture delivered at the Roosevelt Hospital in New York, Dr. Willard Wright, chairman of the Council on Medical Service of the American Medical Association, discussed hospital-physician relationships:

> Certainly, the responsibility of a physician today extends beyond the mere provision of medical care which may be satisfactory to the individual or to members of his family. Today, a member of the medical staff is required to participate in the establishment and enforcement of policies, procedures and regulations which result in individual decisions being tempered and controlled by group judgments. In effect, we have narrowed individual responsibility and instituted collective responsibility, so that the physician's position has changed from that of the undisputed authority to that of member of a health care team. [2]

Hospitals have a right to expect of their doctors a *recognition that the new technology is responsible for some of the changes,* that this new technology is a commendable result of the brain power and motivation of physicians themselves and not a byproduct of administrative bureaucracy. The fact that hardware and ancillary personnel are such that they can only be found in hospitals is a highly desirable reality. The shift from the kitchen table and the little black bag to the physician's office, to the hospital, and then to the medical center is an intrinsic part of medical progress. I believe hospitals should expect their physicians to recognize progress, not to bitterly denounce it as "empire building."

The New Look in Management

The fourth new factor is the new look in management. Progress in management procedures in recent year· has paralleled that in other technical fields. From a shaky uncertain start early in this century, a definite body of knowledge has evolved. This body of knowledge is acquired, not congenital. It is not an incidental acquisition along the road to obtaining competence in other fields. Failure to recognize these simple facts is an important ingredient in some of our present problems.

Herbert Simon, in his book *Administrative Behavior*,[3] reduced to four sentences some of the commonly accepted principles of modern management:

Administrative efficiency is increased by a specialization of the task among a group.

Administrative efficiency is increased by arranging the members of the group in a determinate hierarchy of authority.

Administrative efficiency is increased by limiting the span of control at any point in the hierarchy to a small number.

Administrative efficiency is increased by grouping the workers, for purposes of control, according to purpose, process, clientele, and place.

Doubtless the great majority of hospitals have followed the "Topsy" method of developing an administrative structure; and worse yet, having developed it, they have regarded the result as a frozen sequence of mistakes which cannot be melted down and recast. Since the days of Frederick Taylor in 1911,[4] a whole new body of knowledge has evolved, and new professions have been born, but without much real impact on hospital structuring.

Much of the fault here, and it is a fault, lies with those of us in hospital administration. In general, we have done a poor job in the area of applying proven management techniques to the organization of hospitals. We have made endless excuses but offered no real reasons. If all the excuses were boiled down, in my opinion it would be to this. Many administrators feel that the doctor, as a potential colleague-administrator, has three major deficiencies:

He lacks objectvity and has a tendency toward gun-barrel vision.

He identifies more closely with the aims of groups outside the hospital than those in the hospital.

As a group, physicians tend to close ranks against anyone not exposed to an identical educational background.

This leads to a simple conclusion, then, that the opposite of each of these is what the hospital should expect of the doctor—*a colleague who is interested in all of the patients on all of the services, who holds the economic or prestige aims of his hospital specialty group in secondary position, and who thinks and votes as an individual.*

The Hospital's New Place in the Social Order

My final new item is, to a degree, a composite of the other four. It is the new place of hospitals in the social order.

The place of hospitals has unquestionably changed, and the rate of change will unquestionably accelerate. The hospital's place in our social order is changing because the public wants it to change, and the public will press for and get further change.

Examples of what happens when a professional group attempts to thwart the public's clear choice are plentiful. I cite four.

For 15 years, organized nursing has sought to get nursing education out of hospitals into what they like to term the "mainstream of education." Result: over 80 per cent of all nursing graduates are still products of hospital schools of nursing.

Despite educational campaigns, advertisements in the yellow pages, and personal pleas, the public goes to the emergency department of a hospital rather than face the astringent process of dealing with an answering service. No amount of committee consideration and concern will change this.

A few years ago, a large Blue Shield plan started a campaign to put minor surgery back into the doctor's office where they felt it belonged. It was a dismal failure. People do not want to come stumbling out of an office and grope their way home.

Third party payers have campaigned for years against so-called diagnostic admissions to hospitals. "These procedures can be done in a doctor's office," the public is told. But the public wants the convenience of one-stop service for health for the same reason it wants one-stop shopping centers. This point will not be belabored further. I am aware of the fact that in many areas of health the public cannot have what it wants, but over a period of time, *the public's batting average for getting its way is pretty good.*

Unwillingness to recognize and accept the changing nature of hospitals in the social order is a key factor in many physician-hospital disputes. Earlier, I indicated that because the physician is closer to individual patients than the hospital is, he might well carry the ball for both. Conversely, hospitals are closer to the public and might well be given more responsibility in projecting images and telling the health story.

SUMMARY

A calm, realistic reassessment of traditional approaches to any problem in which hospitals or doctors find themselves bucking public opinion seems to be overdue. Whether hospitals alone do the bucking, or doctors alone do it, or whether it is done together is of no consequence. *The public wants us as one and sees us as one.*

In their efforts to stay close to the public, hospitals should expect their doctors to provide assistance and understanding. This will be no simple task in the coming days of community planning, in the adjustments to Medicare, and with the increasing pressures from without the hospital structure.

Five problem areas have been identified, and ways have been suggested for physicians and hospitals to assist each other in helping find the answers.

BIBLIOGRAPHY

1. Miller, G. E.: Medical Education and the Rise of Hospitals, *JAMA*, 186: 1075–1079 (Dec. 21) 1963.

2. "The Stuart M. Crocker Lectures," Monograph No. 3, published by Roosevelt Hospital, New York, 1964.

3. Simon, H. A.: "Administrative Behavior," 2d ed., The Macmillan Company, New York, 1958.

4. Taylor, F. W.: The Principles of Scientific Management, *Harpers Magazine*, 1911.

12

Hospitals and Public Opinion

By Robert M. Cunningham, Jr

Robert M. Cunningham, Jr., has been editor of
The Modern Hospital since 1951. Earlier, he was
associate editor of *Hygeia*, a publication of the
American Medical Association (now called *Today's Health*). Previously he had been public
relations director of Blue Cross in Chicago and
of the Evanston Hospital Association at Evanston, Illinois. He also served for several years
as consultant in public relations for the American College of Surgeons. Mr. Cunningham is a
graduate of the University of Chicago, where
he received a "Useful Citizen" alumni award
in 1955 in recognition of his community service. He is an Honorary Fellow of the American
College of Hospital Administrators and an associate member of the National Association of
Science Writers.

Some twenty-five years ago *The Modern Hospital* magazine presented
a series of articles on public relations in which the author set forth
the novel concept that hospitals owed their communities some accounting for their stewardship of community resources and, hence, some
information about their operations. The author even suggested that
hospitals might do well to budget for public relations as a continuing,
routine operating expense.

You can imagine what the response was. The prevailing view at the
time was that what happened at the hospital was nobody's business
but the doctors'—and possibly a few trustees'. Toward the rest of the
world the attitude was pretty much, "We'll tell the peasants what we
think is good for them to know, which is nothing."

Of course, all this has changed radically in the last 25 years and
mainly, I should say, in the last 10 years. We live in a Public Relations

Era, and hospitals have long since joined the parade of the press release. The walled fortress has become a bazaar; the quiet zones are laced with Muzak; the aura of mystery that surrounded the old-fashioned doctor has evaporated under the influence of Ben Casey. Patients who are not busy answering questionnaires about the coffee, the nurses, and the color of the draperies are hip-deep in brochures—many of them written with a light touch, as we say, and illustrated with bright little cartoons suggesting that the whole idea of hospitalization is simply hilarious.

Is this good or bad? If it was a good idea 25 years ago to give the public a little information about the hospital, why is it not a good idea now to give a lot of information? Do not all these efforts result in better public understanding of hospitals, and is not better public understanding of hospitals a desirable goal? In fact, is it not an urgent need?

I am not going to quarrel with the desirability of better public understanding of anything, and it is not my intention here to argue that hospitals do not need public understanding and support at least as much as schools and colleges, business, government, or any other segment of our society does. But I do think hospitals need to be warned against expecting too much from improved public understanding or leaning too heavily on the comfortable belief that public misunderstanding is responsible for most of our problems.

At any rate, there is some reason to believe that all the information we have been providing has not notably improved public understanding of hospitals—a circumstance that leads some observers to conclude that there is something the matter with the public, but it may also suggest there is something wrong with the information we have been providing. Certainly there is some evidence that we have not been saying the right things, or at least that nobody is paying attention; and it may be worth while to look at the evidence.

The fact of the matter is that throughout all these years of the Public Relations Era, the years of the bright brochures and press releases and television programs and moving pictures about hospitals and doctors, we do not seem to have come as far as most of us would like in improving public opinion of hospitals and doctors. There are even some gloomy observers who think that public opinion has been deteriorating, instead of improving, in recent years.

Whether this is true or not, I suppose we can all agree that the hosannas we so richly deserve are not exactly raising the roof. Instead, we seem to be increasingly troubled with complaints about our service, about our high costs, and with suggestions that our operations should be investigated by public bodies, if not actually controlled and regulated by public law.

Why does this happen? Why are we getting lawsuits instead of halle-lujahs? As the Russian peasant said near the end of the collective farm meeting when the commissars asked if there were any questions: "If things are really so good, gentlemen, why are they so bad?"

Obviously, there is no clear, simple answer. The reasons are many and complex and interrelated, but perhaps we can sort out a few of them here and shed some light on what the public expects and what we might be doing about it.

One of the reasons nobody seems to be getting the message, in my opinion, is that sometimes the things we have been saying simply do not square with the truth as it is plainly visible to large segments of the population.

For example, the thing we have been saying about hospital costs is that they are going to continue to go up and there is not anything we can do about it because hospitals are a personal service. But then it turns out that a part of our costs—perhaps only a small part but nevertheless a part—has been caused by improper use, unnecessary use, or overuse of our facilities and services, and there is too something we can do about it. We can organize utilization committees of the medical staff to review and supervise admissions and discharges and services and try to keep overutilization at the minimum. This is a good thing to do, but we did not get started until an insurance commissioner kicked us in the shins and made us start.

The thing we have been saying about our plants and facilities is that we need more and more of everything in order to keep pace with the rapid advance of medical technology and the growing population. It then turns out that there are places all over the country where two new hospitals are both half empty and at least one major city where six hospitals are equipped and staffed for open heart surgery, and surgeons say the entire load could be carried by half that many. We are doing something about this now, too. We are organizing area-wide planning councils in an effort to hold down duplication of facilities and services. We have not gone very far with this yet, of course, and it is an uphill task at best. But the fact is we did not do much of anything about it until we got some hard looks, again from insurance commissioners and legislative committees and governors and other public officials.

The thing we have been saying about hospital charges is that we keep them at the absolute minimum consistent with the high-quality service everybody wants and has to have. However it seems that charges for the same service in different hospitals in the same community may vary by as much as 500 or 600 per cent in some cases, and so the things we have said do not always seem to make sense. In fact, there are some rude critics who have stated the proposition in somewhat harsher terms than that. Now we are organizing area-wide and in some cases state-wide groups to establish uniform principles of pricing practice. This is good, but it is also late.

We have been telling prospective employees that the hospital is a desirable place to work, but recently the unions have come along and pointed out, sometimes in 72 point type, that "it ain't necessarily so." We praise our doctors and nurses to the skies as selfless members of dedicated professions, and then it turns out that some of the nurses are following the economic security path right into the union hall and some of the doctors would obviously vote to withhold hospital privileges from St. Luke himself if he belonged to a closed panel, group practice plan.

The thing we always have said, and still say, about our purpose is that we are wholly devoted to the care of the sick and injured, but then we find that all the hospitals in some communities and some of the hospitals in nearly all communities may temper their devotion, or even withhold it on some occasions, according to the patient's color. It also turns out on occasion that what we really mean when we say we are devoted to the sick and injured is that we are wholly devoted to the care of the sick *unless* they are the chronically ill and aged or *unless* they are mentally rather than physically ill.

The trouble is that all these things have been happening in Macy's window. I think the chances are that all these problems are probably insignificant alongside the great accomplishments that have been recorded to our credit—in plant improvement, technological advance, economic practice, personnel training, and many other areas. But nevertheless there are enough problems around so that people sometimes smile when we begin to talk about our accomplishments. It is barely possible that they would pay more attention, or even respect us more, if we acknowledged our problems more readily than we have done and talked about what we are doing to solve them instead of just extolling our virtues.

Another reason we have not been getting a very full return on our public relations investment, it seems to me, is that we are not all saying the same thing, and so the effect of our effort has sometimes been to confuse rather than persuade. The most notable divergence is probably the one between what hospitals are saying and what doctors are saying. In meetings like this (Hospital Medical Staff Conference), and in our professional affairs generally, we make a sharp and proper distinction between the management of medical facilities on the one hand, and the medical care that is rendered in these facilities on the other; but I can assure you that the public makes no such distinction. In the public view, hospitals and physicians are indivisible, and so the problems of hospitals and doctors are indivisible; and yet we constantly reveal ourselves to be far apart in our analysis of the problems and our suggested solutions. To take a simple example, if I am a patient in the hospital and I am dissatisfied with the nursing service, or the food, or the size of my hospital bill, I am not very likely to complain while I am still in the hospital for reasons that were made clear thousands of years ago in the old Hindu proverb: "Before thou fordest the river, O brother, revile not unduly the crocodile's mother!"

Besides, there is nobody to complain to. Management in the hospital is generally invisible from the bedside.

So I hold back until the next time I see my doctor, whom I hold responsible for the whole outrageous episode anyway, and then I render my complaints, whatever they are.

I am sure we all know what happens in many instances: the doctor shrugs and nods his head and agrees with me that it is preposterous, if not downright criminal, the way hospitals charge these days—and look at the service they give you!

I do not suppose there is any way to make absolutely certain that every time the questions are asked the doctors will come up with the right answers—or at least refrain from giving the wrong answers. But I do consider that this is the most neglected area of hospital public relations. Unless we are making some systematic, energetic, continuous effort to give all the doctors both the information and the desire to join the effort to improve public understanding of hospitals, we are overlooking what I think may be the most productive single method of accomplishing this goal.

PATIENT OPINION POLLS

Incidentally, I do not think we should be deceived by the results of our patient opinion polls into thinking that patients are completely satisfied with what they are getting. I have had administrators tell me that 80 per cent, or 85 per cent, or 90 per cent of all the responses to their patient opinion polls were generally favorable. They have interpreted this to mean that patients are generally satisfied with their hospital care, and there are no real problems here.

I think we should be careful about interpreting the results of polls like this. Generally it turns out that out of 1,000 forms or questionnaires distributed, some 300 or 400 are eventually completed and returned. So the fact is that the opinions which are expressed on the completed forms, assuming that they are true, do not constitute a true sample of hospital patients at all. They are rather a sample of hospital patients who are willing to answer a questionnaire from the hospital about their hospital care—and this is something that is vastly different. It tells us absolutely nothing about the feelings and opinions of the 600 or 700 or more patients out of every 1,000 who did not answer the questions. We can speculate all we want about the reasons that they did not answer, but we simply do not know. However, it is at least arguable that their indifference to the hospital's request for information about their feelings reflects something less than total enchantment with the kind of care they received.

Recently, for example, a group of hospitals in one large metropolitan area conducted an extensive survey of patient opinion; some 12,000 questionnaires were mailed out, and approximately 50 per cent were completed and returned.

As always, the overall opinion expressed by the respondents was favorable. Eighty-six per cent of the respondents said their opinion of the hospital generally was good, 11 per cent said it was fair, and 2 per cent said it was poor. Here is a quick summary of some of the other responses:

Ninety per cent of the respondents said the admission procedure was carried out promptly and efficiently, and 85 per cent said the persons who admitted them were "quite pleasant." You understand of course that these were multiple choice questions on printed forms, and "quite pleasant" was the only choice possible which avoided kicking somebody in the shins. Left to their own devices, these patients might readily have thought of some more descriptive phrases.

Eighty-two per cent of the respondents characterized their hospitals as restful and quiet; 86 per cent were satisfied with their room accommodations; 94 per cent said their hospital rooms were either "very attractive" or "all right" (and in this multiple choice context I suggest that "all right" could easily be a pejorative term): 85 per cent said the temperature in their hospital rooms was comfortable and the rooms were "well lighted." That is to say they were not "poorly lighted." The food was hot enough, the quantity of the food was about right, and the people who served the food were considerate and courteous. Seventy per cent of the respondents thought the nurses were really interested in their problems, and 77 per cent thought the response was good when they asked for nursing service.

Here is another result of the survey that you may want to think about pretty carefully: the respondents had been patients in all kinds of hospitals, from big teaching centers to small facilities for neighborhood practitioners, and nearly all the respondents thought they had received the very best, high quality medical care. Perhaps this proves nothing more than what you already know—that there are just two kinds of patients today: those who are satisfied and those who sue.

The questions about financial matters, as might be expected, evoked a somewhat less enthusiastic, but nevertheless generally favorable, response. Sixty-four per cent of the respondents thought the rules regarding payment of hospital bills were all right, and 67 per cent said they understood the charges listed on their bills. Now here is another question, it seems to me, that demonstrates how careful you must be in interpreting the results of patient opinion polls. The fact that 67 per cent of the respondents said they understood the charges listed on their bills should not be confused with an equivalent level of real understanding of the charges listed. This is because for this question the only choice the respondent had was to state that he did not understand the charges listed— a choice that may have seemed to some about the same as saying, "I am an idiot."

As these surveys generally do, the questionnaire concluded with an open-end question in this case asking: "What one thing could the hospital have done to make your stay more pleasant and comfortable?"

Two-thirds of the respondents had something to say here: in about 40 per cent of the responses, what they had to say was interpreted as favorable when they just could not think of anything the hospital might have done to make things pleasanter. One respondent even wrote that he "enjoyed every minute of it"—a reply that may raise a question about unnecessary utilization, if the man was in his right mind.

Some 2,200 responses to the open-end question were judged to be complaints or suggestions. Of these, 27 per cent related to personal comfort or convenience, 21 per cent to nursing service, 15 per cent to food service, 7 per cent to noise, 7 per cent to visitors, and only 6 per cent had anything to do with money. This circumstance rather reinforces my conviction that nobody is as worried about hospital costs as hospital people are, and, just possibly, the best public relations tactic on hospital costs would be to stop talking about them altogether.

Certainly the results of this public opinion survey cannot be interpreted as meaning anything other than that these 6,000 patients were pretty well satisfied with the services provided for them. Whatever the other 6,000—those who did not respond—may have thought, this cannot be added up to anything like the widespread, furious public dissatisfaction with hospitals that we are sometimes led to believe exists.

THE DIMINISHING MYSTIQUE

At any rate, I think there is another and perhaps overriding reason or set of reasons why we do not enjoy the full measure of public confidence that we think our performance should command and that all our public relations efforts have been aimed at achieving. The simplest way to describe it is to say that the doctor and hospital are losing some of their mystique. The reverent awe which set the physician and his associates and his whole environment apart from and above the rest of society has been vanishing in our time and is being replaced by a sophisticated, appraising, and often critical scrutiny, the same cold eye that looks at business, government, labor, and every other element of society as if to say, "What are they up to now, and how much is it going to cost?"

To the extent that this is true, how did it happen?

I suppose, again, there are a lot of reasons. Certainly the growth of prepayment plans has something to do with this. With 160,000,000 people paying for some part of their hospital or medical care on a prepayment schedule instead of by deficit fee, there is a kind of vested or proprietary interest in hospital affairs that did not exist a generation ago. I think this has had, along with its unquestioned and surpassing good effects, this little side effect of somewhat diminishing the glamour or mystique. Certainly the same kind of effect may result eventually from the further vesting of public interest in medical and hospital affairs represented by Medicare and federally aided public and medical assistance programs.

But I think the most important contributing cause of the diminished mystique has unquestionably been the constant advance of medical science and the consequent proliferation of medical technology, resulting in inevitable changes in the emotional tone or climate of the medical environment. The traditional one-to-one relationship of doctor and patient, with total responsibility on one side and total confidence on the other, is still the prevailing relationship in medical practice; but it is simply not the only relationship any more. The processes of medical care are shared today among specialists, consultants, assistants, technologists, technicians, and others; and this means the responsibility is necessarily shared to some extent, and the confidence is divided accordingly. I think most people understand instinctively that there are gains as well as losses involved here. Most people understand, for example, that the antibiotic is an excellent substitute for the cool hand on the fevered brow, and most people understand that the spectrophotometer is an improvement on the naked eye. But there is also some emotional loss, without any doubt, and by that much the patient-physician relationship and the patient-hospital relationship have been altered—the appraising look has been substituted for the worshipful gaze.

WHAT CAN BE DONE ABOUT IT?

I am not sure exactly what can be done to ameliorate the effects of these changes, but I am sure that the place to begin is not in the brochure but at the bedside. As a practical matter, for example, I would suggest a concerted effort on the part of everybody involved to cut down the number of consultants, assistants, residents, junior residents, interns, clerks, and medical visitors from Chile who come into the hospital room to palpate the spleen.

Of course, this is not going to be accomplished. The parade into the patient's room is going to grow, not diminish. Nobody is going to reverse the progression of medical technology. Medicine will become more specialized, mechanized, transistorized over the years rather than less so, and the resulting problems having to do with changes in emotional tone and response will become more severe rather than less so. The father-child relationship between doctor and patient, or the deity-communicant relationship, is vanishing along with the old-fashioned family doctor—the community savant who could read Greek and play the violin as well as deliver babies, set fractures, and cure pneumonia. The physician today is so busy keeping up with his specialty that he scarcely has time to learn English, let alone Greek; and the physician who delivers babies does not set fractures, and the one who sets fractures does not cure pneumonia. Thus the love and respect that were once lavished on one man have been fragmented and diluted, almost to the vanishing point at times; and this is the core of the problem.

Our first obligation, it seems to me, is to understand what is happening. These are not problems to be solved by public relations techniques; they are deep-rooted changes in the social organism. They need to be studied and analyzed, not just by questionnaires but by specialists in the social and behavioral sciences engaging in serious, continuing long-term research supported by hospitals and clinicians. Several projects of this kind have already been undertaken in individual institutions and communities. We need many more of them, perhaps for many years, before we shall ourselves fully understand all the effects of the "industrial revolution" in medicine that is taking place in our time. We still do not understand all the effects of the technological revolution that began in industry more than 100 years ago.

I am hopeful that the results of such studies might point the way toward changes in our public posture that would be in line with the changes that have occurred in our professional performance. The reason I am hopeful is that I think people are smarter than we generally give them credit for being when we keep trying, as we have often done, to make the physician in the proliferated, specialized medical technology of today project the public image of the old-fashioned, Greek-speaking family physician and community savant. No more can we make the modern, businesslike, specialized, transistorized hospital project the public image of the old-fashioned, benevolent, charitable, religious asylum. I believe just as strongly as any that benevolence and charity still exist in our hospitals, but today these appear to be recessive rather than dominant traits. To make other people understand that charity and benevolence can exist side by side with data processing machines, linear accelerators, and physiologic monitoring systems, we have first to demonstrate that this is possible; and I am not sure we have done it completely as yet. When we do understand it, and then demonstrate it, public understanding will come along inevitably. I believe this because I believe in a principle that is firmly rooted in our political society and that was stated in its simplest terms by Thomas Jefferson 180 years ago: "Given right information," he said, "the people make right judgments."

Our faith in the principle is strained at times, but I believe it will stand up. We ought to give it a chance.

Part II

Clinical Services of the
Hospital Staff

13

Full-time Service Chiefs

By Victor Richards, M.D.

Victor Richards is chief of surgery at the Presbyterian Medical Center and at the Children's Hospital, both of San Francisco. He received the M.D. degree and his surgical residency training at Stanford University, and he now serves as clinical professor of surgery at Stanford University School of Medicine and also at the University of California School of Medicine. Formerly, he was professor and chairman of the Department of Surgery at Stanford. In 1965, he completed a three-year term as chief of staff at the Presbyterian Medical Center. Dr. Richards is a member of the American Board of Surgery, representing the Society of University Surgeons. He is a member of Surgery Study Section B of the National Institutes of Health and is also a member of the Review Committee on Continuing Medical Education of the American Medical Association.

The Guide Issue of *Hospitals, JAHA,* August 1, 1965, gives the following data for the Presbyterian Hospital and Medical Center of San Francisco: Beds, 242; Admissions, 8,938; Census, 188; Bassinets, 30; Births, 874; Newborn census, 9; Payroll, $2,902,000; Personnel, 559.

Hospitals exist to serve the public interest by the prevention and treatment of disease or, in more positive terms, by the provision of optimal health care for the community. Thus, their aims are identical with those of medicine, and the relationship between physicians and hospitals should be viewed in the broadest social and educational perspectives. The public rightly demands of both hospitals and physicians the answers to several questions:

What are the medical needs of the community in this period of rising
   expectations and growing affluence?

How many physicians are required to meet our changing medical needs?

How should these physicians be educated, and, in particular, how can
   they be kept abreast of the swelling flood of new knowledge and
   difficult techniques?

How can physicians and hospitals best work together to bring important
   advances in medicine to the community, to preserve the quality of
   medical care, and to provide the quantity of medical care required
   inside and outside the hospitals?

In our larger communities, particularly those with universities, the
impetus to seek solutions to these challenging problems will arise from
new and refreshing relationships between the universities and the community hospitals and between the community hospitals and their medical
staffs.

THE VISION OF 1932

In 1932, Dr. Ray Lyman Wilbur, a past-president of the American
Medical Association, a former Secretary of the Interior, and a former
president of Stanford University, stated three major recommendations
in the report of the Committee on the Costs of Medical Care.[1] The Committee recommended (1) that medical services, both preventive and
therapeutic, be furnished largely by organized groups of physicians,
dentists, nurses, pharmacists, and other associated personnel, *organized
preferably around a hospital for rendering complete home, office, and
hospital care* [italics mine]; (2) that the costs of medical care be placed
on a group prepayment basis through the use of insurance, through the
use of taxation, or through the use of both of these methods; and (3) that
the study, evaluation, and coordination of medical services be considered
important functions of every state and local community, that agencies
be formed to exercise these functions, and that coordination of rural
and urban services receive special attention.

These recommendations lay dormant for 30 years, but the concepts
became national issues in the 1960's largely as a result of the rising cost
of medical care and the shortage of physicians for a growing population.
The medical profession has become increasingly concerned with the
ability to attract bright young people of high integrity into its ranks,
with their undergraduate medical education, their graduate education
in hospitals, and particularly with the continuing education throughout
their life's practice. The proper utilization of scientific advances not
only makes medicine more costly but also requires lifelong study by the
physician. The optimal environment for this lifelong education is the

hospital. The kind of hospital environment required for excellence of patient care includes the teaching of interns and residents, continuing education of the hospital staff, and research, both clinical and basic.

THE COST OF EXCELLENCE

Like many good things, excellence costs money. Hence, it is not surprising that in excellent hospitals the cost of patient care has increased remarkably, and hospitals have had to become concerned about hospital-physician relationships. The costs of house staff and the support of research have been increasingly borne by the hospitals. New contractual relationships have had to be established with physicians specializing in radiology, laboratory medicine, anesthesiology, radiobiology, and other specialties. The prevailing conditions of private practice and the fee for service indemnity insurance have encouraged the use of hospital facilities, which, of course, contributes to the rising community costs of hospital and medical care. Hospitals have become more deeply involved in medical education, and this requires the establishment of new contractual relationships between certain key teaching personnel on the medical staff and the hospital. Teaching hospitals have naturally developed closer affiliations with other educational institutions in the community. To implement educational programs for interns and residents, private hospitals had to assume the burden of the cost of care of medically indigent patients incident to teaching. Hence, rising hospital and medical costs have become a national issue which fomented far-reaching federal legislation.

THE 1965 REALITY

The 1932 vision of "medical care for the American people" reported by the Committee on Costs of Medical Care is about to become a reality. Prepaid insurance provides medical care for an increasingly larger proportion of our population, and now for those over 65 through the Medicare Act. The study, evaluation, and coordination of medical services will be increasingly important in every state and in every local community if the goals envisaged by the President's Commission on Heart Disease, Cancer, and Stroke are attained.

Patients are beginning to shift their identification from the solo physician to the hospital center. Physicians are being forced to group themselves together with dentists, nurses, pharmacists, and other paramedical personnel, and the hospital is emerging as the principal institution for rendering complete medical care. Excellence of patient care in the clinical setting of the hospital requires the best knowledge available from teaching and research, and the image of the hospital is becoming that of a health and educational center rather than a disease-oriented institution. Many physicians are coming to feel that hospital-based groups will enjoy advantages over independent ones.

Three major changes in our social and economic structure emerged in 1965 which will affect immeasurably our hospitals: (1) the passage of Medicare, with a new national and governmental stake in the community hospital; (2) legislation supporting Regional Medical Programs for Heart Disease, Cancer, and Stroke, stressing cooperation among hospitals and medical centers and other health facilities; and (3) the changing image of the hospital as a health center, and reciprocally, the patient's weaker identification with the solo physician. These developments involve the hospital staff more deeply in research and education and point to the need for more serious consideration of full-time service chiefs in an effort to achieve their goals.

THE CHANGING RELATIONSHIP BETWEEN UNIVERSITIES AND HOSPITALS

Since the days of Hippocrates, the teaching of clinical medicine has involved a student, a teacher, and a patient—the three meeting at the bedside for a useful learning experience. The necessity of this one-to-one-to-one relationship has not changed over the centuries.

The traditional clinical teaching material in university hospitals was the indigent medical patients. The patient who was unable to pay for medical care relinquished his identification with an individual physician and accepted medical care by an unknown group of physicians who related themselves to him in various capacities. The patient willingly accepted the premise that he could be used as a teaching subject by any or all members of the group, with the sole proviso that in exchange the group would furnish good medical care cost-free. This source began to dwindle in the 1940's under the impact of prepaid health insurance.

With the spread of insurance and prepayment plans, *university hospitals have begun to accept insurance patients and other private patients.* The teaching patient—whether indigent, private, or third-party payment —still identifies himself to a large extent with the group to whom he entrusts himself for medical care rather than with an individual physician.

The moral issue is simple and clear. The teaching patient receives optimal medical care regardless of his ability to pay, and the physician-in-training is permitted to render care to the patient and assume increasing responsibility to the point of full responsibility as his training progresses. This is true because the teaching group gives tacit assurance that the care of the patient will not be jeopardized by the student physician. It thus becomes morally indefensible for the group to render anything less than optimal total care to the patient, and it becomes morally defensible for the physician-in-training to assume total responsibility for the care of the patient with the sanction and support of the training group. *The legal issue* is not entirely clear, but the physician-in-training usually is a licensed physician and duly qualified to practice medicine. *The economic issues* remain clouded, for many insurance companies and some groups still feel that the physician-in-training is not entitled to a fee for professional services, either for himself or for the group. These economic issues become increasingly important as prepaid health insurance coverage increases.

As more and more patients become insured, new dimensions in group practices in university hospitals and in teaching community hospitals will necessarily evolve if adequate clinical teaching material is to be found for the education of physicians. The problem for university hospitals is particularly complex since traditionally they have not engaged in the private practice of medicine. Of necessity, new relationships must be worked out between universities and teaching community hospitals.

BASIC BIOLOGY VERSUS CLINICAL BIOLOGY IN THE UNIVERSITY SETTING

In the university setting, research has been increasingly emphasized in recent years, and academic advancement in many universities is primarily related to research attainments. Basic research is at a premium—concurrently, emphasis on teaching has dwindled. The application of new and basic scientific knowledge to patient care is best initiated in the university setting, but it requires a new breed of clinician who can best be called a clinical biologist. This new kind of clinician also has a place in the community teaching hospital with its trend toward greater specialization combining clinical research and patient care. The trend is especially noticeable in fields such as hematology, endocrinology, and cardiovascular diseases. The application of basic biological knowledge to optimal bedside care requires the education of more clinically oriented biologists and the diffusion of these men into community hospitals.

THE NEED FOR PROFESSORS OF CLINICAL MEDICINE

The application of new knowledge to patient care in community hospitals is best accomplished through physicians who are primarily dedicated to education—the clinical professors—and they can work as well in the setting of a teaching community hospital as a university hospital. The clinical professor may be supported by the clinical biologist working in a highly specialized field, but the bulk of day-to-day clinical practice and clinical teaching does not lie within special research spheres. The teaching of broad clinical medicine must be encouraged and supported if the educational needs of the community are served.

THE NEED FOR UNIVERSITY LEADERSHIP IN RELATING COMMUNITY TEACHING HOSPITALS TO THE UNIVERSITY

The dwindling source of clinical teaching material in university hospitals, the orientation of many university physicians toward research rather than practice, and the general desire of the faculty to maintain individuality, freedom, and independence—these conditions will inevitably force the universities to change their relationships to community hospitals. The orientation of the university hospitals will remain toward teaching and research with service as an important but secondary function, while the orientation of the community hospital will remain primarily toward service, with teaching and research of secondary importance. If educational needs at all levels are to be fulfilled, a closer relationship must be established between the two institutions. These relationships will be educationally sound if the universities assume a proper role of leadership. Educational influences and scientific advances can then be translated into patient care to the advantage of all concerned. Great economic advantages will accrue to the universities, for university hospital construction costs will be minimized by the utilization of existing community hospital facilities. Further, the cost of patient care incident to teaching will also diminish through the use of community hospital patients.

The moral issue remains clear. Teaching enhances the quality of medical care regardless of the patient's ability to pay. Organized professional groups should be established in university and in community hospitals alike so that fees can be legally received from any source, for all professional services rendered in the total care of teaching patients. The disposition of the funds would be according to a predetermined plan of the group.

The economic and educational advantages of relationships between universities and community hospitals are indeed great. It is hoped that universities will soon relate themselves to the mainstreams of medicine and community interest in more meaningful ways.

THE CHANGING ROLE OF THE PRIVATE HOSPITAL AND ITS STAFF

Private hospitals must also reorient themselves if they are to discharge their new responsibilities for health care. First, those in larger communities must attain sufficient size either by themselves or through mergers with others so that optimal patient care, with the many specialized services this implies, can be provided economically. The emerging image of the hospital community health center will require development on a community-wide basis. Increasingly, patients will receive the highly specialized care which demands expensive facilities and equipment and, most important, fully qualified physicians and paramedical personnel will be on duty in the hospital on a 24-hour basis. To provide these difficult, expensive, and specialized services economically will require organized professional groups supported by hospitals of adequate size, usually ranging from 500 to 700 or more beds. Hospitals will then become true centers of excellence.

Certain highly technical but necessary specialty units must be supported on a community-wide level to avoid expensive and needless duplication. The artificial kidney, organ transplant units, and cancer immunology units are some examples. Community support is also appropriate for out-patient facilities and for special treatment units within the hospital which are related to community health problems, for example, units for the care of nervous and mental disorders and for alcoholism.

Standards of excellence can best be achieved through group associations within the hospital environment where there are invigorating currents of teaching and research flowing directly into the mainstream of clinical practice. This is not to say that only specialists will practice in the hospitals, for it is clear from the experience in England that proper arrangements for the family physician within the hospital setting are imperative. In the ideal hospital, family physicians and specialists will work together harmoniously, with their respective roles more clearly defined.

Not all physicians on the staff will be interested in or capable of participating in the enlarged educational and research aims.

FULL-TIME SERVICE CHIEFS

In the ideal community teaching hospital, a nucleus of full-time service chiefs in the major departments will be essential. They will furnish stimulus, guidance, and administration of education, research, and patient care. In exchange for a way of life which would permit dedicated men to identify themselves with the mission and purposes of the hospital and to emphasize teaching and research, new contractual relationships must be established between them and the hospital. They can accomplish their goals only if their time and energy are utilized most efficiently, and this requires that they be geographically full-time in the hospital setting. Their background and capabilities should qualify them for joint appointments with universities. In this manner, interrelationships between two institutions will be facilitated and strengthened. The full-time chiefs would carry responsibility for education within the hospital at all levels, and in addition they would give leadership and guidance to research.

Payment of Full-time Service Chiefs

In essence, there are three sources of income for the full-time chief of service. In some instances, the hospital may pay the full salary. This method is most likely to be found in the areas of radiology, radiobiology, laboratory services, and other specific technical areas. In some instances, the university may pay a part of the salary in recognition of educational services to medical students and residents in affiliated programs. In other situations, the full-time chief may be permitted to conduct within the hospital a limited private practice, usually only consultation practice. In any case, he is geographically full-time in the hospital.

The question is frequently asked whether it is proper and just for the hospital to support full-time chiefs of service and other educational activities out of hospital income. The income, of course, comes from the charges to patients, who thus actually bear the burden of the hospital's educational expenses. Are these costs properly charged to patient care? They are entirely proper if the quality of patient care is improved by these additional services. There is little doubt that hospitals oriented to education and research are better able to serve the community needs in both the quality and the quantity of medical care. The standards of medical care are invariably higher in an educational atmosphere, and this in turn attracts promising young physicians for training and subsequently for community service.

The cost of these educational services is indeed small in comparison to the benefits. For example, in a hospital with an average daily census of 500 patients, an additional charge of $1.00 per day would provide $500.00 per day in additional income, an ample amount to support the activities of five full-time service chiefs. It must be emphasized that flexibility of arrangements may exist so that the full financial support need not come from hospital funds.

SUMMARY

The opportunities for full-time service chiefs are rich with promise. They constitute a challenge to physicians who have the intelligence and good will to establish new relationships within the hospital and between the hospital and the university so that new scientific knowledge may be used more effectively to meet the health needs of the community.

BIBLIOGRAPHY

1. Wilbur, R. L.: "Medical Care for the American People," the Final Report of the Committee on the Costs of Medical Care, The University of Chicago Press, Chicago, 1932.

14

The Chief of Medicine

By John C. Leonard, M.D., and
Robert S. Liggett, M.D.

John C. Leonard was the director of medical education at Hartford Hospital from 1947 until his death April 26, 1966. His position was the first of its kind in the United States. He held many important posts during his very active career, including associate director of education programs for rural hospitals of the Commonwealth Foundation, associate director of the Bingham Foundation, and associate director of the Joseph H. Pratt Diagnostic Hospital in Boston. He received the M.D. degree from Yale University and served there as clinical professor of medicine. Dr. Leonard was a member of the Advisory Committee on Internships of the AMA Council on Medical Education, a member and chairman of the AMA Residency Review Committee in Internal Medicine, and chairman of the AMA Committee on Postgraduate Medicine. He was vice-president and regent of the American College of Physicians and had been Governor of the College for Connecticut.

The Guide Issue of *Hospitals, JAHA,* August 1, 1965, gives the following data on Hartford Hospital: Beds, 800; Admissions, 30,584; Census, 723; Bassinets, 150; Births, 5,411; Newborn census, 82; Total expenses, $15,207,000; Payroll, $10,626,000; Personnel, 2,082. There are three other short-term general hospitals in Hartford with 144 beds, 189 beds, and 654 beds. The population of Hartford in the 1960 census was 162,178.

Robert S. Liggett is now the full-time director of medical education at Saint Luke's Hospital in Denver. He was formerly the chief of medicine, and the chief of staff at this hospital. He is clinical professor of medicine at the University of Colorado School of Medicine, and president of the Colorado Society of Internal Medicine. He received the M.D. degree from Washington University; he is a diplomate of the American Board of Internal Medicine, and a Fellow of the American College of Physicians.

(ED. NOTE: *This chapter has been prepared by Dr. Liggett from a tape recording of a discussion seminar at the Estes Park Conference in October, 1965, led by Dr. Liggett and the late Dr. John C. Leonard.*)

The chief of medicine is responsible for the administration and co-ordination of activities of his department and for cooperation with other departments. It is important for him to make ward rounds and to keep in touch with the service professionally because without the image of a competent clinician he cannot retain the respect of the house staff. By example he must inspire the house staff to achieve rapport with patients, for only in this way can meaningful histories be obtained.

QUALIFICATIONS

The Joint Commission on Accreditation of Hospitals states: "A good Chief of Service must have professional competence, administrative adequacy and, in addition, he must have quality . . . Quality means besides the above, compassion, skill, economy, understanding, sympathy, integrity and character." [1]

There are other attributes of a good chief of medicine. He must be a stable, experienced individual but not so old that he is looking toward retirement. He must not be lazy. He must be a clinician who is devoted to the importance of good patient care. It is estimated that administrative duties require from 35 to 40 per cent of his time. If there is a medical school in the area, he should have a teaching appointment on the faculty.

When prospective interns visit a hospital, they want to know who will teach them. Although chiefs of services are not directly responsible for house staff procurement, their influence will be positive or negative, perhaps unknowingly.

A prime requisite of a chief of service is *time* to devote to his duties; volunteer and part-time chiefs are at a decided disadvantage as compared to the full-time chief.

THE FULL-TIME CHIEF OF MEDICINE

The need for a full-time chief of medicine is becoming increasingly apparent, and the larger the hospital the greater the need, for administrative as well as for educational reasons. Specialty boards are becoming more and more demanding, and it is well established that residency review committees look with favor upon programs headed by full-time chiefs.

Perhaps most smaller hospitals (of 400 beds or less) and especially those without house staff should not seek full-time chiefs of services because they are expensive. However, the need for a program of continuing education and for a program of quality control may justify such an appointment even in small hospitals and in the absence of house staff. The most important requirement is unreserved support of the hospital attending staff. Without this, even the most promising program will collapse.

The sources of full-time chiefs of medicine are generally restricted to one or two possibilities: pick one of your own young men of proven competence or go shopping in the academic field.

The economics of the position of full-time chief of medicine and the cost of programs of medical education were discussed at some length. A reference to a statement of the late Allen Gregg of the Rockefeller Foundation is rather startling, namely, that a hospital should be willing to pay up to 10 per cent of its budget for a good program of graduate education. Other estimates quoted varied from $3\frac{1}{2}$ to $6\frac{1}{2}$ per cent of the hospital budget. Hartford Hospital estimates their internship program alone costs them about 75¢ per patient day, and the combined intern-resident programs cost about $1.50 per patient day.

The salary of the chief of service should be approximately the same as the income of the average practitioner in the same specialty in the community. It is emphasized that there should be no general dissemination of information regarding individual salaries among hospital-based physicians.

Should the chief of medicine be allowed practice or consultation privileges? The consensus is that he should be permitted to see patients in consultation but not practice. He should charge a fee for his service which should go into the education fund. It is felt that the privilege of consultation should be extended to all full-time hospital-based physicians, and their fees should likewise be assigned to the education fund.

FINANCING MEDICAL EDUCATION

The financing of programs of medical education in the community hospital may be sought from a variety of sources. Insurance carriers, recognizing that medical care is better in hospitals with aggressive teaching programs, are increasingly willing to absorb a portion of the cost. Hospital auxiliaries should be encouraged to raise funds for this purpose, and affluent patients should be asked to make contributions or set up trusts for the endowment of graduate medical education.

Asking the attending staff to finance their educational program through contributions or assessment is frowned upon because physicians are already plagued by too many appeals for financial support. However, some hospitals do have a plan where the staff pays at least part of the salary of a director of medical education.

The question is raised concerning the need for a director of medical education in a hospital that has full-time service chiefs. In this situation, the primary function of the director of medical education would be to get everyone to work together for the welfare of the hospital and overall program and to prevent each department from developing isolated selfish interests. The director of medical education should function in the non-university hospital somewhat as a dean functions in a university hospital.

CONTINUING EDUCATION

Finally, emphasis is repeatedly placed upon the continuing education of the staff as one of the greatest needs of medicine. It is stated that this area alone furnishes sufficient reason for the employment of full-time chiefs of medicine and directors of medical education.

BIBLIOGRAPHY

1. Chiefs of Departments or Chiefs of Service, *Bull. Joint Commission Accreditation Hospitals,* No. 30 (Aug.) 1962.

15

The Chief of Surgery

I.

By Luther C. Carpenter, M.D.

Luther C. Carpenter is a general surgeon practicing in Grand Rapids, Michigan. He is a native of Michigan and a product of the University of Michigan where he received the A.B., M.D., and M.S. in surgery as well as his surgical residency training. He is a diplomate of the American Board of Surgery and is a Fellow of the American College of Surgery. At the Blodgett Memorial Hospital in Grand Rapids, he has served on many committees and was chief of surgery from 1951 to 1954 and chief of staff from 1954 to 1957. He has been a member of the Board of Trustees of the Commission on Professional and Hospital Activities since its inception in 1955, and he is currently the president of the board.

The Guide Issue of *Hospitals, JAHA,* August 1, 1965, gives the following data on Blodgett Memorial Hospital: Beds, 420; Admissions, 16,251; Census, 330; Bassinets, 66; Births, 2,475; Newborn census, 35; Total expenses, $5,721,000; Payroll, $3,597,000; Personnel, 988.

(ED. NOTE: *In this chapter, two general surgeons who have served as chief of surgery in their respective hospitals describe their experience and give their own philosophy of the duties and responsibilities of this office. Their viewpoints in many respects are quite similar; the variations in experience and emphasis in two successful departments provide background for hospitals similarly situated.*)

The modern chairman of a department of surgery is an anachronism. So declares George D. Zuidema, M.D., Professor of Surgery at Johns Hopkins University School of Medicine. "He is expected to possess the classical qualities of 'the professor,' a man of superb technical competence and clinical ability, all-knowing, fatherlike, an educator emanating new ideas of medical education, a research scientist without peer, an administrator, writer, lecturer, and traveling committee man."

Few if any such individuals exist today. While Dr. Zuidema was obviously discussing the problems of a chairman of surgery in a large university medical center, many of his remarks may be applied equally well to the problems in a community hospital.

Since the majority of hospitals in this country are non-profit, community hospitals not affiliated with a medical school, the chief of the surgical service in such hospitals will be discussed here. Over three-quarters of the internships and more than half of the residencies available are offered by non-affiliated hospitals. Moreover, non-affiliated hospitals have four times as many beds as affiliated hospitals. These data emphasize some of the real responsibilities of the community hospital.

The functions and responsibilities of the community hospital have widened. The hospital is now (1) the center of medical care for the geographic community; (2) the center of medical education and training for physicians, both house staff and practitioners; and (3) a center for medical research. The chief of surgery is responsible for the quality of surgical care rendered by his staff, for the continuing education of both the house and attending staffs, and for the development of research—all of which are growing so complex that it is becoming nearly impossible for a single individual to run a surgical department well. Let us then discuss the qualifications of the chief. Should he be elected or appointed? What should be his tenure of office? Should he be paid? What are his duties?

QUALIFICATIONS

The days of selecting a new chief by rotation, by default (being absent at the time of election), or as the result of a popularity contest are over. What should be his qualifications?

First, he must have professional excellence. He must be a successful practitioner of his specialty who commands the respect of his coworkers. He must be well trained, knowledgeable, technically skillful, and he must use sound judgment.

Second, he must have administrative ability. It is physically impossible for one man to carry out all of the duties and functions of his department. He must therefore be a good organizer and must be able to delegate authority and motivate others to perform many tasks. He must be able to make decisions and to enforce them.

Third, he must be dedicated to an active, vigorous training program which should include the continuing education not only of the house staff but also of the staff members in his department.

Fourth, he must be interested in research. This requires a knowledge of the past and an open mind for progress. He must have intellectual curiosity to serve as a catalyst and a stimulant to others to perform basic and clinical research. Nothing is more restrictive than a chief who maintains the status quo.

SELECTION

How should the chief of surgery be selected? He may be appointed or elected. In either event, his selection must be confirmed by the governing body. If appointed, he may be selected by the chief of staff, by the administrator, or directly by the board. If elected, he may be selected by staff vote or by vote of his department. The most common and certainly the most democratic method is by vote of the department. He is then more likely to receive cooperation from the members of his department as their elected representative.

TENURE

What should be his tenure in office? This depends on his ability, his willingness to serve, and the availability of replacements. A one-year term is too short to permit the chief to learn all of his duties and to implement a positive program. Yet if he proves incapable, the quicker he can be replaced the better. At the other extreme, self-perpetuation leads to dictatorship, stifles the interest and ambition of others, and vitiates cooperation. A capable man should hold office for a two- or three-year term and be eligible for re-election.

REMUNERATION

Should the chief of surgery receive remuneration? There is a trend toward part- or full-time salaried chiefs of departments. This, I believe, is a mistake, at least in most community hospitals. The strength of our staffs has been in the voluntary contribution by the individual member. This is one of the responsibilities a staff member assumes as a reward for becoming a member of his department. As soon as an individual is paid for services, he becomes a "hired hand." This may lead to hospital control of his department; it may reduce the amount of voluntary services rendered by others; and it may stifle interest and responsibility and lead to inertia in the department. If the chief is a capable leader and is able to delegate authority, the tasks need not be so burdensome as to require remuneration.

DUTIES

What are the duties of the chief of surgery?

Administrative Head. He is the administrative head of his department. He presides at all business meetings, appoints committees to perform essential duties, and serves as an ex officio member of all committees. He recommends individuals to the chief of staff to represent the department on standing staff committees. He is a member of the credentials committee to select new members and to recommend change of status— advancement, restriction of privileges, withdrawal of privileges, or retirement. He must enforce the hospital's bylaws, rules, and regulations. He must cooperate with the operating room supervisor in recommending new equipment, improvements, and supplies and in maintaining a smoothly functioning operating room suite.

Responsibility for Professional Care. The chief of surgery is responsible for the quality of care rendered by members of his department. He must see that there is a critical review of work done, an analysis of all complications, a survey of infections, a frank discussion of mortalities, and, in short, an internal audit of surgical care in his department.

Education. The chief of surgery must be an educator. He is responsible for the training of house staff and for furthering the education of the attending staff members in his department. He must see that the teaching of surgery is properly organized and presented by all methods available: operating room instruction, teaching rounds, case presentations, journal club discussions, and numerous other aids to modern education.

The chief of surgery must stimulate the younger members of the department to prepare for responsibility and for advancement. He must encourage all members of the department in continuing education on as broad a base as possible.

CONCLUSION

It is obvious that the chief of surgery must be selected carefully. To perform all of the duties required is a real challenge and a time-consuming job. Yet with proper organization, delegation of authority, and the cooperation of his fellow members he renders to his community and profession a real service—a service which need not be too burdensome and which can be very rewarding.

II.

By Kenneth C. Sawyer, M.D.

Kenneth C. Sawyer is in the private practice of general surgery in Denver, and he is chief of surgery at Presbyterian Hospital. He received the M.D. degree from the University of Colorado where he is associate clinical professor of surgery. He is a diplomate of the American Board of Surgery and a Fellow of the American College of Surgeons. He is a delegate to the American Medical Association and a member of the AMA Council on Medical Education. These are but a few of the many posts in which he serves.

The Guide Issue of *Hospitals, JAHA,* August 1, 1965, gives the following data for Presbyterian Hospital in Denver: Beds, 290; Admissions, 11,-765; Census, 254; Bassinets, 54; Births, 1,856; Newborn census, 21; Total expenses, $4,-402,000; Payroll, $3,013,000; Personnel, 722.

I am chief of the surgical service in a private hospital which is respected for the high quality of its patient care, which consistently fills its complement of interns and residents, and which, in spite of a progressive, successful building program, still has a bed shortage. I shall outline the program that we follow to obtain the individuals necessary to maintain the high standards we expect of our surgical service.

SELECTION

The chief of surgical service in a private hospital may be selected in several ways: (1) appointment by the chief of staff; (2) selection by the medical advisory board; (3) election by the staff members of the department concerned; (4) election by the general hospital staff.

The position of chief of a service should not be an honorary one. The chief should be appointed rather than elected since the most popular man obviously may not be the best administrator. The Council on Medical Education of the American Medical Association suggests that adequate continuity is desirable and leads to stronger and more effective programs.

RESPONSIBILITIES

In our hospital, as in others, the responsibilities of a department head fall into five main categories:

1. Responsibility for building and maintaining a staff dedicated to adequate patient care and quality of work
2. Responsibility for determining the privileges and restrictions of members of the staff
3. Responsibility for graduate and continuing education
4. Responsibility for research
5. Responsibility for a medical library

Responsibility for Building and Maintaining a Staff. The service chief cannot discharge his duties and responsibilities without a staff of physicians who have proper qualifications as to medical education and licensure. The staff must also be limited to physicians whose professional and moral integrity are unquestionable; who are proficient in their chosen fields of practice; who give personal attention to their patients; and who are willing to assume responsibility as a group for providing adequate instruction to each other and to the house staff.

Each specialty chief and department head must choose a small group from the general staff to participate in the administrative duties and to help with professional aspects of the service.

To maintain the highest possible standards of work, the service chief conducts weekly group conferences and monthly statistical meetings. At these conferences, which are well attended, morbidity and mortality findings are discussed in a friendly but candid manner.

Operative cases with minimal pathology and those presenting probable defects in diagnosis or management are evaluated by the tissue committee, which consists of chiefs of all clinical services, the chief pathologist, and the radiologist. With an effective service chief, a well functioning staff, and constant attention to the equipment and physical plant we can assure the best care possible to the patients in our hospital.

It is a policy on our surgery service to call frequently upon our colleagues for help in dealing with seriously ill patients, when there is a questionable diagnosis, or whenever there is doubt concerning the proper procedure. It is the responsibility of the department head to see that this sequence is adhered to rigidly.

Responsibility for Privileges and Restrictions. The second charge to the chief of surgery concerns the privileges and restrictions of those working in the department. This can be difficult in a private hospital; but the problem must be met head on, and it can be resolved by evaluating and clearly defining the potential of each new staff member and frankly discussing the findings with him.

In our hospital, as it should be in all hospitals, a general practitioner is not categorically restricted in surgical privileges. The general practitioner, the "family doctor," should be required to perform only those procedures he can do well. As with other physicians, his work in surgery is evaluated by the staff, and decisions regarding his competence are made by the service chief.

The main pitfalls are encountered in dealing with very young and very old practitioners. When a young man comes to the staff, his obligations, privileges, and restrictions are clearly described. If he does not voluntarily ask for guidance, an established staff member is assigned to assist him in the operating room and observe his competence. Frequently, the older man who has been an outstanding surgeon for many years and who has been a substantial contributor to the teaching program and to the many hospital building funds fails to realize or refuses to recognize that he is no longer a technically efficient surgeon. A compulsory retirement age is inadvisable, and I know of few private hospitals that enforce the rule if they do have one. We are obligated to these senior men. We tactfully help them with their operations; and most of them soon realize that they have passed their peak, and they send their patients and friends to other staff members. Unfortunately, there are exceptions; and when the surgical chief tells these men that they can no longer operate, "hell hath no fury like an outmoded surgeon."

Responsibility for Continuing Medical Education. Graduate medical education for interns and residents and continuing medical education for mature surgeons are important functions in the community hospital and are essential to better patient care. For the private hospital not affiliated with a medical school, there is abundant opportunity to develop outstanding intern and residency programs. Many non-affiliated community hospitals are able to provide the varieties of educational environment desired by significant numbers of medical school graduates. It behooves us, as men who derive our livelihood and professional stimulus from private hospitals, to establish effective educational programs. The quality of these programs is in direct proportion to the leadership provided by the department heads.

House Staff. To maintain an adequate graduate program, interns, residents, and the staff are given opportunities both to observe and to participate in total patient care. In order that this may be accomplished, they should follow an optimal number of patients through their full course in the hospital and in the out-patient department.

The intern training program in general surgery features diagnosis and preoperative and postoperative care. The value of this experience to the intern is in inverse proportion to the time spent in the operating room, although much good teaching can be done at the operating table. The dressing of wounds and determination of fluid requirements are an important part of the intern's experience and give him an opportunity to note the effects of the surgical procedure he has observed. This assignment should extend into the out-patient clinics.

Work in the operating room constitutes a vital part of the training of the surgical resident also. He must be given enough progressively graded operative responsibility to acquire proficiency in technique and judgment so that, upon completion of his training, he is able to take the responsibility for the diagnosis and treatment of any major surgical challenge.

It is a staff obligation to furnish enough cases for the senior resident to have full responsibility for a minimum of 150 major surgical procedures. Private cases may be used to augment his experience, provided the patient is aware of the arrangement. This is best accomplished on an individual basis. If the resident is introduced as a member of a team and the patient knows that an operation is a team effort, the resident can be given responsibility commensurate with his ability.

The journal club is an effective tool for stimulating the attending staff and house staff to become familiar with current literature. In our hospital, these meetings are conducted as social affairs. They are held monthly in the homes of members of the teaching staff and are occasions to which all surgical staff members look forward.

A director of medical education enhances the training of the house staff. In cooperation with the chairmen of the clinical departments and the hospital administrator, he is responsible for the integration of all educational activities in the hospital. This does not mean, however, that staff members can delegate their teaching responsibilities to him.

Bedside teaching is emphasized on our surgical service; all agree that this is the most important phase of intern and resident instruction. Formal teaching bedside rounds are held three days each week, and working ward rounds with the attending physician, the residents, and the surgical interns are conducted at the bedside each afternoon. If the attending surgeon is unable to take part in the rounds, his previously assigned alternate leads a detailed discussion of each patient. It is the responsibility of the department head to see that the history, physical examination, and admission notes are written by the intern and are commented upon and initialed by the resident and by the attending physician.

Conferences. Clinico-pathologic conferences are held each month. These conferences, conducted by the pathology department in cooperation with the clinical department heads, enhance the interest of the attending physicians and the motivation of the house staff. This is well documented since 50 to 75 per cent of the active staff always participate. Our hospital is blessed with pathologists who are excellent teachers and who work hard to make the programs attractive.

At monthly departmental meetings, deaths on the service are critically reviewed. Management and alternative proposals for treatment are discussed for each case. The department also attempts to present at least one interesting live case.

Weekly x-ray conferences, held jointly with other departments, are conducted by the department of radiology.

Perhaps the most stimulating conferences are the grand rounds held at 7:00 Saturday morning. This is the epitome of both graduate and continuing medical education. It is mandatory for the house staff, and the auditorium is well filled with attending men. Surgical rounds are held the first week of the month and medical grand rounds on the third week. Tumor conferences are held on the second and fourth weeks.

Responsibility for Research. An important factor of both graduate and continuing education in any hospital is the encouragement of the residents and staff to engage in investigative work. Those who pursue a research problem receive a stimulus which can be obtained in no other way. Our hospital, like most, has facilities available to the house and attending staffs for both basic and clinical research.

Responsibility for an Active Medical Library. An adequate medical library is an essential facility in the community hospital. Textbooks and monographs must be kept up to date, and a full range of appropriate medical journals should be available for all specialties in which training is being conducted. The medical library should be directed by a qualified medical librarian who can stimulate library research and assist in the preparation of reports.

16

The Chief of Obstetrics and Gynecology

I. IN THE PRIVATE HOSPITAL

By Wilbur F. Manly, M.D.

Wilbur F. Manly is chairman of the Teaching Committee and was formerly chief of the department of obstetrics and gynecology of St. Luke's Hospital in Denver. He received the M.D. degree from Stritch School of Medicine and was a resident at Chicago Lying-In Hospital. He is a diplomate of the American Board of Obstetrics and Gynecology. He is associate clinical professor of obstetrics and gynecology at the University of Colorado School of Medicine.

The Guide Issue of *Hospitals*, *JAHA*, August 1, 1965, gives the following data for St. Luke's Hospital: Beds, 449; Admissions, 17,797; Census, 392; Bassinets, 60; Births, 2,047; Newborn census, 33; Total expenses, $6,462,000; Payroll, $4,020,000; Personnel, 963.

The chief of obstetrics and gynecology in the private hospital holds a position that differs in many respects from that in a university hospital. In most private hospitals, the position has limited tenure of one to three years. The organization is more democratic and involves less hierarchy probably because the majority of work is done by men of comparable training, experience, and ability. In contrast, the university medical school department may be likened to a benevolent dictatorship in which a "party line" is developed prior to the actual treatment of any specific medical entity. The major function of the department is educational in

155

contrast to the private hospital's primary responsibility to the care of the patient.

The American College of Obstetrics and Gynecology has developed a guide listing the duties and areas of staff activity for the chief of obstetrics and gynecology.[1] The following is extracted from this manual of standards.

A. Duties of the chairman of the department
  1. The chairman of the department must:
     a. Be interested in organizing and developing the department.
     b. Be given the authority to establish and enforce specific departmental policies.
  2. His duties should include the following:
     a. Establish departmental rules and regulations.
     b. Submit recommendations for staff appointment and dismissal.
     c. Develop and supervise training programs for house staff.
     d. Schedule and supervise teaching and service responsibilities of the staff members.
     e. Appoint appropriate committees.
     f. Serve as consultant and arbitrator should differences of opinion arise over policy or patient care.
B. Areas of staff activity
  1. The size of the hospital and the degree of medical specialization determine whether departmental activities are assigned to committees or whether they are the personal responsibility of the chairman.
  2. The following areas are considered to be appropriate departmental committee activities for large services:
     a. Executive and administrative.
     b. Out-patient clinic.
     c. Tissue or operative review committee.
     d. Infection control.
     e. Therapeutic abortion and sterilization.
     f. Consultation for other ward services.
     g. Nursing.
     h. Nursery.
     i. Medical records.
     j. Staff conferences.

These activities will vary in localities and may depend to a large extent on the degree of emphasis on a house staff teaching program.

The role of the private hospital in the education of interns and residents faces almost inevitable escalation. Nearly all social programs aimed at improving the well-being of the indigent may remove some of these patients from charity institutions to the private hospital. Medicare programs may be the first to transfer patients in large numbers from university hospitals. (ED. NOTE: *There are varied opinions concerning the effect of Medicare and other social programs on the availability of teaching material in university hospitals. An opinion contrary to that expressed here is found in Chap. 30, where Dr. Price expresses fear that potential programs similar to those proposed by the President's Commission on Heart Disease, Cancer, and Stroke may divert patients away from the small community hospital to the medical centers.*) The demand for increased numbers of medical graduates will pinch the university hospital with its lowered inventory of teaching material. (ED. NOTE: *The diversion of patients from university hospitals by Medicare and similar programs may be more than offset by the increasing trend toward private patients seeking care in university hospitals.*) If one accepts the maxim that higher quality care is found in hospitals that offer education programs, then the obvious conclusion is that the best possible educational programs should be developed in private hospitals. In this light, the following steps for strengthening the department should be considered:

1. Lengthen the tenure of the chief of the department to a minimum of three to five years with provisions of reappointment.

2. Create a departmental executive committee of perhaps three members, and give the committee authority to act. The usual executive and credential committees at the hospital level have only one representative from the obstetrics and gynecology department, yet these committees are the final authority in evaluating the quality of work and the qualifications for staff appointment.

3. Prepare for an expanded teaching role.

   a. Establish prenatal teaching facilities for student nurses, medical students, and interns. If obstetric clinic facilities are not available, perhaps the private offices of staff members may be used. (ED. NOTE: *It is quite improbable that a preceptor type of prenatal experience in physicians' offices would suffice for resident training.*)

   b. Allocate clinic beds for teaching cases referred by attending physicians to the house staff for care.

   c. Indoctrinate the hospital administration as well as private patients to a cooperative role in medical education.

   d. Develop a teaching program that emphasizes the strong features of a department. Many private hospitals would do better by concentrating on participation in the education of medical students and interns, leaving the residency programs to the university hospitals. Affiliations may be arranged for the rotation of residents to the private hospital for limited periods rather than offering one good year of approved residency. (ED. NOTE: *Some medical educators have proposed that medical schools assume some of the teaching responsibilities for house staff in private hospitals through full-time faculty members recruited specifically for teaching programs in these hospitals.*)

   e. Provide opportunities for continuing education of the staff and require their active participation. A conference committee should arrange monthly scientific programs at a departmental level to provide current, informative, and stimulating discussions rather than didactic, junior-level lectures. Departmental business meetings should be held at a separate time to avoid having administrative matters infringe on the scientific session. Death and morbidity reviews should be part of the business meeting rather than the scientific sessions. (ED. NOTE: *The primary objective of meetings of the staff required by the JCAH—either general staff meetings or departmental meetings—is improvement in the care and treatment of patients in the hospital, with the agenda "limited largely to a review of current or recent cases in the hospital. Scientific programs not associated with the work of the hospital do not meet this requirement."* Hospital Accreditation References, *1964 ed., American Hospital Association, Chicago, Ill.*) Weekly small group seminars with the house staff furnishing the basic presentation are also stimulating. One or two staff men on a rotational basis should be responsible for directing the discussion and providing guidance. A monthly review of current obstetric and gynecologic literature is also a worthy part of this program.

4. Encourage the development of combined obstetric and gynecologic facilities. The use of a portion of the postpartum floor for selected clean gynecologic cases has been fully documented as to safety and convenience. The nursing staff develop gynecologic skills that are difficult to match in any other area of the general hospital. There should be an elastic arrangement whereby some of the gynecologic beds may be reclaimed during times of large obstetric demands, thus allowing a reasonably full usage of the bed capacity and reducing the need for temporary transfer of personnel during slack times. It also helps in the adjustment of staff when a hiatus occurs because of unexpected resignations or untimely deaths.

5. Review all the labor room pathology. The traditional method of reviewing only those cases with questionable results leaves much of the potential teaching material unused. A workable method embodies the completion of short forms on all abnormal cases. These are reviewed by the conference committee for educational possibilities.

CONCLUSION

The chief of the department of obstetrics and gynecology in the private hospital has many areas of responsibility—the patient, the continuing education of the medical and nursing staff, the student and house officers to whom he must give direction and education as well as counsel, and the hospital administration whose interests must be considered in the total picture. Much time and wisdom are required from this man and in many instances the task is becoming too great for the busy practitioner to handle effectively. The time is probably not too distant when the teaching private hospital will have a full-time chief in each of the major clinical departments as well as a full-time director of medical education.

BIBLIOGRAPHY

1. "Manual of Standards in Obstetric-Gynecologic Practice," 2d ed., American College of Obstetricians and Gynecologists, Chicago, 1965.

II. IN THE UNIVERSITY HOSPITAL

By Clyde L. Randall, M.D.

Clyde L. Randall is professor and chairman of the department of obstetrics and gynecology at the State University of New York at Buffalo. He received the M.D. degree from the University of Kansas and served residencies in pathology and surgery in Kansas City before a residency in gynecology at the University of Buffalo. He is past president of the staff of Buffalo General Hospital. He was a member of the AMA Residency Review Committee for Obstetrics and Gynecology for six years and has been a director of the American Board of Obstetrics and Gynecology since 1960, serving as secretary-treasurer of the Board since 1964.

In the university hospital, the chief of obstetrics and gynecology has six major areas of responsibility—patient care, departmental function, resident education, hospital staff function, community welfare, and the development of the specialty.

Responsibilities for Patient Care

Records. The chief of obstetrics and gynecology should have concern for the quality and adequacy of patient records. He should personally make notes on patients' records and see that each one is completed promptly. He should honor consultation requests and personally request consultations when indicated. He should maintain a continuing review of current records and express dissatisfaction in conferences when records are inadequate. He should encourage a continuous survey and evaluation of the quality of patient care by the staff and house staff.

Rounds. By personal example the chief should indicate the importance of daily rounds by the attending physician. He should have concern for the patient's complaints while noting the manifestations of her disease. He should avoid using bedside rounds to display personal knowledge of the patient or her disease. It is well to discuss the patient's complaints at her bedside, but her disease in the conference room. He should review the orders; the resident who routinely orders everything is usually not displaying competence or judgment.

Conferences. The chief must encourage objective discussion of complications as well as unusual cases. If his attitude is tempered by a conviction that "there but for the grace of God . . . ," he is able to point out effectively where different management might have made the difference. A chief's display of the importance of depending upon consultants—whether internist, radiologist, surgeon, or pathologist—is as important as emphasizing the occasional advisability of interpreting the consultant's recommendation in the light of aspects of the problem best understood by the obstetrician-gynecologist.

Responsibilities for Departmental Function

The chief is largely responsible for departmental esprit de corps. To develop a cooperative effective group, there must be no hint that policies are determined by an unofficial group that are "in" on the real decision making. Issues in which differences of opinion may be anticipated should be discussed in meetings open to all department personnel. It is important to reach a consensus that will have popular support, and a departmental executive committee may not be the most effective group. A better group might be an "administrative committee" on which paramedical personnel in the department are represented—head nurse, social worker, business office representative, one or more secretaries—along with representatives of the clinicians who utilize the hospital's facilities as well as the physicians of academic and administrative rank within the department. Such a committee develops the ability to discuss issues freely and is an effective way to minimize feuds among personnel. Otherwise, unexpressed complaints may interfere with the effectiveness of departmental function.

In larger hospitals, and on larger services, it may be well to have a committee of the nurses and personnel primarily concerned with the gynecologic service separate from the obstetric committee. Luncheon meetings provide an informal atmosphere and occupy little additional time away from duty.

When a laboratory service or another clinical department has a complaint about the behavior or practices of members of the obstetric-gynecologic department, the departmental administrative committee provides an opportunity for a spokesman of the dissatisfied group to express his complaint; and the group will likely be able to effect whatever changes of policy or practice that may seem indicated.

Responsibilities for Resident Education

One of the chief's primary interests must be the development of a good residency program. Providing an opportunity for the resident to gain an adequate clinical experience is as important as the chief's efforts to present an organized "teaching" program. No approach to the residency is likely to be more effective than the chief's participation in the residents' daily problems of patient care and administration. Failure to attend and participate in rounds and conferences is likely to result in the residents feeling that they "got nothing out of the chief."

An impressive schedule of didactic teaching conferences "for the residents" usually suggests a lack of a true teaching atmosphere.

Perhaps the most difficult achievement for the chief is to strike a balance between an emphasis on patient care and the study of the patient's disease. Failure to achieve proper emphasis of both is likely to occur where the departmental program is dominated by research or where there is little or no research and residents are wholly occupied in the care of patients. Overemphasis on patient care at the expense of keeping aware of scientific progress related to the specialty can occur where there is responsibility for the care of a heavy service load, as well as in those institutions in which the residents are largely occupied as assistants in the care of private patients. It is not easy to maintain a desirable balance, but it is perhaps the chief's most important teaching responsibility.

Responsibility for Hospital Staff Function

Participation in the administrative duties of the hospital staff is both an obligation and a privilege. It is important for the chief of obstetrics and gynecology to participate in the committees of the staff charged with credentials, records, discipline, public relations, and long range planning, to mention a few.

Responsibility for Community Welfare

In those situations in which the hospital is the only one or the dominant one in the community, the chief of obstetrics and gynecology may be responsible for maternal welfare within the community. He is likely to be involved in organizational efforts to assure public education, a community consciousness of the importance of the annual pelvic examination, the importance of adequate prenatal care, and healthy working conditions where women are employed. No less responsibility must be assumed by the chief of obstetrics and gynecology in a larger urban center, where cooperation with the chiefs of other hospitals in the community may achieve improved conditions through a pooled effort.

In a prosperous community particularly, the chief of obstetrics and gynecology is in daily communication not only with patients but with other citizens. Tact and perception are necessary if the chief is to avoid the development of relationships which, while very pleasant, can take too much of his time and seriously interfere with his effectiveness as a chief. Few have the ability to spend much time "at the club" and at the same time run a "tight ship" in the hospital.

Responsibility for the Development of the Specialty

Local, regional, national, and international organizations of obstetrician-gynecologists provide almost unlimited opportunity to participate in programs and develop a wide circle of professional friendships. An individual physician may become influential in shaping policies which determine the privileges and responsibilities of the obstetrician-gynecologist. When one observes those who become influential in their specialty, one is impressed by certain characteristics which seem typical and perhaps required in such a role. The leader in a specialty must keep well abreast of the times; he delegates responsibility yet honors and fulfills his own responsibilities. He never tires of the "leg work" and continues to serve on committees of his hospital; he does not shirk community obligations, and he continues to present papers at medical meetings. What a chief should do may be too much to expect of one man. Obstetrics and gynecology is fortunate to have many willing to assume the varied but interesting responsibilities of the chief of service.

17

The Chief of Pediatrics

By Robert M. Heavenrich, M.D.

Robert M. Heavenrich is in private practice in Saginaw, Michigan, where he is chairman of the department of pediatrics at the Saginaw General Hospital. He received the M.D. degree from Columbia University and was pediatric resident at Mt. Sinai Hospital in New York. He is a diplomate of the American Board of Pediatrics. He is alternate chairman of District V of the American Academy of Pediatrics and past chairman of the Academy's Hospital Care Committee.

The Guide Issue of *Hospitals, JAHA,* August 1, 1965, gives the following data on Saginaw General Hospital: Beds, 300; Admissions, 11,131; Census, 235; Bassinets, 63; Births, 1,653; Newborn census, 22; Total expenses, $3,532,000; Payroll, $2,363,000; Personnel, 584.

Other hospitals in Saginaw are: Saginaw County Hospital (long-term), 308 beds; St. Luke's Hospital, 239 beds; St. Mary's Hospital, 242 beds; Veterans Administration Hospital, 217 beds. The population of Saginaw in the 1960 census was 98,265.

The chief of the department of pediatrics has the usual responsibilities of the head of any hospital department. Yet because hospitals are adult oriented, he has an added role. Because his patients are more vulnerable physicially, biologically, and emotionally and because they may be a source of infection or contagion to the hospital or the community, his problems are compounded. Because his department is in essence a department of general practice limited to a specific age group and involving all the disciplines of medicine, he has broader problems than other relatively isolated departments, such as orthopedics or gynecology. He must effect coordination, cooperation, and communication with the other departments that are also involved in the care of the young patient. And more than any other department chief he must be in contact not only with the family of the patient but also with the entire community of which the patient is a segment. Just as he must consider the needs of the family in relation to the patient's hospitalization, he must also be concerned with the impact of the family's role and reaction on the patient himself. Finally, the focus of the department of pediatrics is broader than others because care of the child is not based merely on restoration to health or correction of defects but is also directed toward optimum growth and development of all areas: physical, emotional, intellectual, social, and even moral.

UNIQUE RESPONSIBILITIES

The chief of pediatrics must present the needs of child care to the hospital and the community, to the rest of the medical staff, to the nursing and ancillary staffs, to the administrator, and lay boards. Initially he is a consultant in planning and organizing the department on the basis of demography and patterns of illness in the community. The chief, in cooperation with the board and other community agencies, must decide what part of the population will be served by his department and what diseases will be accepted for treatment. He must consider with the board which physicians are qualified to admit and care for patients and to give pediatric consultation. If he feels that his staff is not competent or that the hospital is not equipped to handle certain cases, he should work with the administrator to see that these patients are transferred elsewhere. Yet he should constantly try to upgrade the quality of care available through teaching, research, and acquisition of equipment and personnel.

The chief is responsible to the chief of staff or medical director for the functioning of his department, the clinical work it embraces and for the general supervision of all medical work. He makes decisions on medical matters. He establishes rules of child care in the hospital, some of which are made especially because of the patients' size, incapacitation, lack of communicability, dependency, and susceptibility to accident or infection from other patients. He establishes rules for isolation and accident prevention. He must be certain that equipment appropriate for children is available in his department as well as ancillary departments. It may be possible to provide educational facilities so the child will not miss time from school. Reminding the pharmacy, diet kitchen, and central supply of specific problems of children is also the concern of the chief of pediatrics. He must see that the emergency room is prepared to handle the inevitable cases of contagion. He must apprise everyone from the admission clerk to the cashier of the differences between child and adult patients and of the differences between the needs of the patient and the patient's parents.

Quality of Care. The chief of the department is responsible for constant review of adequacy and quality of care and appropriateness of hospitalization; he is a one-man utilization committee. But the indications for hospitalization and treatment of a child may be entirely different from those of an adult with the same symptoms. Diarrhea of a day's duration may be catastrophic to the small infant yet hardly faze the adult. A child might be discharged on the day of surgery for hernia or tonsillectomy, whereas the adult would be obliged to stay longer.

Standards of Care. The chief should frequently take inventory of his department and review standard procedures. He should familiarize himself with public health regulations which involve his department. In some states, as in Michigan, the State Department of Health not only licenses the nursery but also has prepared a *Hospital Manual*[1] as a guide to the hospital. The manual, *Care of the Newborn,*[2] published by the American Academy of Pediatrics, is recognized internationally as the authority on nurseries. The Academy also has published *Care of Children in Hospitals,*[3] and an *Evaluation Check List Based on Care of Children in Hospitals,*[4] which are of great help. Some state departments of health provide hospital consultants who offer service to hospitals upon request.

To satisfy child needs, the general hospital routine may need to be varied, for example, to permit parents to "room in" or to visit at all hours or even to let the child wear his own pajamas. The chief of pediatrics can point out to other physicians that often their adult patients regress to a younger stage and behave like babies under the stress of their illness or operation.

Educational Programs. The chief of pediatrics is usually responsible for pediatric training of interns and residents. He may also serve as consultant for in-service education of nurses and other personnel. He should encourage the pediatric house staff to contribute their knowledge and skills to other services, such as their techniques with intravenous treatment and fluid balance, and invite other departments to give advice and consultation on pediatric problems. The relationship with the department of obstetrics should almost be symbiotic. Perinatal mortality and morbidity conferences should be held conjointly in every hospital that has an obstetrics department and a nursery.

The chief should cooperate and encourage the use of hospital facilities in training of personnel in social work, public health, and educational activities of other community agencies. In one hospital, all city, county, and visiting nurses are required to attend weekly Pediatric Conferences.

These meetings keep the nurses alert to changes in pediatrics and keep the hospital mindful of the social, economic, and community aspects of the patient's care.

RESPONSIBILITIES OUTSIDE THE HOSPITAL

The emergency room and out-patient departments are links between the public and the hospital, and the chief of pediatrics must see that they are properly equipped and that the personnel is properly trained and oriented to the care of children. The chief should help to establish alternatives and supplements to inpatient care, to define which cases require hospitalization, and to make sure the benefits of hospitalization will not be lost after the patient is discharged. Furthermore, he must be certain that children will not expose the community to contagious and infectious diseases as was seen during the days of the "hot staphylo-coccus." He usually functions in close cooperation with the local and state health departments: his department must report cases of contagion as well as cases of battery. In some states, congenital anomalies are likewise reportable. In this way, health departments and pediatric departments may jointly identify incipient epidemics and possible clusters of anomalies. Catastrophe plans may be developed and tested with the health department. The injured minor, especially when separated from his family, creates complex problems.

The chief of pediatrics must continually review his department's role in the community. As a leader in child health, he is expected to be a resource person to other agencies and to spearhead the development of facilities outside the hospital, which are sometimes extensions of the hospital, for the total care of the child population.

HOSPITAL COSTS

Traditionally and perhaps inevitably, pediatrics has always been an expensive department with the lowest average per cent occupancy. Yet the hospital must assure the community that the needs of any and all children can be handled at any time, even in epidemic or catastrophe. The nursery must be able to handle all newborns on demand. The department must be flexible and thus is expensive. The administrator and board may need to be reminded that the small child is helpless and requires more hours of nursing care than adults. The child is more susceptible to sudden change or accidents and needs closer supervision. The infant has poorer immunity and is more likely to have contagious and infectious disease, requiring more time and expensive isolation. The hospital may need to be reminded that the personnel handling children are more numerous than in other departments, and therefore there can be no saving on space, personnel, or salaries. The needs of the patient demand the most skilled help, and it is a platitude that the strength of the department is as great as its poorest worker.

PUBLIC RELATIONS

There are no better public relations than parents who are happy with the care given their children, or conversely, no greater detriment to the image of a hospital than when a child has suffered physical, biologic, or emotional trauma. The chief of the department of pediatrics who maintains good public relations is a great asset to the administrator and board because it is a relatively easier matter to raise money for the welfare of children than it is for adults.

LEGAL PROBLEMS OF THE MINOR

The department chief must be knowledgeable of the legal aspects of the minor patient, the rights of parents and guardians, and the role of the courts. The chief must be certain that the legal problems of the newborn nursery are understood and that the law is followed in the care, protection, and anonymity of the minor mother, the illegitimate child, and the child placed for adoption. His department must conform with recent phenylketonuria legislation, sharing the responsibility with the private physician, the director, and the lay board.

SUPPORT BY STAFF

One man cannot fill all of these roles. The chief should surround himself with competent aides to whom many of his responsibilities may be delegated. He should see that his staff and the pediatric point of view are included in committees such as accident, bed utilization, diet, education, catastrophe control, executive, emergency room, pharmacy, public relations, library, infection, joint conference, nursing, out-patient department, planning and equipment, record, tissue, hospital auxiliary intern-resident, and volunteer. One of his staff members should represent the problems of the child patient in each of the other departments.

ADMINISTRATIVE SKILLS OF THE CHIEF

In some hospitals, there are problems as to who should qualify as chief of pediatrics; how should he be chosen; and how long should one person hold this position. These are problems for each hospital to decide, even at the departmental level. Since more and more pediatric beds are being used for surgery, it has been suggested that the position of the chief alternate between a pediatrician and a surgeon. But we feel the head of the department of pediatrics should whenever possible be a board certified pediatrician. His training emphasizes not only the healing of the sick and injured, the pathophysiologic problems of growing children, but also the preventive and social aspects of child care.

That doctors have adequate innate ability in the problems of hospital management, administration of a pediatric department, executive skills, the art of teaching, social skills, group dynamics, fiscal planning, and budgeting is apparently presumed. Medical school curriculums are already too full for us to add these areas, and training will have to come in postgraduate experience, such as that offered by the University of Colorado. The school should be given credit for filling the void.

With the decreasing ratio of pediatricians to an increasing child population, there is a great need for recruitment of men and women for this specialty. The chief of the department is in an opportune position to assist in this function. His attitude and that of his staff may also be effective in recruiting other personnel and volunteers for his department. People who care for children have a maternal attitude toward the children; they have anxieties much like mothers, and they expect the chief to listen to and not minimize their complaints. And they expect him to be both paternalistic and authoritative.

Finally, the last role of the chief of the department is to train a successor and to establish such a smooth organization that his succession can be accomplished with ease and efficiency.

SUMMARY

There is sometimes a tendency to minimize the department of pediatrics—as if the diminutive patient warrants less concern. Let it be remembered that in the public's eye what happens to a child in a hospital is often a dramatic picture of what happens to adults in the same institution. The nursery and the pediatric sections are critical areas where events happen explosively. The chief of the department is constantly aware of this. He wishes empathy from the rest of the hospital; he wishes to reciprocate understanding of their problems. Yet he knows, and they know, that pediatrics is usually the happiest and most satisfying department in the hospital.

BIBLIOGRAPHY

1. "Hospital Manual," a guide to accompany "Rules and Minimum Standards for Hospitals," Michigan Department of Health, Lansing, Michigan.

2. "Standards and Recommendations for Hospital Care of Newborn Infants," American Academy of Pediatrics, Evanston, Ill., 1964.

3. "Care of Children in Hospitals," American Academy of Pediatrics, Evanston, Ill., 1960.

4. "Evaluation Check List Based on Care of Children in Hospitals," American Academy of Pediatrics, Evanston, Ill., 1962.

18

The General Practice Department

By Stanley R. Truman, M.D.

Stanley R. Truman is a general practitioner in Oakland, California. He received the M.S. and M.D. degrees from the University of California. He holds membership certificate number 1 in the American Academy of General Practice, and he was the first secretary and one of the early presidents of the Academy. He was a commissioner on the Joint Commission on Accreditation of Hospitals for nine years. He was chairman of the AMA Committee on Medical Practices and a member of the AMA Maternal and Child Welfare Committee. He is a delegate to the California Medical Association and on many committees, and he is a trustee of the California Physicians Service. He is the author of many articles on the practice of medicine and doctor-patient relations.

Increasing specialization in all areas of medicine continues. With it is the growing concern of the public, the profession, and educators over the need and the demands of the patient for a first contact physician with a broad spectrum of skills. Many specialists are engaging in an "aside" general practice from various motivations.

It appears to many that the best solution of this problem is to continue to train a group of physicians in the area encompassed by the present field of general practice, with modifications as time and local medical needs dictate. This group of doctors, general practitioners, must be fully integrated into the stream of medical practice if the quality of medical care is to be maintained at the highest level. No area of practice is more important than hospital care, and general practice should enhance the team aspect of it.

WHY A GENERAL PRACTICE DEPARTMENT?

A department of general practice can contribute materially to team-work in hospital care as well as utilize the abilities of the general practitioners in staff and hospital functions. General practitioners shuffled into various specialty departments without a departmental voice of their own may feel outnumbered and overpowered and thereby lose their feeling of responsibility. With a department of general practice, the general practitioner has a full and equal interest in all aspects of medical care in the hospital, and he willingly accepts his share of responsibility. It has often been reported that general practitioners are more strict in their concern for quality of care than their specialist colleagues are.

Some hospitals obviously do not need a department of general practice because of size or limited number of specialists. Teaching hospitals may have no general practitioners on their staff, but most community hospitals have staffs composed of varying mixtures of general practitioners and specialists. It appears ridiculous that a category of physicians should lack the mechanism of organization that would give them representation and responsibility in staff affairs. The department of general practice is an arm of the staff organization established to work with other departments of the staff and hospital organization to improve intraprofessional relationships, give general practitioners a voice in staff affairs and official representation, utilize their community contacts, increase their loyalty and effectiveness, and assist in elevation of standards of care. The department should be tailored to hospital and community needs.

THE GENERAL PRACTICE DEPARTMENT IS NOT A CLINICAL SERVICE

A clinical department or service is one to which patients are sent for care by the members of that department. Tonsillectomies go to the Ear, Nose and Throat Service; hernias go to the Surgical Department; fractures go to the Orthopedic Department; heart attacks go to the Medical Department. But the general practice department is unique. *No patients are sent to the general practice department.* There is no clinical service to send them to. If three fractured wrists are going to be cared for by three different categories of physicians—an orthopedist, a general practitioner, and an industrial surgeon—all three patients will go to the Orthopedic Service, and the doctors will work under the rules, regulations, and authority of that service.

DEPARTMENT MEETINGS

How often should the general practice department hold meetings? They should be held as often as necessary to conduct the business of the department. If this can be done in one meeting a year, that is all that is needed. One hospital holds two meetings a year: at one, officers and representatives are elected, and at the second meeting the entire department sits as a committee of the whole to consider the qualifications of new candidates and to make recommendations to the credentials committee. Another department of general practice meets monthly for clinical meetings held jointly with the department of internal medicine. Still another department meets monthly with other departments on a rotating basis and finds this a broad educational experience. I know of one department that has never met, all their business being conducted by correspondence. I believe that every one of these different departments is pleased with its own arrangement and is fulfilling its requirements and needs.

Will the Joint Commission on Accreditation of Hospitals accept attendance at general practice department meetings? The Joint Commission on Accreditation of Hospitals will give credit for meetings at which review of clinical material in the hospital is performed. Credit is not given for attendance at business meetings. The commissioners have voted twice *not* to give credit for meetings of the general practice department where review is conducted by the department of general practice alone. The obvious reason for this is to prevent the development of two categories or standards of medical practice. If it is desired to hold the department of general practice together for clinical review, the problem can be solved readily by holding joint sessions with other departments. If the department wants to review its cases of pneumonia, hold a joint meeting with the department of internal medicine; if it wants to study its cases of carcinoma of the bowel, have a joint meeting with the Surgical Department. The majority of general practitioners prefer to attend meetings that seem likely to contribute the most for their time and effort or to those that appeal most to their current interest. Therefore most staffs designate the number of meetings that must be attended but leave the selection to the individual doctor.

TEACHING ACTIVITIES

In most hospitals the general practitioners take very little active part in the teaching program. However, the specialists who are actively teaching usually constitute a small percentage of the total staff membership. Teaching requires a special talent and interest. It may be acquired, but in the training of general practitioners there has been little opportunity to develop this talent. Specialists are exposed more often to teaching experience—residents teach interns, second-year residents teach first-year residents as well as nurses and other paramedical students. During this process there is selection by talent, by success, and by experience. Some have blamed economic factors for the scarcity of general practitioners in teaching activities. I can see zero correlation between income or economic bracket and interest, time spent, or ability to teach among those who are active in the hospital's educational programs. It is logical that the specialist has deeper knowledge and greater skills in his own limited field than the general practitioner, and therefore, he is likely to be called upon more often for teaching assignments.

RELATIONSHIP TO OTHER DEPARTMENTS

What is the relationship of the department of general practice to other departments? The structure, functions, and relationship of a general practice department to the rest of the staff should not follow a rigid pattern but should be tailored to meet the needs of each individual hospital.

For example, in the simplest structure of a departmentalized hospital, there are four departments: surgery, medicine, obstetrics and gynecology, and general practice. Each department elects its officers and a representative on the executive committee. The executive committee consists of the officers of the staff and the representatives of the departments. Members of the executive committee meet with the board of trustees or sit on the joint conference committee. All major committees—credentials, audit, tissue, record, and others—have representatives from each department. In all these functions, the department of general practice is represented. As mentioned before, there is no general practice clinical service to which patients are assigned, but each general practitioner has privileges in each of the clinical departments according to his ability, training, and experience as determined by the credentials committee and approved by the executive committee and the board of trustees.

RESTRICTION OF PRIVILEGES

It is sometimes said that general practitioners are afraid to form a department for fear of having blanket restrictions imposed upon them. How realistic is this? Neither I nor my colleagues in the American Academy of General Practice are aware of any hospital in which blanket restrictions have been imposed on general practitioners as a group where the general practitioners have made a real effort to contribute their share to hospital affairs and to correct the deficiencies, if any, of their fellow members. There should be some blanket rules, but these should be impartial and should apply to all physicians on the staff. All doctors should be observed before giving them privileges and staff membership; all doctors should keep adequate records and should have their records reviewed. Physicians should be given privileges to do only those things for which they are qualified, and this should apply to *all* physicians.

CONCLUSION

Whatever else we do, we must strive to keep all physicians in the mainstream of medicine. There must be frequent contact and communication between all of us. Of course, the danger of isolation between the research scientist and the practicing physician is apparent, but there is also danger that some specialties are becoming so involved in their own fields that they may not be able to contribute all the talents and advances in their fields to the maximum advantage of the patient.

The public needs and demands the knowledge and broad skills of the general practitioner; the public needs and demands the complex skills of the specialists; and the public needs and demands that we shall all work together as a smooth running team for the greatest benefit of the patient.

Part III

Administrative Functions of the Medical Staff

19

Accreditation of Hospitals

By John D. Porterfield III, M.D.

John D. Porterfield became the director of the Joint Commission on Accreditation of Hospitals in 1965. He has had a long and distinguished career in public health, preventive medicine, and hospital affairs. He comes from a medical family and is the son, grandson, and nephew of physicians. He received the M. D. degree from Rush Medical College of the University of Chicago, and the M.P.H. degree from Johns Hopkins University. He had a distinguished career in the United States Public Health Service, culminating with five years as Deputy Surgeon General, from which post he retired in 1962. From then until assuming his present post, he was coordinator of medical and health sciences of the University of California (university-wide).

Through the combined influence of organized medicine, medical schools, and state licensing boards, physicians have long been concerned with the maintenance of high standards of medical practice. Hospital personnel have also sought high standards through the programs of national and state hospital associations and the programs of societies composed of special categories of hospital personnel.

Nevertheless there was a gap unfilled, a need unmet. This came to light around 1915 when the American College of Surgeons found that many of the candidates appearing before it seeking fellowships were unable to provide the case histories documenting their required experience. The candidates' defense was that hospital records were so incomplete that it was almost impossible to prepare the case reports required by the College.

The Development of the Joint Commission on Accreditation of Hospitals

The American College of Surgeons, concerned with this difficulty, surveyed conditions in a large sample of hospitals. They found that not only were the records so incomplete as to prevent adequate case summaries, but that other conditions surrounding the hospital experience of candidates for surgical specialty left much to be desired. To correct this situation, the American College of Surgeons established a program for standardization of hospitals in late 1917. While particularly devoted to surgical practice in hospitals, the program was broad enough in its application to encourage improvement in other aspects of patient care.

The essential feature of this program was the development and adoption of basic standards. These were not directly concerned with the quality of surgical practice since it was expected that this matter had the continuing attention of those responsible for post-graduate training programs. The standards addressed themselves rather to the conditions surrounding surgical practice in hospitals which would strengthen, support, and make more certain a high quality of patient care. They dealt therefore with such things as the safety and sanitation of the physical plant; the clear establishment of authority and responsibility for the activities of the hospital; the maintenance of clinical records so current, so complete, and so pertinent that continuity of patient care was assured; the provision of competent clinical services, such as laboratory and radiological services, nursing services, and dietary services; and the establishment of active medical staff committees which would review the work carried on in the hospital and document their review in such a way as to provide material for useful medical staff education programs.

These standards were then used to measure conditions actually existing in hospitals. Beginning at about the end of World War I, the program continued for well over 30 years. It had been understood from the beginning that the standards would be those considered minimal for the provision of safe, effective patient care. In the early years, only a small percentage of the hospitals surveyed were found to meet the minimal standards to a sufficient degree to be accredited. Very gradually, the situation changed and ever higher percentages of the hospitals surveyed were found to conform to the standards. At the same time, the program became better known and more popular so that each year a greater number of hospitals requested this review by the American College of Surgeons, for accreditation became an important mark of prestige.

About mid-century it became apparent that the accreditation program had grown to the point where it required a broader base of support—both in policy and financially. After long and careful negotiation, *the Joint Commission on Accreditation of Hospitals was formed in 1952* with the support of the American College of Surgeons, the American College of Physicians, the American Hospital Association, and the American Medical Association. A carefully balanced corporation was created with representation from each of the supporting organizations. The Joint Commission adopted as its code of standards those which had served the American College of Surgeons program for so long and it prepared to extend its services to meet the growing demand.

That the founding fathers were wise in their deliberations has been shown by the flourishing career of the Joint Commission. Changes have been made as time has passed, but each has been an orderly evolutionary change. From an original use of traveling representatives of each of the member organizations, the Joint Commission now uses almost exclusively its own full-time staff of trained physician-surveyors. From a survey program supported by assessments derived from the member organizations, the Joint Commission now has field surveys supported by cost-based fees charged to those hospitals seeking accreditation. Member assessments continue to support the expanding central function of study, training, and information. Canadian hospitals and Canadian representation originally on the Joint Commission have now withdrawn to form their own similar program under the Canadian Council on Accreditation of Hospitals.

The minimum standards, adopted from the American College of Surgeons program, have continued to be held out as just that—standards essential to permit a high quality of institutional patient care. The total number of hospitals seeking an accreditation survey has increased every year. So, too, has the percentage of hospitals given accreditation, so that by 1965 it could be reported that 85 per cent of the registered hospital beds in the United States were in hospitals accredited by the Joint Commission.

Amendments have been made to the Joint Commission standards since its beginning, but they have been approached gradually and adopted cautiously. The entire program is geared to a careful and comprehensive attempt to improve conditions, recognizing that it works in that sensitive interphase between a specially constructed, manned, and operated physical facility and the activities—part science, part art —of a highly trained professional staff.

The Changing Role of the Joint Commission—1965

Such were the circumstances in 1965—a milestone year as it would prove—before many forces initiated the beginning of profound changes in the Joint Commission on Accreditation of Hospitals, its methods of operation, its relations, and its total role in the intricate scheme of American health activities.

Only one serious flaw had developed in all those years of growth and acceptance. This was epitomized in the report of a study commission by one of the member organizations which had been charged with a full investigation of the Joint Commission and its activities. After thorough review, this study endorsed the purpose, procedures, and activities of the Joint Commission with but one serious criticism—*the Joint Commission was not well enough known, particularly by hospital medical staff members,* and the fault lay with the Joint Commission which should publicize itself and its program more effectively to physicians.

It was true that the program of the Joint Commission was least well known to physicians, and it was natural that most communication was with hospital administrators. As full-time executives, they had the responsibility for application for the survey, arrangements for the survey visit, and implementing the Joint Commission recommendations. The part-time chief of the medical staff was less directly aware of what accreditation actually entailed, and he knew more than most of the private practitioners composing the hospital's attending staff.

Physicians, almost always pressed for time and with their primary interest focused on their patients and the performance of their uniquely professional pursuits of diagnosis and treatment, generated little sympathy for the source of demands that clinical records be completed and that medical staff committee work be done and documented. These were the less glamorous aspects of medical practice, little dwelt on in medical school curricula. To most physicians the entire activity of the Joint Commission seemed to be an inspection operation concerned not with patients and their welfare but rather with the bookkeeper compulsiveness of completed forms and closed charts.

The Joint Commission recently added to its standards *a new requirement that each medical staff must have an accreditation committee* which would be aware of the true nature of the program and would keep the rest of the medical staff informed. But in 1965 it was still not clearly understood by many medical staff members, in spite of three of the four sponsors of the Joint Commission being professional medical associations, that the fundamental purpose of the Joint Commission and the validity of its standards are in the interests of an improved quality of institutional patient care. Although the situation is much improved over previous years, this continues to be one of the more serious problems seeking solution. As 1965 ended, a number of events conspired to bring the Joint Commission on Accreditation of Hospitals into a period of increased activity and accelerated change.

Federal Medical Act

Although the Joint Commission standards have been used for some years as a benchmark of quality by third-party payers for services in hospitals, the enactment of the federal Medical Act did two things. It established a network of state "certifying" agencies, which would survey hospitals and certify them as maintaining substantial compliance with a set of standards adopted by the federal government as the third-party payer for a substantial group of beneficiaries. *It also established the voluntary standards promulgated by the Joint Commission as the ceiling beyond which federal standards could not go.*

This federal action also spurred the Joint Commission to adopt a new standard which had been under consideration for some time and which calls for the *hospital medical staff to review not only the quality of services rendered in the hospital but also the appropriate utilization of the hospital's resources.* The Joint Commission had long eschewed any consideration of the fiscal side of hospital medical care. But the new requirement gives official recognition to the necessity of an efficient use of the hospital's resources so that all who require the benefits of hospitalization might find it more easily available, so that professional and technical services often in short supply will be directed to the individuals who will benefit most from them.

The greatest significance of the creation of a network of state certifying agencies is that now for the first time in this country there will be a nation-wide, stable, uniform program supporting minimum standards for hospitals. Coming as it did at a time when the work of the Joint Commission, and its predecessor, had already led to a fairly general conformance with minimum standards in the nation's hospitals, the network of state certifying agencies opened the way for the Joint Commission to consider progression to a higher order of consideration, the development of "optimum achievable" standards. The provision of federal law that hospitals accredited by the Joint Commission be considered a priori to be certifiable by the state agency under the Medicare program fits neatly into this consideration.

Currently, the Joint Commission is attempting to review and renovate all parts of its program and is instituting a searching study of its standards and their interpretation and application. The purpose is twofold: to make the language of its standards more precise and clearer, to remove ambiguities, and to illuminate their purpose without inadvertent change in their conditions; and at the same time, to retest the continuing validity of the scientific facts on which each standard is based, to determine the contemporaneous nature of each requirement, and to consider the propriety of raising each standard to call for more than the minimum conditions essential for quality patient care. It is planned that this exhaustive review of Joint Commission standards will be completed during 1967.

The Principal Areas of the Joint Commission's Program

The Joint Commission considers its program to have three principal areas: the development of standards, an informational program to publicize and interpret these standards, and a consultation-evaluation program by which hospitals may be measured against the standards. To the major project of standards review, the Joint Commission has added a study to improve its information program with primary emphasis directed toward the medical profession.

A number of approaches are being used to strengthen and improve the consultation-evaluation program. A larger field staff of physician-surveyors is being recruited to provide more prompt service to applicants, to permit more flexible survey schedules, and to allow longer times for surveys where this is indicated or desired. At the same time, the initial orientation period for physicians joining the staff has been extended and improved; the annual in-service training period for field staff is being lengthened and intensified; and arrangements have now been made to give better consultation service to the field staff during the course of the year's work.

A more fundamental question is also being explored. Recognizing the criticism that has been leveled at the Joint Commission survey, that it is more concerned with the mechanisms surrounding good patient care than it is with the direct substance of the care given, the Board of Commissioners is studying the desirability and feasibility of converting to a "peer team" approach. The full-time staff physician of the Joint Commission would continue to check physical plant, hospital organization, patient records, and medical staff function documents. However, he would be joined by one or two practicing physicians from other hospital staffs who would spend the survey period with the hospital's medical staff, discussing the actual content of the medical practice carried on in the hospital. Several state medical and hospital associations have joined such a practice review. The question is whether this is best done at the state level, or should it also become a function of the national voluntary program.

Accreditation of Extended Care Facilities

In January, 1966, the Joint Commission assumed the new responsibility of a national accreditation program for extended care facilities, specifically nursing homes and domiciliary homes. This came about from the merger of several competitive programs when the Board of Commissioners expanded its number to include representation from the American Association of Homes for the Aging and the American Nursing Home Association as non-member participating organizations. This program has only begun, but hopefully it will bear the same benchmark of quality for the increasingly important extended care facilities that it has meant in the past for hospitals.

Accreditation of Other Health Facilities

Nor has the concept of broader coverage stopped there. The Joint Commission is studying a new basic form of organizational structure that will permit extension of the accreditation service to other activities which combine a specialized facility with a professional health service.

Interest has been expressed in services to rehabilitation centers, home health services (providing multiple services), group practice facilities, and college health services, if solid foundations can be laid. Expansions of this nature are being contemplated in the growing recognition that close cooperation among the various categories of health facilities and services is needed if the most useful and most efficient provision of medical care to the American people is to be assured.

To better carry the responsibilities of today and to prepare intelligently for the responsibilities of tomorrow is the dual goal of the Joint Commission on Accreditation of Hospitals, highly sensitive as it is of the role it bears as a voluntary, professionally based joint operation.

20

The Executive Committee

By Phillip T. Knies, M.D.

Phillip T. Knies is the president of the Medical Advisory Board and chairman of the department of medicine at Mount Carmel Hospital in Columbus, Ohio. He received the M.D. degree from Ohio State University and is a diplomate of the American Board of Internal Medicine. He has been on the faculty of Ohio State University since 1934 and is now professor of medicine at that institution. Dr. Knies has chaired many staff committees at Mount Carmel Hospital and has extensive staff organizational experience. He is a Fellow of the American College of Physicians.

The Guide Issue of *Hospitals, JAHA,* August 1, 1965, gives the following data on Mount Carmel Hospital, Columbus, Ohio: Beds, 419; Admissions, 14,668; Census, 373; Bassinets, 55; Births, 3,428; Newborn census, 37; Total expenses, $6,039,000; Payroll $3,460,000; Personnel, 882.

This chapter reviews the composition, duties, and opportunities of the executive committee of the medical staff and refers to the position and orientation of the executive committee in respect to the board of trustees, the hospital administration, and the attending staff.

Pertinent general principles have been reviewed in *Hospital Accreditation References*, 1964 edition, published by the American Hospital Association.[1] In attempting to define requirements and suggesting approaches applicable to hospitals of all sizes, backgrounds, and orientations, this reference suggests median methods of attaining the desired ends. Variation in application of these methods may reflect differences in sponsorship, central purpose, method of growth, background of staff, and at times, personalities which have affected the establishment and internal development of hospitals. Also contributing to variation in executive committees has been an incomplete knowledge or appreciation on the part of many staffs, administrators, and boards of trustees of the basic principles of medical staff organization or the attempt to assure or maintain certain prejudicial advantages without regard to the unity of hospital purpose.

Despite these differences, however, reasonable and effective function of the executive committee has been accomplished to attain the primary purpose of best possible patient care. The Joint Commission on Accreditation of Hospitals has considered this fact in accrediting many hospitals despite their widely differing organizational detail. To require these hospitals to adopt stereotyped forms of medical staff organization might well delay coordinated effectiveness of the several components of a hospital.

On the other hand, in view of the federal interests in individual hospital organizational patterns and functions, many misunderstandings would probably be avoided by the adoption of generally understood concepts and terminology, and changes involved need have no real detrimental effect on function. Our principal concern is the attainment of necessary medical staff functions, in the present context in reference to the executive committee, rather than an obsession with trivia including titles, offices, and provincialisms. Certain principles are applicable in all circumstances.

BASIC PRINCIPLES OF ORGANIZATIONAL PATTERNS

A primary principle is a *clear understanding of the origin and scope of authority, the delegation of authority, and the limitation of such delegation* as established by its purpose. The source must actually possess the authority it purports to delegate, and delegation must consider the propriety and competence of the delegate. In the community general hospital, private or public, the governing board or board of trustees is the source of all authority, with the exception of medical authority which is inherent in the hospital's staff of physicians. The executive committee of the staff has as one of its principal responsibilities the coordination of these primarily complementary authorities with the derivation of principles and of specific applications to attain administrative methods and ends to achieve the purposes of both authorities harmoniously and without violence to either. To this end, in the evolution of medical staff bylaws, rules, and regulations there must be specification of whence comes what authority, to whom it is delegated, and the intended purpose of the delegation.

A second coordinate principle is the *definition of channels*. When authority or responsibility is delegated from one individual or body to another, the responsibility for reporting back is in the precise reverse direction. While there may be exceptions in which an individual or committee to whom a specific responsibility has been delegated may be directed to make report to another than the appointing authority, it is more desirable for the delegated committee or individual to report to its authority, which in turn can endorse that report to its ultimate destination. If for any reason of expedition this principle of approval and endorsement cannot be followed, there should be at least an information report to the appointing authority so that its own records may be complete. If, then, a modification of the report is considered advisable, such modification can be forwarded to the originally designated recipient.

If, for example, a board of trustees of a hospital requests recommendations from the physician staff of that hospital for the operation of its emergency room, the general staff might delegate to a committee the investigation of the problem, the preparation of a report, and the forwarding of that report to the hospital administrator. In these instances, two channels of reporting back will be disregarded unless the delegated committee sends to the general staff a copy of its reports and recommendations to the administrator, and the general staff in turn forwards that report with such additions or exceptions as it may desire to make to the board of trustees which originally delegated responsibility for the investigation and report to the general staff. Differences may be arbitrated and adjusted by the executive committee or in accordance with local determination by a joint conference committee, if this body exists in addition to the executive committee. In some instances this role of joint conference committee will reside with the executive committee. The purpose of this discussion, however, has been to point out the appropriate channels of feedback.

It may be contended that staff members do not receive their individual authority to practice medicine from the hospital board of trustees or the administrator but rather from a state board of medical examiners. Outside the hospital, that is true without modification, but the members of the staff do receive authority from the board of trustees to practice medicine in that hospital and, collectively, to function as a staff. This does not prevent the individual members of a hospital staff, or the staff as a whole, from exercising the privilege and obligation to originate opinions, recommendations, exceptions, or reports of accomplishment to the board of trustees or to the administrator along defined channels. Again, these channels should be anticipated, designated, and respected.

A third principle is that *the responsibility to establish, supervise, and assure the satisfaction of a function must include the authority to regulate it*. A pertinent statement is included in *General Principles of Medical Staff Organization*,[2] published by The American Medical Association, which points out that "Without the authority to supervise and to designate responsibilities and privileges, the assignment of responsibility for quality would be an empty delegation." A staff must have the authority to enforce compliance with its rules so long as the principles of the rules have been approved by competent administrative authority. Along with the authority to enforce such compliance, there is also the obligation to do so, either by itself or by superior authority. A medical records committee, for example, must have the assurance that the executive committee not only has the authority to insist, but it will in fact insist on compliance with approved rules and regulations; otherwise the work of the medical records committee has very little meaning.

POSITION AND AUTHORITY OF THE EXECUTIVE COMMITTEE

It is pointed out in the *Hospital Accreditation References*[3] that ". . . the governing board is morally and legally responsible for all that occurs in the institution." Obviously, such broad responsibility must be accomplished by wise delegation, ordinarily in part to the executive committee. In the same source,[3] it is noted that the most authoritative body of the medical staff is the executive committee in representing the governing board or board of trustees on the one hand and the medical staff on the other. No dichotomy will result, however, if the entire hospital organization is considered as one. This is recognized in the statement, "There must be a clear and well defined relationship between the medical staff and the administration. Preferably, this occurs at the level of the executive committee of the medical staff. . . ."[4] While some might wish to debate whether the executive committee is properly an agent of the board of trustees or of the medical staff, the fact is that whatever relationship exists must do so with the approval of the board of trustees. This relationship is best determined by joint deliberation, taking account of the inherent purposes and responsibilities of both the board of trustees and of the general staff. In this manner there will be assured a greater likelihood of attaining all goals. There is actually no conflict in purpose.

COMPOSITION OF THE EXECUTIVE COMMITTEE

The structure of the executive committee must take into account the details of delegation of authority and of operation within a specific institution. Thus, in determining the members of the executive committee, the general principle of effective representation may be strained in hospitals in which the chiefs of departments are appointed by the administrator or board of trustees. Since these appointed chiefs of departments may constitute a sizable proportion or even a majority of its membership, the executive committee should include an adequate number of representatives elected by the staff to assure effective staff representation. This assumes that the freely elected officers and representatives of the staff are sufficient in number and are appropriately chosen for competence and responsibility to assure effective staff representation. These assumptions, unfortunately, are not always satisfied. It is in this connection that an adequate slate of candidates for election to office is ordinarily presented by a responsible nominating committee which will exercise careful choice in presenting at least two candidates for each office and will assure the willingness of all candidates to accept office if elected. This does not prevent the nomination of additional candidates from the floor in a general staff meeting.

The executive committee does not bear this name in all hospitals. In some, including the one of my own most intimate association, the executive committee is termed the *medical advisory board*. This name derived from a long-standing and very effective staff organization, even though for many years definitions had not been committed to writing. In others, as described by K. J. Williams, M.D.,[5] the executive committee is known as the *medical advisory committee*. Subtly, to myself and apparently to Dr. Williams and to the Canadian counterpart of the American Joint Commission on Accreditation of Hospitals, these names are more descriptive of major function than is "executive committee." The chief importance of names is that of communication and mutual understanding; and although these alternative terms have at times required explanation to accreditation authorities, we are again reminded that chief concern is for function and accomplishment. With the reservation that a different name, even though with slightly different connotation, may pertain, continued reference in this discussion will be to the executive committee.

The size of the executive committee may vary. While it may consist of eight to ten members in a medium-sized hospital, it may consist of as few as five, or as many as twenty, depending on the size of the hospital, the degree of its administrative suborganization, and the specialization of its staff.

The terms of office should be sufficiently long to permit adequate continuity, usually two, three, or four years, with the election or appointment of a half, a third, or a fourth of the membership of the executive committee every year.

If the advisory nature of the executive committee is the principal determinant, its members may be predominantly appointed by the authorities seeking the advice, i.e., the board of trustees or administrator. Tenure of office under these circumstances may not conform with periods of election by the general staff. However, appointments should be for designated periods in order to facilitate change and to take advantage of the individual capacities of successive appointees. Even then, it is the opinion of some that no limitation should be placed on an appointee succeeding himself for any period of time in which his advice is considered desirable and his function is effective.

Whether the members of the executive committee are elected or appointed, the understanding by the general medical staff of hospital problems and policies would be increased when membership on the executive committee has been extended to a reasonable number of the general staff, at the same time insisting on competence and active participation in accordance with principles carefully defined in the bylaws. Thus, it is important to orient oncoming generations of the general staff to the responsibilities and activities of the executive committee by having among the staff a number of emeritus members of the executive committee to guide staff opinion on the basis of their own past experience. It is also necessary to assure the stability of the executive committee through tenure sufficiently prolonged to eliminate rapid turnover and to control maverick attitudes.

Such differences in the composition of executive committees emphasized the comment by Dr. K. J. Williams[5] that medical staff organization is a place for both democracy and oligarchy. He notes that while the fear of dictatorship may be a basis for objection to the long continuation of executive committee members in office, "Caesarism has more often been produced by the failure of a weak organization than by the success of a strong one."

Wide variation in the constitution of executive committees is illustrated in the following three examples of hospitals in which the author holds staff membership:

Hospital A: Executive committee comprised of:

> Chairman, elected by general staff
>
> Chairman-elect, elected by general staff
>
> Vice-Chairman (ex officio), elected by general staff
>
> Three general staff members at large, one of whom is elected annually for a three-year term by the general staff

Hospital B: Executive committee comprised of:

> President of medical staff, elected by medical staff
>
> Secretary of medical staff, elected by medical staff
>
> Chairmen of six clinical departments, elected by general medical staff
>
> Director of medical education, employed by board of trustees
>
> Hospital administrator (participating), appointed by board of trustees

Hospital C: Executive committee comprised of:

Chairmen of eight professional departments, appointed by board of trustees through administrator

Director of medical education, employed by board of trustees through administrator

Members of staff at large, usually two, appointed as elder statesmen by board of trustees through administrator

President of general medical staff, elected by staff annually from list of candidates approved by administrator

Chairman of credentials committee, appointed by administrator

Administrator and associate administrator (ex officio) appointed by board of trustees

RESPONSIBILITIES OF THE EXECUTIVE COMMITTEE

The derivation of the executive committee as indicated above determines to some degree its responsibilities. In one situation it may attend to virtually all of the business of the general medical staff; in another, only that which is specifically delegated to it. In still another, in which the executive committee is entirely appointed with the exception of the president of the general staff, the committee serves only to advise the administrator and conducts none of the business of the general staff. In the first two organizational patterns, all of the activity of the executive committee, except that which is confidential, is reportable to the full medical staff for its information and confirmation. In the third pattern, the activity of the executive committee may be reported to the general staff, either by the chairman of the executive committee or by the president of the general medical staff who is the staff representative on the executive committee. In any event, it must again be emphasized that any such form of staff organization is subject to approval by the governing board or board of trustees.

Thus, the executive committee has a responsibility to the general medical staff as well as to the governing board or board of trustees. Some have feared this double representation as reminiscent of the two-faced head of Janus. It will be recalled that the countenances of those two faces were quite different, and it is possible that the purposes and responsibilities of the executive committee may be unclear unless the committee clearly recalls the origins and natures of its responsibilities as consultative, deliberative, and advisory, with reference not only to the overall conduct of the hospital but also to medical professional practice and ethics. Only the board of trustees holds ultimate responsibility in the one direction; and only the general medical staff, under appointment by the board of trustees, possesses and can exercise responsibility in the other. The two meet in the executive committee which serves to correlate both interests which, after all, are not divergent. Both must be subserved in full coordination if the common interest of both the board of trustees and the general medical staff are to be implemented for the best possible care of patients.

In its role as the major quality control mechanism for the practice of medicine in hospital, the executive committee has certain specific responsibilities:

1. The formulation, coordination, and application of general policies throughout the several divisions and echelons of the staff and staff function. In these connections, the administrator requires the advice of the executive committee to avoid difficulties on the bases of aggressive or indolent departments, services, or individuals. The executive committee has the responsibility to advise standards and their specific implementation for the welfare of the entire staff, for the hospital as an institution in the community, and for the benefit of all patients.

2. The reception and evaluation of committee reports. These may be transmitted directly when the executive committee has appointed the individuals or subcommittees submitting the reports as extensions of the responsibilities of the executive committee, or they may be presented to the executive committee by the administrator or by the president of the general staff, depending on their origin. As a result of critical evaluation of such reports, the executive committee is in the position to make recommendations to the administrator or to the staff in matters of combined medical and administrative importance. Recommendations may pertain to the privileges or discipline of individuals, the obligations of clinical sections, the activities of and within departments, or may consider proposals by the administrator, the board of trustees, or the general staff. In general the executive committee should avoid the prerogatives of administration and should allow the execution of policy to fall to those charged with that responsibility.

3. The expression of its opinion and recommendations to the administrator, the board of trustees, or the general medical staff on matters legitimately falling within its interest. The role of the executive committee in planning for the hospital belongs here, in clear recognition that hospital planning takes more into account than structure. The executive committee is in a unique position to evaluate staff responsibility and participation. Utilization reviews, presently under intensive country-wide refinement, have ordinarily included executive committee evaluation of reports from the tissue committee, medical audit committee, infection committee, and others. Such particular responsibilities of the executive committee are not diminished in meeting federal requirements.

4. Keeping careful and permanent records of the deliberations and actions of the executive committee, to document the background and details of judgments reached and of recommendations offered. These records should be confidential and limited to review by authorized persons, including the members of the executive committee who, in turn, should have the grace of discretion.

5. Proposing actions which commonly place responsibilities on individuals or groups. These responsibilities must be clearly defined and indicated to those who should have the advantage of knowing the pertinent thinking of the executive committee. This notification may be made a responsibility of the secretary of the executive committee, of its chairman, or of the hospital administrator. Lack of such notification, including pertinent background, is frequently the cause of ineffective execution.

6. Preparing a follow-up report on its recommendations to indicate the degree to which they have been implemented and whether they have served their intended purposes. A basic obligation to the executive committee in all of its relationships with the total hospital organization is complete frankness on the part of boards of trustees, councils, administrator, departments, services, and individuals, without which the executive committee cannot reach equitable and appropriate judgments. Fairness and candor is equally essential on the part of the executive committee, without which its efforts may be impaired by misunderstanding, suspicion, and prejudice.

In its proper function the executive committee, perhaps more than any other group in the organization of the staff or hospital, can either perpetuate desultory mediocrity or encourage progressive excellence.

BIBLIOGRAPHY

1. "Hospital Accreditation References," 1964 ed., American Hospital Association, Chicago, 1964.

2. "General Principles of Medical Staff Organization," p. 3, American Medical Association, Chicago, Dec., 1964.

3. "Hospital Accreditation References," 1964 ed., p. 17, American Hospital Association, Chicago, 1964.

4. Ibid., p. 64.

5. Williams, K. J., and Osbaldeston, J. B.: The Hospital Medical Advisory Committee—The Cabinet of the Medical Staff, Canadian Med. Assoc. J., 92:1117–1124 (May 22) 1965.

21

The Joint Conference Committee

By Keith O. Taylor

Keith O. Taylor is professor and director of the course in hospital administration at the University of California. He received the M.B.A. in hospital administration from the University of Chicago and has been the assistant administrator at Peralta Hospital and administrator at Children's Hospital, both in Oakland, California. He is a Fellow of the American College of Hospital Administrators.

Committees of all types apparently exist for one of four basic reasons —to make decisions, to advise on the making of decisions, to avoid making decisions, and to serve as a form of communication link for information regarding policies and current or proposed activities. Committees may function properly at the decision-making, advisory, and informational levels provided they are constituted in such a way that all members participate realistically and are not dominated by one or two members and, most important, that they remain aware of the committee's real reasons for existence, its functions, and its relationships.

Committees to avoid decision-making are usually appointed when someone who should make a decision prefers not to and passes this responsibility to a group whose members are chosen for their certainty of inaction or their willingness to assume the unwanted decision responsibility. Such committees can generally be classified as dysfunctional for everyone except the buck-passer. But any other committee can be dysfunctional when it is poorly constituted, poorly chaired, tedious in deliberation, or uncertain about the reasons for its existence. The old story about a faculty committee in a school of architecture provides a good example of dysfunction. The faculty was evenly divided on the question of whether to have a new building or remain in the old one. After two years of deliberation, the committee came up with a solution. First, a new building should be built. Second, the new building should be constructed from the materials of the old building. Third, classes should continue in the old building until the new building was completed.

Any considerable experience in committee work provides adequate examples of the good and the bad, the functional and dysfunctional committees. Dysfunction, in terms of the many demands on time in an organization, becomes a serious matter.

COMMITTEE ACTIVITIES

Despite the importance of the joint conference committee, especially in hospitals where it is the sole or major instrument of communication among the medical staff, administration, and board, the level of function will inevitably vary depending on the committee membership and its concern with the proper activities of the committee.

Decisions as to membership and to some extent the function of the joint conference committee reside with the individual hospital, but the pertinent activities have been rather carefully delineated by the Joint Commission on Accreditation of Hospitals.

> The Joint Conference Committee is a discussion committee of the governing board and the medical staff. It has no intrinsic authority; if allowed to become an action group, its usefulness will at once be jeopardized.

Purposes

Its purposes, all directed toward better patient care, should be at least three:

    a. Communications to keep board, staff and administration cognizant of pertinent actions taken or contemplated by one or the other. These should be reported to the committee even though they do not require action by more than one component of it. Open communications through the Joint Conference Committee will emphasize the importance of prior knowledge of all affected groups before action is instituted and will thus prevent misunderstanding.

    b. Planning. Plans for growth and inevitable change in the hospital organization should be considered by this committee.

    c. Problems. Issues which arise in the operation and affairs of the hospital affecting all parties should be brought to the committee for consideration.

Organization

While the Joint Conference Committee may be organized in any of several ways, the following, which is only a guide, is offered as an example:

   a. The Joint Conference Committee of the governing board and the medical staff should be composed of equal numbers of representatives elected or appointed by the governing board and the medical staff. The administrator should be ex officio member of the committee.

   b. The chairman of the Joint Conference Committee may be alternated between representatives of the governing board and of the staff.

   c. The Joint Conference Committee should meet at regular intervals no less frequently than four times per year, and should meet on call when necessary.

   d. The committee should feel free to invite to its meetings persons within or without the hospital who can contribute from their specialized knowledge or experience.

   e. A formal agenda should be prepared from suggestions of the members and submitted to all members of the committee in sufficient time before the meeting.

   f. Minutes should be kept by the secretary and should be maintained in the permanent records of the hospital.

   g. A resume of the minutes of the Joint Conference Committee should be presented at meetings of the governing board and at meetings of the medical staff.[1]

A statement and preamble on the Joint Conference Committee provides the basic reasoning of the Commission's objectives for this committee.

STATEMENT ON THE JOINT CONFERENCE COMMITTEE:

The Standards for Hospital Accreditation of the Joint Commission on Accreditation of Hospitals state that the governing body of a hospital should establish a formal means of liaison with the medical staff. Although the method used to accomplish this is a decision to be made locally, the Commission considers the establishment of a Joint Conference Committee a preferable plan. The Boards of Trustees of the American Medical Association and the American Hospital Association have approved the following statement which should be of help in the formation of such a committee:

Preamble

As the art and science of medicine have become more complex and more comprehensive, hospital services, of necessity, have followed suit in an effort to produce maximum results from medical progress. For this reason and because of the other joint and separate responsibilities which physicians and hospitals have in providing medical care and hospital services, organization and cooperation are essential.

These responsibilities cannot be discharged with maximum effectiveness without proper liaison between doctor and hospital, the doctor being represented in an organized manner by a medical staff and the hospital by its governing body and that body's designated representative, the administrator.

In addition to, but not in conflict with, regularly established lines of authority and responsibility, there should be a common ground where these two groups can meet in order that there may be mutual understanding of each other's activities and problems. A suitable medium for this interchange of information and discussion is the Joint Conference Committee.

This document seeks to encourage the development and to strengthen the role of the Joint Conference Committee of the Board of Trustees and medical staff. It urges the establishment of such Joint Conference Committees because it believes that they will bring to bear on major decisions which must be made in the hospital a full measure of broad experience, intelligence and responsibility.

Such a Committee should be a part of the organizational structure of every hospital. It should exist even where there is medical staff representation on the governing board. The representatives of this committee meet—not as representatives of the departments from which they were chosen—but as members of the committee as a whole in the interest of the patient, the physician, the hospital and the community.[2]

Dr. Anthony Rourke, at the first University of Colorado Conference for Chiefs of Staff in 1964, provided some additional thoughts on the Joint Conference Committee. He stated:

It is in this committee that matters directly related to medical-hospital interest may be discussed in greater detail, in a more intimate group because of its size and in a more open manner. Such matters as snow removal, leaking roofs, inefficient boilers and steam pressure to the mangle need not take up the physicians' valuable time. Consequently, greater attention can be given to trends to be expected in obstetrics, for example, or the need for expanding laboratories and x-ray, utilization reviews, and medical education.

Many joint conference committees have fallen by the wayside because a non-imaginative agenda of nit-picking failed to challenge intellectual capabilities of important people. The agenda, then, should be formulated with care. The administrator should be the repository for suggestions made by individual members between meetings. In addition to suggested items, he should add stimulating ideas of his own because he is in a position to see areas in which board and medical staff cooperation could be fruitful.

While the governing board has ultimate responsibility for medical care in the hospital, it must delegate such responsibility to its medical staff; in delegating, however, the board must not relegate responsibility and forget it. There is no better place for follow-up than through a sophisticated joint conference committee with a professional accounting report made at each meeting.[3]

At the same meeting, Floyd Mann offered some important ideas on how committees can play an important part in the interlinking roles essential to organizational coordination.[4]

ANALYSIS OF MINUTES OF COMMITTEES IN THREE HOSPITALS

An analysis was made of the committee minutes in three hospitals, varying in size from less than 100 beds to over 300 beds, and the results are presented in Table 21-1. These minutes suggest linkage by noting requests for information from or recommendations to various segments of the hospital. The functioning of the committee is itemized under subjects considered and activities, with the latter further categorized as information, recommendation, request for information, and decision avoidance. Information includes discussions based on presentation by one or another of the committee's component groups and frequently involves no action. In some cases, however, it may result in later recommendations to the board, administrator, or staff. The informational aspect, and presumably the recommendation aspect, fit well within the Joint Commission's recommendations for this committee. The avoidance of decisions was noted only a few times and was related to the discussion of seemingly important matters, but the inaction was obvious over a considerable period of time. Analysis of a greater number of joint conference committees would probably establish the incidence of dysfunction in these committees as extremely low. But doubtless there may be some dysfunction not apparent in the minutes. Final decision-making by a committee presumed not to be a decision-making body was noted a few times only but appeared at least once in each hospital.

The frequency of meetings varied. The committee of one hospital met 13 times in two years; in a second hospital, 11 times in two years; and in a third, 15 times in three years. Matters considered by the committees have been tabulated under 25 subject headings. The frequency with which these subjects appeared in committee minutes is as follows: (1) most frequently, equipment came up for discussion 20 times; (2) in second place the requirements of Joint Commission appeared 12 times; (3) in third place emergency room organization and procedures appeared eight times. Fourth place was shared by several subjects: specialist contracts, physical plant, hospital activities, nursing relations, and nursing education, each with seven entries. Other topics were medical library and educational objectives.

On the whole, the three committees studied appear to be good committees, carefully organized and with discussion recorded from many members; but significant differences in committee action appear even in this small sample. Although discussions on equipment were the most

TABLE 21-1. The Functions of the Joint Conference Committee as Shown by an Analysis of the Minutes of the Committees in Three Hospitals of Varying Size (Less Than 100 Beds to More Than 300 Beds)

RANK	SUBJECTS	TOTAL ENTRIES	HOSPITAL			ACTIVITIES For information only; for consideration and recommendations to board, administration, or staff; for final decision-making.
			A	B	C	
1.	Equipment	20	8	12		7 Information 1 Information-Board 1 Information-Administration 3 Information-Staff 3 Recommend-Board 1 Recommend-Staff 1 Request other Information 1 Final Decision (procedural) 2 Avoid Decision
2.	Joint Commission on Accreditation of Hospitals Requirements, Visits, etc.	12	8	1	3	3 Recommend-Staff 3 Recommend-Administration 1 Recommend-Board 5 Information
3.	Emergency Room Organization & Procedures	8	7	1		1 Information 1 Information-Board 1 Information-Administration 4 Recommend-Board 1 Avoid Decision
4.	Medical Staff Appointments	7	3		4	2 Information 1 Information-Staff 2 Recommend-Board 2 Final Decision
	Specialist Contracts	7		5	2	2 Information 3 Information-Staff 2 Recommend-Board
	Physical Plant	7	4	2	1	5 Information 1 Recommend-Staff
	Hospital Activities e.g., New Departments, Home Care, etc.	7		7		4 Information 1 Request Administration 2 Avoid Decision
	Nursing Relations—2 and Nursing Education—5	7	5	2		4 Information 2 Information from Staff 1 Recommendation to Board
5.	Intern-Resident Programs	6		1	5	2 Information 1 Recommend-Board 1 Recommend-Administration 1 Recommend-Staff 1 Request-Administration
	Medical Records—Policy	6		1	5	1 Information 1 Recommend-Board 1 Recommend-Administration 1 Recommend-Staff 2 Final Recommendation: Policy Delinquency

TABLE 21-1 (cont'd)

RANK	SUBJECTS	TOTAL ENTRIES	HOSPITAL			ACTIVITIES For information only; for consideration and recommendations to board, administration, or staff; for final decision-making.
			A	B	C	
	Medical Staff Bylaws	5	3	1	1	1 Information from Administration 1 Information only 1 Information-other 2 Recommend to Staff
6.	Hospital Bylaws	5	2		3	2 Information 1 Information from Board 1 Information from Administration 1 Information from Staff
	Medical Staff—Staff Officers	5			5	2 Information 1 Recommend-Staff 1 Recommend-Board 1 Final Decision: Rules for Procedure
	Special Legal Problems	5	3	1	1	2 Information 2 Information-Outside 1 Information-Administration
	Employee Health Program	4		4		1 Information 1 Information-Staff 1 Information-Other 1 Avoid Decision
7.	Visiting Hours	4	4			1 Information 2 Recommend-Board 1 Information-Other Sources
	Board's Responsibilities and Authority	4			4	1 Information 1 Recommend-Board 1 Recommend-Administration 1 Recommend-Staff
	Joint Conference Committee Meetings Composition	4	1		3	1 Recommend-Board 3 Final Decision
	Medical Staff Committee Appointments	3			3	2 Recommend Board 1 Final Decision
8.	Tissue Committee Activities	3	3			1 Information 1 Recommend-Board 1 Recommend-Administration
	Intra-Hospital Affairs	3			3	2 Information 1 Request Outside Information
	Board-Administration-Staff Organizational Relationships	3			3	3 Information Only
9.	Assistants in Surgery	2	1	1		1 Information 1 Recommend-Staff
	Bed Utilization	2		2		1 Information 1 Recommend Staff
10.	Medical Library	1		1		1 Information
	Educational Objectives	1	1			1 Information

frequently recorded item, the total of 20 occurred in only two of the hospitals (8 and 12 times respectively). In some cases, avoidance of decision seemed to be the reason that equipment matters were before the committee. The one final decision made by a committee was on purchasing and stores procedure. The preponderance of the discussion about equipment raises the question as to whether the committees were busy with inconsequential minutiae, but most of the discussions involved medical and surgical equipment, several items being both costly and controversial.

Discussions of accreditation revolved about standards and the imminent approach of a survey. There were eight discussions in one hospital, three in a second, and one in a third. The hospital with eight entries was anticipating an inspection visit, while the third hospital with only one entry did not indicate any concern with its accreditation status.

The third most frequent topic—emergency room organization and procedures—was centered in one hospital where seven of the eight recorded discussions occurred.

Medical staff appointments were discussed in only two hospitals. In one, the matter of final decision on appointments rested with this committee. Recommendations came to this joint group from the credentials committee and staff; although the full board could presumably overrule the committee, such a veto seems unlikely. Decision-making by the Joint Conference Committee is not in accord with recommendations of the Joint Commission on Accreditation of Hospitals, but there may be real merit in discussion of staff appointments by this body which includes responsible members of both the staff and the board.

The infrequent appearance or absence of some subjects is significant and suggests that these committees lost some opportunities to consider both immediate and long-range planning on utilization, educational matters, hospital and medical staff activities, medical staff–nursing staff relationships, and the effects of Medicare on the hospital.

There was indication in the extensive minutes that joint conferences actually involved joint deliberation. In all three hospitals, meetings were more frequent than the minimum quarterly sessions recommended by the Joint Commission on Accreditation of Hospitals.

FURTHER STUDIES

In a further study made in 1966, detailed reports on board-staff-administration liaison were obtained from 17 hospitals—six of 100 beds or less, six between 100 and 250 beds, and five above 250 beds in size. Of these hospitals, 14 utilized the joint conference committee, and 3 used other methods of liaison. Of these latter three, it was interesting that one fell into each of the three size categories, and they were located in three different sections of the country.

Information was obtained on committee composition, frequency of meetings, committee functions, and whether the committee reviewed medical staff reports on quality of medical care. Opinions were also sought as to whether the committee meetings were considered to be useful to the hospital. A summary of these data follows.

Size of hospital:
Under 100 beds... 5
100 to 250 beds... 6
Over 250 beds... 3

Sponsorship:
Voluntary non-profit.. 10
District and government... 4

Length of time committee has been organized:
Over three years.. 12
One to three years.. 2
Less than one year.. 0

Frequency of committee meetings:
Monthly... 5
Quarterly... 5
Less than quarterly... 4

Committee membership:

Five members................... 4

Six members................... 1

Seven members............... 4

Eight members................ 2

Nine members................ 1

Twelve members.............. 1

Fifteen members.............. 1

NOTE: In 10 of the 14 hospitals there was an equal number of board-staff members. In three other cases there was one more staff member than board member, and in one there were six more staff than board members. The administrator served as a member of all 14 committees.

Committee function:
Information only... 0
Advisory.. 14
Decision making in special cases...................................... 5

Review of medical staff reports on quality of medical care:
Regularly... 2
Occasionally.. 5
Not at all.. 7

Committee meetings are considered valuable:
Seldom.. 0
Most of the time.. 7
Always.. 6

Of the topics discussed in the 14 committees, the number one subject in the three hospitals studied in 1965, equipment, again appeared as a common topic, being discussed by 11 of the 14 committees. But equipment was discussed frequently in only 1 hospital, infrequently in 10, and not at all in 3.

Accreditation matters, last year's number two topic, was again commonly discussed (7 hospitals). Other common topics were physical plant (10 hospitals), routine hospital activities (8 hospitals), accreditation matters (7 hospitals), quality of care (7 hospitals), and long range planning (7 hospitals). Special legal problems, specialist contracts, medical staff bylaws, the emergency room, utilization review, community relations, and Medicare were also common topics.

The extent and importance of discussions cannot be determined from these data, although frequency of discussion provides some suggestion of committee interests.

Specific answers to the question, "Which topics were considered most significant in committee deliberations?" provided a considerable number of items. The order of frequency with which they were mentioned is shown in the following list. It is of interest that Medicare, the most frequently mentioned, was missing from the 1965 list.

Problems associated with Medicare
Professional problems including appointments, privileges, and discipline
Long-range planning
Quality of hospital care
Community relations
Hospital programs and activities
Accreditation matters

Board-staff relationships
Emergency service
Educational objectives
Utilization
Medical records
Building programs
Nursing
Board responsibility and authority
Equipment

BIBLIOGRAPHY

1. "Hospital Accreditation References," pp. 14–15, American Hospital Association, Chicago, 1961.

2. *Ibid.*, pp. 13–14.

3. Rourke, A. J. J.: Essential Committee Functions, *Hospital Prog.*, 46:74–77 (Jan.) 1965.

4. Mann, F. C.: Achieving an Effective Staff, *Hospital Prog.*, 46:91–95 (Jan.) 1965.

22

The Credentials Committee

By Anthony J. J. Rourke, M.D.

Anthony J. J. Rourke is a hospital consultant in New Rochelle, New York, and is a frequent contributor to the hospital literature. He received the M.D. degree from the University of Michigan. He was active in hospital administration from 1937 to 1952 at Columbia Presbyterian Medical Center, the University of Michigan Hospital, then at Stanford University Hospital. He was the director of the Hospital Council of Greater New York from 1952 to 1954. Dr. Rourke is a past president of the American Hospital Association and also served on their Board of Trustees. He was a founding commissioner of the Joint Commission on Accreditation of Hospitals from 1951 to 1954. He is a diplomate of the American Board of Preventive Medicine.

The governing board of every hospital is legally and morally responsible for all the activities, professional and otherwise, which occur within its institution. Among these responsibilities is the quality of medical care, and closely related to this is the appointment of members of the medical staff. Appointments involve rank, department, and delineation of privileges.

Obviously, a group of laymen without training in medicine cannot fulfill this responsibility. Therefore they must delegate the problem of medical staff evaluation and recommendation to a qualified credentials committee. While they must delegate, they should never relegate and forget. The governing board must be assured that the members of the committee realize the responsibilities they are assuming, that they are willing to wholeheartedly accept them, and that they are willing to report back periodically that their mission is being accomplished.

COMMITTEE MEMBERSHIP

In the majority of hospitals the members of the credentials committee are appointed by the chief of staff, or the president of the medical staff, or the chairman of its executive committee (or medical board). Many bylaws call for the approval of the president's appointment by the executive committee of the medical staff. The four major departments—Medicine, Surgery, Obstetrics and Gynecology, and Pediatrics—should be represented on the committee. Members should be selected on the basis of their maturity and previous experience on other hospital committees, and with an eye to their vision and wisdom. Many feel that the minimum term should be three years. If the president also appoints the committee chairman, the selection is taken out of a popularity contest. The chairman should always be a physician; however, dentists should also be eligible to serve on the committee.

FUNCTIONS

In brief, the functions of the credentials committee are invesitgational and advisory. *It is not an action committee; it makes recommendations* only to the executive committee and the governing board in accordance with prevailing medical staff bylaws. It should never be assigned disciplinary or punitive powers.

Procedure. The greatest problem seems to revolve around the methodology under which this committee carries out its function. There is more than one right way. The following are suggestions which have been tried and found satisfactory:

1. Accept only completed applications. It is the function of administration to see that the application is properly and completely filled out. Be sure that it states:

    a. Educational background.

    b. Other training.

    c. Other staff appointments.

    d. Professional attainments (boards, societies, etc.).

    e. Medical license number.

    f. Narcotics registration number.

    g. Three references (character and/or professional).

    h. Signatures of two sponsoring members of the active staff of the hospital.

    i. A statement that the applicant, if appointed, will abide by the medical staff bylaws, rules, and regulations at all times.

2. Require a separate self-evaluation form, filled out by the applicant, which indicates:

    a. Rank being requested.

    b. Department sought.

    c. Privileges requested.

3. Conduct an investigation of the applicant. (ED. NOTE: *The Circulation and Records Department of the American Medical Association offers a service to hospitals and other organizations in which a physician's credentials are verified for all matters pertaining to education, training, and licensure. There is no fee for this service, and forms on which to request information may be secured from Robert A. Enlow, Director of Circulation and Records Department.*) Information needed includes:

    a. Confirmation of his educational background by telephone or by letter to his medical school and to the hospitals of his training or affiliation.

    b. Confirmation of licensure and specialization by use of available directories.

    c. Identification of persons listed as references. Are they classmates, fellow interns, or luncheon club members? Or do they represent previous chiefs of staff, directors of clinical departments, members of governing boards, or administrators?

    d. Consultation with the head of the clinical department in which the applicant is seeking appointment.

4. The credentials committee should make a recommendation to the executive committee no later than two months after the receipt of each new application. The recommendation may be:

    a. To accept and appoint, designating recommended rank, department, and delineated privileges.

    b. To reject.

    c. To defer. When the recommendation is to defer, a second recommendation to accept or reject should be made at the next regular meeting of the executive committee.

5. Record minutes of each meeting, listing date, attendance, time started, matters discussed, and time of closing. Each set of minutes should be signed by the recorder (a member of the committee) and be approved at the next meeting.

6. Meet at least twice each year and more often if indicated.

7. Investigate the making of recommendations for all reappointments as well as for new appointments, as charged in the bylaws. In making recommendation for reappointment, the committee should consider:

    a. Attendance at staff and committee meetings.

    b. The quality of medical records.

    c. Any comments regarding the staff member from the record, tissue, or utilization committees.

    d. Recommendation of the head of the clinical department to which the staff member belongs.

STEPS OF APPOINTMENT

It might be well to list the route of an application for medical or dental staff privileges which results in appointment. The application is:

1. Received by the administrator and checked for completeness.
2. Referred to the medical staff and recorded in the staff minutes.
3. Referred to the executive committee of the medical staff and its receipt recorded.
4. Referred to the credentials committee.
5. Referred to the executive committee with recommendation for appointment, indicating rank, department, and privileges.
6. Posted on the bulletin board in the staff room for two weeks.
7. Referred to the governing board for action.
8. The applicant is notified by the administrator of the governing board action.

The bylaws governing the creation of the credentials committee and a discussion of its activities can be dull and uninteresting. However, the activities of the credentials committee may be constructive, exciting, and profound in the impact on the community if they move out of the mundane and take on new life and approaches.

RECRUITING OF STAFF

The arrival of new physicians in a community is often the result of much happenstance. No one appears to assume responsibility for finding the specific man to fill a specific vacancy or need. While a credentials committee is spending all its time clearing another surgeon there may be a crying need for a specialist in pediatrics. While doctors may arrive in town to join others, the need may be for some independent practitioners to better serve the community.

Seldom does one hear a discussion of which intern or resident should be brought back to the staff for appointment because of his knowledge, personality, or leadership qualities. There is very little contact between hospital staffs and professors at medical schools or directors of clinical departments of teaching hospitals to the end of finding the right doctor to fill a need.

There is need for a comprehensive and balanced medical staff in every hospital commensurate with the size of the hospital. Balanced between what? General practitioners and specialists? Leaders and followers? Short-rangers and long-rangers? Teacher-practitioners and practitioners? Youth and maturity? Is the staff balanced also in terms of wisdom and compulsion? Acceptance and doubt? No more important function can be assigned to a credentials committee than that of evaluating the medical staff as a whole—its qualities, its composition, its deficiencies, its future—in addition to the function of dealing with the applications and reappointments of individual physicians.

23

The Medical Audit

By Vergil N. Slee, M.D.

Vergil N. Slee has been the director of the Commission on Professional and Hospital Activities since its inception more than ten years ago, and he also was the originator and director of the pilot study in the 15 hospitals of the Southwestern Michigan Hospital Council, which was the forerunner of the Commission's Professional Activity Study (PAS). The phenomenal growth of the programs of the Commission can be largely attributed to his vision and energy. He received the M.D. degree from Washington University and the M.P.H. degree from the University of Michigan. He is a Fellow of the American College of Physicians and a Diplomate of the American Board of Preventive Medicine. Before becoming the director of the Commission, he was Administrator of Pennock Hospital in Hastings, Michigan, and concurrently the health officer for Barry County, Michigan.

(ED. NOTE: *An earlier version of this paper appeared in* The Modern Hospital *in November 1961, and is reprinted by permission.*)

A few years ago the medical audit was viewed by the majority of physicians in this country with fear and suspicion. The phrase "medical audit" conjured up a threat of inspection and criticism. There are pockets in the country where this attitude remains; but most medical staffs agree that a medical audit is a good thing and every hospital should have one. As a matter of fact, the pendulum has now swung so far that many hospitals have appointed an audit committee so that at least on paper the mechanism will exist.

There is eagerness to take advantage of the rising popularity of this movement. At one time or another, virtually every constructive endeavor in the hospital field, from the accreditation survey to a study of hospital costs to a study of hospital housekeeping, has been labeled a medical audit. This misuse of the term and the resultant confusion may seriously harm the medical audit and deprive medical staffs of a most useful tool unless the situation is remedied.

DEFINITION OF A MEDICAL AUDIT

In 1954 our group began to investigate medical audit methodology in collaboration with a research project of the American College of Surgeons. One of the most useful results of this study has been the development of a clear, workable definition of a medical audit, one which circumscribes the territory encompassed by a medical audit so that the process can be clearly understood by the medical staff of a hospital. Furthermore, it can be seen that the task attempted by a medical audit, as we have defined it, is a manageable task and one which has clear, positive rewards for the physician participating.

Figure 23-1 lays the basic groundwork for the definition of the medical audit and presents the chain of events which results in medical care. When we are practicing medicine and providing medical care, we are utilizing medical knowledge which has been disseminated through the educational efforts of the medical community. As indicated in the diagram, the great bulk of medical knowledge used in daily practice comes from research; relatively little is contributed from the physician's own practice. The research arm of medicine is constantly providing us with better and better ways of investigating, diagnosing, and treating patients. Since a medical audit, by definition, excludes the research arm of medicine and restricts itself to the application of medical knowledge in the delivery of medical care, the scope of a medical audit is clearly shown.

There is a strong temptation to confuse a medical audit with retrospective clinical research. One result of this confusion in earlier years was

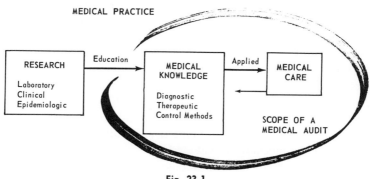

Fig. 23-1

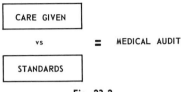

Fig. 23-2

"end result" auditing, which was based on the concept of using the long-term effect on the patient to evaluate the medical care. No workable method of monitoring daily clinical practice by review of its end result has ever been devised, nor is it likely to be. Often years must pass before a judgment can properly be made as to the true end result of therapy. One must give relative values to length of life, suffering, and physical and psychological disability. Furthermore, there is no practical method of obtaining long-term information on patients. Considering the difficulties attendant upon development and maintenance of a successful cancer registry, it seems unlikely that one could ever mobilize similar information systems for tonsillitis or the normal delivery.

More to the point is the fact that careful study and evaluation of end results is a part of clinical research which must be done under far more controlled and objective conditions than may be obtained in clinical practice. We depend upon research to provide a constantly growing and changing body of medical knowledge. We depend upon the medical audit to test the effectiveness of our medical education processes and at the same time help combat obsolescence in the practice of medicine.

The medical audit matches the care given against medical knowledge (Fig. 23-2). The medical audit thus involves the evaluation of the quality of medical care. This statement does not constitute the full definition, however, and before the definition can be completed, this concept of quality must be explained.

The term *quality* as used in the definition of a medical audit refers to the degree of conformity with standards, with the best of medical knowledge, and with accepted principles and practices. We often paraphrase this by saying that the accepted principles and practices are those of the textbooks. To most people this is a well-understood description. Occasionally, however, the inference is drawn that this means standardization at the university hospital level of complexity, with medical student-type histories and physicals and every diagnostic procedure available from the laboratory and x-ray department. This interpretation is surprising because the student is always made acutely aware in his medical training of the importance of insuring that fundamental things are done for every patient, that a certain minimum battery of steps and procedures are taken for each specific type of patient, but that both investigation and therapy are tailored to the individual patient. It is this conformity with standards of excellence which is intended when one speaks of "textbook standards." This is nothing more or less than the standards that each physician would like to have met when he or a member of his family is the patient and which he honestly would like to meet in his own daily practice.

At this point it might be well to counter a common objection to the medical audit, the contention that it will rigidly standardize the practice of medicine. One answer is that the fundamentals of good care should be applied to all patients; there is no excuse for sloppy care, for failure to take an adequate history or to examine the patient. The second point is that the physician is entirely free to treat the patient the way he feels the patient should be treated so long as he can qualify his departure from the usual or traditional practices in a particular case. Failure to give the ordinary or expected care through neglect or carelessness cannot, of course, be tolerated.

The second segment of the definition that needs attention is *medical care*. We use this phrase in a restrictive sense and include in it only those elements of care which are provided by or at the specific direction of the physician. The quality of nursing care, the reliability of laboratory determinations, and the efficiency of the admitting procedure are excluded from the definition to delimit more clearly the scope of the medical audit. We are perfectly willing to grant that a medical audit may uncover problems in all of these areas and that these problems must not be ignored; however, the medical audit is responsible only for passing its observations on to the responsible component of the medical staff for transmittal to the hospital administration.

The definition of the medical audit cannot be completed until we find out what kind of care was given so that it can be matched against the standards. Medical research provides for us information about the *things which must be done* in order to provide the best end results. What we need then, after a description of the patient and his problems, is information as to the things done in response to the patient's needs, the *diagnostic efforts exerted*, and the *management employed*. Direct observation is employed when surgery is done under supervision and during teaching rounds; but here the subjective element is large, and such activities are too sporadic to be relied upon for a medical audit. For this purpose, the only practical information source is the clinical record.

We are now ready to complete the definition of a medical audit: *A medical audit is the evaluation of the quality of medical care as reflected in medical records.*

This definition sometimes elicits comments that the result is the audit of medical records, not of medical care. Although when it is first initiated a medical audit may merely measure the records and not the care, this will come as no surprise to physicians conducting the medical audit.

The experienced physician will not confuse a poor record with poor care. If the first result of a medical audit is to bring about improvement of medical records, this is itself beneficial because good records are an essential part of a good medical practice.

The success or failure of a medical audit may well depend on the staff's understanding of the definition given. Many medical staffs attempting a medical audit have failed because of their impression that the purpose of the review of clinical records is to gain new medical knowledge. Under ordinary circumstances, the physician reads charts either to help him care for individual patients or to add to his knowledge of the effectiveness of various diagnostic or therapeutic procedures. When such knowledge does not come out of the medical audit, the physician may think that the medical audit has been misrepresented and the whole process may be rejected. This may be avoided with a clear statement of the purposes and targets of the medical audit, followed by periodic examination of the process to make sure that retrospective clinical research is not creeping in.

The definition of a medical audit is valid whether it is done by an external auditor or by the medical staff itself as an *internal* (within the medical staff) medical audit. External medical audits are not common and are not increasing in frequency for a number of reasons. Internal medical audits however are becoming permanent activities of hospital medical staffs. Most of the comments which follow refer to the internal medical audit.

PROCEDURE

Much of the resistance to a medical audit has been based on the idea that it is a process of detecting bad practice, or as Dr. Robert Myers has said, "for catching rascals." No medical audit could survive if this were its sole or even its major purpose. An internal medical audit is only incidentally concerned with policing and disciplinary action. The internal medical audit is finding favor and enthusiastic acceptance because it is one of the most highly motivated and best developed forms of continuing medical education. The educational value will vary greatly, however, depending upon the methodology employed.

Establishing an Internal Medical Audit

The medical audit is best carried out by *committees* within the medical staff. The traditional single committee is not recommended. Obviously a single committee must represent the various medical disciplines and specialties. Equally obvious, there is work to be done. One of the advantages of rank in the medical staff, as elsewhere, is that tasks which may be burdensome can be delegated to juniors. The typical single committee, then, will be made up of younger members of the staff, one each from medicine, surgery, pediatrics, obstetrics, and the department of general practice, with perhaps the pathologist and radiologist thrown in for good measure. When the committee faces the task of reviewing care, the surgical cases are then placed squarely in the lap of the young surgeon, the medical cases with the young internist, and so on. We now have a group of one-man junior subcommittees attempting to function. The young man, seeking to establish himself in the staff and build a referral practice, is not likely to voice criticisms of his seniors, or even question their practice, when in so doing he is completely alone. This produces a situation which is not likely to be productive.

In contrast, a two- or three-man subcommittee on each of the major clinical services utilizes the existing departmental structure of the medical staff which is based on specialty training and interest, and this small group can intelligently and productively discuss the topics falling within its jurisdiction. Thus, the process can become interesting rather than terrifying.

General practitioners as well as specialists are expected to participate in the medical audit. A medical audit is not a method by which the specialists review and criticize the generalists; it is a review of the practice, not of the practitioner.

An exception to the departmental committee structure is indicated for certain topics which cut across departmental lines. Perhaps the best example of this is diabetes which may be found in patients throughout the institution. Here, an ad hoc interdepartmental committee going over the problem of diabetes once every year or so would be the answer.

Another point of procedure which is important to educational effectiveness is that the wise staff reviews *clinical topics* rather than a random selection of cases. A random sample, presenting a wide variety of cases, can only be frustrating to the physician whose normal pattern of medical study is to concentrate on one topic at a time. But a series of cases drawn from a single topic permits this normal pattern of medical study to be followed and the process becomes efficient and stimulating. The clinical grouping may revolve around diagnosis, or operation, or investigative routine, or some other topic of clinical importance and interest. The individual practitioner is de-emphasized, and the process capitalizes on the clinical interests of the medical staff members.

Obviously the small medical staff composed largely of general practitioners cannot structure its medical audit within the clinical departments. However, the same principles may be applied. The review of care may be rotated through the medical disciplines from meeting to meeting, considering a medical topic one month, a surgical the next and so on, and making sure that all of the types of patients cared for in the hospital are reviewed periodically.

The goal of the medical audit is the maintenance of the highest quality of medical care. It does not exist for the purpose of compiling statistics or writing reports about the quality of care, but some sort of measurement of care must be made so that evidence can be presented which either supports satisfaction with current practice or defines need for improvement. The medical audit must be concerned both with the standards of care to be met and also with the retrieval of information from medical records.

The medical audit process. The process itself is really quite a simple one. The first step is for a committee faced with the auditing of a clinical topic to *adopt the standards* which it will expect of the medical staff. (Note that the assignment is not to *set* standards since this is a function of the research branch of medicine.) The first step in this process is to review the literature, and this in itself is an extremely important educational component of the medical audit. Further education occurs in the committee discussion which follows, and this is reinforced by the necessity for reaching final agreement on realistic standards which can be expected under the particular hospital situation involved. In the process of adoption of standards, the committee may accept or reject the contentions that a patient in the hospital suspected of pneumonia deserves a chest x-ray; and that if the first one is positive, a second one should be taken to confirm resolution of the pneumonia and determine the presence or absence of underlying pulmonary pathology. The committee considering a pediatric topic may agree on an age above which the taking of blood pressure should be routine. This does not mean that the staff is making up these standards in a vacuum. It is merely reviewing its own knowledge of good medical practice, supplemented when necessary by review and further study, so that the same criteria may be applied to the care rendered by all of the staff members.

The suggestion is sometimes made that the American College of Physicians, or the American College of Surgeons, or the Joint Commission on Accreditation of Hospitals, or the Commission on Professional and Hospital Activities, or some other body should publish sets of standards for the treatment of various conditions in hospitals. To us this does not seem a wise course of action although statements such as those of the American Academy of Pediatrics on the care of children and those of the American College of Obstetrics and Gynecology on maternity and gynecological care are most helpful. American medicine does not need outside agencies to impose standards upon the local medical staff. The typical medical staff has all of the knowledge it needs for enumeration of standards of good practice, or it can easily brush up on current thinking. Furthermore, the process of reaching agreement on standards is a very important educational facet of the internal medical audit. The medical staff of an individual hospital needs standards which are more sensitive to changes in medical thinking than those promulgated by national agencies. And the medical staff which conscientiously accepts this responsibility sets standards considerably higher than those they would tolerate from an outside agency.

The wise medical audit committee will *put its standards in writing* for future reference and for their educational value with other members of the staff.

Once the standards have been adopted, the committee must *review the care which has been rendered and test it against the standards*. Reference to reviewing the care that has been rendered has no qualifying phrases such as "part of the care" or "to some of the patients." There is a clear-cut understanding that *all* of the care will be of the highest quality, and this necessarily means that all of the care will be monitored.

With this recognition of responsibility comes the immediate idea of having medical staff members read all medical records to see if the care appears to have been acceptable. No one is expected to read his own charts. Many medical staffs following this course of action meet failure because of two problems. The first problem is that the sheer burden of work is enormous. Careful and thoughtful case review and evaluation are time consuming. Medical staffs pursuing this course usually end up reviewing *all cases except certain types*, such as normal deliveries, normal newborns, T&A's, cases of certain doctors, and cases which are clearly all right. (It is very difficult at times to find out who determines that cases are all right—often this is the decision of the record librarian.) If the staff continues to pass every chart in front of a reviewing physician, the process degenerates into a perfunctory check for signatures and for the presence of history and physical examination. Such clerical checking is rightfully the duty of the medical record department and an unforgivable misuse of the talent and skill of the physician.

The second problem involved in reading all of the clinical records is that it may not be possible to see the woods for the trees. Recurrent significant problems such as failure to take blood pressure may not be noticed. One or two deficient charts seen by each of a number of reviewers may not look like much of a problem to any single reviewer, yet all deficient charts may belong to one physician or one service or occur in one type of patient.

An alternate solution to the problem of retrieval of information from medical records is the use of statistical profiles and descriptions of care given. The traditional hospital statistics are likely to give such a broad picture as to be essentially worthless in evaluating quality. For example, the kinds of patients, their ages, complications, and treatments are completely obscured in the average length of stay for a clinical service or individual physician. The use of such statistics may actually do more harm than good.

The Professional Activity Study and the Medical Audit Program

The need is to build a bridge connecting these two extremes. Such a bridge exists in the Professional Activity Study (PAS) and the Medical Audit Program (MAP) which together form a medical information system. (ED. NOTE: *Detailed information on this system may be obtained from the Commission on Professional and Hospital Activities, Ann Arbor, Michigan.*) This bridge permits reasonable attention to be paid to the entire medical practice without requiring physicians to read every individual clinical record.

The solution to the problem of auditing all of the care lies with refined statistical profiles and with case abstracts. Abstracting is not a new technique to medicine; however, its application to medical auditing is recent. Abstracting makes information compact and manageable and gives a quick summarization of the parent document. Review of abstracts help to locate documents which the reader wishes to study in detail and eliminates the need for referring to the original whenever the information required has been included in the abstract itself. In PAS and MAP, the abstracted information is transferred to punch cards and then to magnetic tape. Subsequent electronic handling of the information further reduces the work load on the physician and on the medical record librarian.

The information bridge. Such a bridge works in this way. Statistical views of the medical care are supplemented by a variety of more detailed statistics, utilizing a concept called *progressive magnification.* Smaller and smaller segments of the hospital's activity are shown in greater and greater detail and involve each clinical department, each disease and operation group, each specific diagnostic classification and surgical procedure, and the individual physician and surgeon. Each statistical report is supported by listings of individual cases so that all cases contributing to a given statistic can be located, and the story of each patient can be reconstructed and his care reviewed in detail.

All successful medical audit techniques depend on the same principles: condensing the bulky clinical record and reviewing cases in various clinical groupings on the basis of diagnosis, operation, investigative procedure, therapy, department, physician, or other axis of medical importance. Unique features of PAS and MAP include a single standardized abstract for all kinds of cases, extensive use of automation in the handling and display of the information, the availability of interhospital comparisons to serve as bench marks, the elimination of a good deal of clerical work in the record department, and the depth to which one can investigate the individual case without recourse to the original record.

Armed with a medical record information source of this nature, the committee is able to proceed in a logical fashion, first obtaining an overall view of the care and then inspecting various areas in more detail. This insures that no areas escape scrutiny, and yet the task is one which the medical staff, with the assistance of the medical record librarian, can continuously perform.

Requisites for a Successful Internal Medical Audit

There are three requisites for a successful, effective, and efficient internal medical audit:

The hospital must convert its medical record department into a modern information center. This demands a change in emphasis from filing to retrieval. Automation must replace manual methods. Their personnel must become skilled in data retrieval, presentation, and analysis. They must be ready to help the medical staff and administration solve information problems on demand, and they must also use initiative in displaying information so that the medical staff can see the care as it is provided in the institution.

The physicians themselves must learn techniques of utilization review and medical auditing, processes not taught in medical schools or residencies. Here as with every skill, there exists a body of technical knowledge which can make the task simpler, more efficient, and more effective. Training is now available both in the development of criteria or standards against which care can be measured and in the use of information in statistical and coded form in order to handle large quantities of data rapidly. Only when the medical staff, as well as the record department, is prepared, can the staff perform its accepted duties with maximum effectiveness and minimum effort.

The medical staff must be efficiently organized. In the past, each new task has been handled by the addition of a new committee, with resulting duplication of effort and loss of efficiency. The Joint Commission on Accreditation of Hospitals recognized this problem in Bulletin #40 issued in December, 1965,[1] which amends the medical staff function standard by rephrasing Section 3 of the chapter on "Organization of Medical Staff." This section, previously entitled "Committees," is called "Administrative Functions," and the staff is now permitted to organize in any way it sees fit so long as the functions are carried out and "provided effectiveness can be demonstrated by the documentation of activities."

Since a medical audit is concerned with the quality of all of the care in the institution, it must necessarily be concerned with appropriate surgery, formerly the concern of the tissue committee; with wise use of blood, commonly the area of the transfusion committee; and with proper use of beds and services, formerly the concern of the utilization committee. With reorganization permitted by the new Joint Commission standards, the trend toward consolidating a number of functions within the framework of a comprehensive medical audit may accelerate since this is a logical medium for handling all quality control functions which depend on medical records for information. This development is particularly welcome at the time when the Medicare Act might well have imposed two other committees on the medical staff to handle the review of utilization.

EDUCATIONAL ASPECTS

The medical audit procedure establishes a continuous, self-energizing process which will demand the continuing evaluation of standards themselves, the continuing review of care, and the continuing appraisal of that care. The result is an extremely dynamic, highly motivated educational system which revolves around the experience of the medical staff itself in caring for its own patients. Often the discrepancies between the ideal practice as represented by the standards and the actual performance of even the best of medical staffs are most stimulating.

The committee itself profits most from the medical audit. In order to share the benefits and also to complete its function in quality control, the committee, which is a fact finding body, must record not only the meetings held, topics considered, and standards used, but also its findings. This information must be forwarded through proper medical staff channels to the department and executive committee levels, whether the findings are complimentary or whether they point up problems. The rest of the staff is apprised on both the audit activity and the findings. Often formal educational programs in the medical staff are triggered.

The responsibility of a medical audit is fulfilled when it has uncovered the facts, recorded and transmitted them. No disciplinary power should be given to the committee nor should any be assumed by the committee. The finding of less than desirable quality of practice, particularly by an individual, should be dealt with by the appropriate higher echelon, which may be the department or the executive committee. The first step must be independent verification of the audit findings for the protection of both the individual and the committee. Only then should action, if indicated, be taken.

The staff must satisfy the governing board that there is proper attention to the quality of care, for the board carries the basic responsibility for the public trust. This may be achieved by judicious reporting of the audit methods employed, of the findings, and of resulting action.

In addition to information about the quality of the medical records and of the care provided, *a medical audit may turn up information about problems in other parts of the hospital.* For example, nursing care may come in for some criticism or suspicion; a question may be raised about the accuracy of laboratory determinations; x-ray routines may appear inefficient. It may be discovered that there is an unwarranted delay in getting reports of laboratory, x-ray, and other procedures into the clinical record. Administrative practices in the hospital may be suspected of interfering with most effective medical care. Although further investigation in these areas is not the function of the medical audit, these findings must not be ignored. Medical staff and administrative organization must be developed which can receive and act on these collateral findings.

SUMMARY

An internal medical audit is a continuous process carried out year after year as a part of the life of the medical staff. It is a source of satisfaction to the staff to observe changes in practice and the application of new techniques and methods and the abandonment of old. The hospital can take pride in the promptness and thoroughness with which medical advances are put into actual practice. While a medical audit may not change the course and direction of medical progress, it may shorten the time required for patients to receive the benefits of the latest medical knowledge.

The medical audit springs from medicine's own drive to ensure for the next patient better care than that given to the last. The evaluation process itself is highly motivated, continuous education for the physicians on the committees, and the findings of the audits are springboards for the staff's formal and informal education programs.

The medical audit is here to stay. Originating as a method for detecting problems, it has now evolved into dynamic, effective continuing education. Furthermore, methodology has been developed by which a medical staff can conscientiously monitor all the care, and the audit process itself can be refreshing and stimulating.

BIBLIOGRAPHY

1. Bulletin of the Joint Commission on Accreditation of Hospitals, Bulletin No. 40, Joint Commission on Accreditation of Hospitals. Chicago, December, 1965.

24

The Mechanics of Medical Audit

By Kenneth J. Williams, M.D.

Kenneth J. Williams is the medical director of Saint John Hospital in Detroit. He was a high-rigger in logging camps in British Columbia for several years before entering the University of Manitoba Medical School from whence he received the M.D. degree. After eight years of private practice in British Columbia, he entered Yale University and earned the M.P.H. degree in Hospital Administration in 1959. He was medical director of St. Joseph's Hospital in Hamilton, Ontario, for five years, during which period he was a surveyor and field representative for the Canadian Council on Hospital Accreditation and consultant medical director to three other hospitals. He is a Fellow of the American College of Physicians and a member of the American College of Hospital Administrators. He is also consultant medical director to the Hospitals of the Sisters of St. Joseph of Nazareth, Nazareth, Michigan.

The Guide Issue of *Hospitals, JAHA*, August 1, 1965, gives the following data on Saint John Hospital: Beds, 292; Admissions, 15,606; Census, 282; Bassinets, 80; Births, 4,798; Newborn census, 58; Total expenses, $5,182,000; Payroll, $3,140,000; Personnel, 735. (*Ed. Note: Since this issue of* Hospitals, *Saint John Hospital has opened up a 200-bed addition, bringing the total bed capacity to 500.*)

The history, philosophy, definition, misconceptions, and advantages of the medical audit are well set forth in Chap. 23 by Dr. Vergil N. Slee entitled "The Medical Audit." He lists the three requisites for a successful, effective, and efficient internal medical audit, viz.: (1) an effectively organized medical staff, (2) a medical record department functioning as a modern information center, and (3) a medical staff knowledgeable in the techniques of medical auditing. This chapter will deal with these three requisites in some detail.

ORGANIZATION OF THE AUDIT COMMITTEES

Genuine interest and dedication of physicians not withstanding, many medical audit programs often fall into limbo because of a failure to spell out succinct terms of reference and to provide for follow-up and coordinating mechanisms. A staff's medical audit program can best function on a decentralized basis. The actual auditing of professional activities on disease, operation, investigation, and therapy bases is carried out by departmental audit subcommittees. These subcommittees, each consisting of two or three members from the particular department and including general practitioners, report to and are coordinated by the main medical audit committee (Fig. 24-1).

Main Medical Audit Committee

This committee should consist of the chiefs or the vice-chiefs of the clinical departments and the department of general practice. The supervision of the quality of medical care rendered within a clinical department is the prime responsibility of the chief of that department. With all the numerous duties a department chief must discharge, it is not recommended that the chief or vice-chief participate in the audit program at the subcommittee level. His presence on the main medical audit committee affords him the necessary opportunity to know what is going on

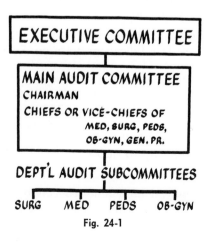

Fig. 24-1

in his department without having to become involved in all the details and minutia. This group, the main audit committee, receives regular reports from the audit subcommittees and, in turn, through its chairman reports directly to the executive committee—the body which must accept responsibility for the professional practices of the medical staff as a whole and report on same to the governing authority of the hospital.

The main medical audit committee is not a disciplinary body. It does not summon members of the staff to appear before it. It is a fact-finding group which, on the strength of the information it receives, may recommend that a department direct attention to a particular facet of practice. For example, the department of medicine's audit subcommittee, while reviewing the manner in which congestive heart failure has been handled, may find that there is an unusually high percentage of patients receiving intravenous fluids. The main audit committee on receiving this information might recommend that both the departments of medicine and general practice discuss these findings, coupled with a presentation on the management of congestive heart failure, at their respective departmental meetings. On the other hand, the main audit committee, mindful of its coordinating function, might first decide to ascertain the extent of the utilization of intravenous fluids in other departments and in other diagnostic categories. It is conceivable that their findings would warrant an educational approach being made to the entire staff rather than to just one or two departments.

This main audit committee, while initiating audit studies and serving as an interlocking mechanism for the departmental audit subcommittees, must also be alert to the need for instituting follow-up studies to measure the effectiveness of the educational messages previously beamed out to the staff.

The executive committee of the medical staff should recognize the main audit committee as one of its most important committees. Criteria should be established for the selection of the individual to serve as chairman. The chairman of the main audit committee should not be encumbered by other staff duties. He should not serve as a chief of a department or chairman of other committees. He must have some permanency of office, at least two to three years, to permit him to become knowledgeable in the necessary techniques and to follow up on the various studies he and his committee initiate. It is essential he have the skills to plan, direct, and coordinate the efforts of the main audit committee and the subcommittees reporting to it. This is not a role for the hard-nosed crusader type of individual. On the contrary, it is far more desirable to possess an inquiring mind, the patience and tenacity to follow through, and the ability to use the soft-sell educational approach. The hard-sell approach, *if needed,* should emanate from the executive committee of the staff.

Terms of Reference

The following terms of reference, excerpted from the *By-Laws of the Medical and Dental Staff* of Saint John Hospital, Detroit, are recommended for the effective functioning of this key committee.

> Composition. The medical audit committee shall consist of the chiefs or vice-chiefs of the departments of surgery, medicine, obstetrics-gynecology, pediatrics, and general practice, and another member of the staff appointed by the executive committee to serve as chairman. There shall be an audit subcommittee for each of the departments of surgery, medicine, ob-gyn, and pediatrics.
>
> The duties shall be as follows:
> a) To review, analyze, and evaluate the clinical practice of the medical and dental staff in all areas of the hospital.
> b) To maintain through its own auditing procedures a continuing appraisal of medical care as practiced in the hospital.
> c) To direct, coordinate, and follow up the work of the departmental audit subcommittees and to receive at monthly intervals reports in writing from the aforementioned subcommittees.
> d) To submit to the executive committee each month through its chairman a written report outlining the work done.
> e) To audit professional activities on disease, operation, investigation, therapy, and individual physician bases.
> f) To evaluate medical care as one basis of the medical and dental staff's overall program of continuing education.
> g) To make recommendations to the executive committee regarding the establishment, maintenance, and improvement of professional standards within the hospital.
> h) To meet at least monthly and keep minutes of all such meetings.
> i) It shall have access to all records and PAS-MAP abstracts pertaining to any aspect of clinical practice.

Departmental Audit Subcommittees

The departmental audit subcommittees are the teams carrying out the detailed audit of professional activities. Each team or audit subcommittee has a captain, usually selected by the medical director (chief of staff) in conjunction with the respective department chief. There should be an audit subcommittee for at least the departments of medicine, surgery, obstetrics-gynecology, and pediatrics. Depending on the extent of departmentalization, there may be other subcommittees. Inasmuch as the department of general practice is not a clinical department, the auditing of the work of general practitioners is carried out by the appropriate specialty departments. The audit subcommittees of the departments of medicine, pediatrics, and obstetrics-gynecology should include general practitioners.

It is advisable to keep the composition of these audit subcommittees fairly small, preferably three to four members on each team. It takes time for them to become versed in the techniques to be used and to become familiar with the potential of the medical information at their disposal. The appointments to these subcommittees should therefore be for at least a two-year period.

Although the main audit committee directs and coordinates the work of these teams the captain and members of each team should be encouraged to initiate their own projects. They are, after all, the group which will eventually become most familiar with the various techniques to be used.

In the interest of good communications there has to be a degree of parallel reporting by the captain of each audit subcommittee. In other words, as well as reporting in writing to the main audit committee each month, he should also maintain direct contact with his department chief. True it is the chief (or the vice-chief) who sits on the main audit committee and will therefore have an opportunity each month to hear what the audit subcommittee for his department is doing. However, the department chief should not have to rely solely on this mechanism to be kept abreast of the projects which the members of his department are carrying out.

THE MEDICAL RECORDS DEPARTMENT AND MEDICAL INFORMATION SYSTEM

The Orthodox Approach

The time-honored approach to medical auditing has been for the audit committee to call for the medical records pertaining to a particular disease entity and to proceed to review them. More often than not this amounted to aimless wandering through mountains of charts without any uniform approach by the various members of the committee, or without first having recognized the need to have predetermined criteria at hand. Understandably, such hit-and-miss methods could not long sustain the interest of busy physicians. Another frequently used and less sound approach has been to review a small random sample of records and then to draw broad, general conclusions regarding the patterns of practice of an entire medical staff. Such methods are fraught with pitfalls and leave much to be desired.

Latterly the need to *first establish criteria* for auditing medical care as reflected in the medical record has been recognized. Yet this alone is *not* the answer. The busy and well-intentioned physician members of the audit committee, armed with uniform criteria and confronted with the task of thumbing through great piles of medical records for a single disease entity, still find some very basic questions unanswered: How is it possible to find the time to do this? How can this approach even begin to audit all the care? Is there not some streamlined approach which will permit us to get a broader view of medical practice which cuts across diagnostic borders, etc.?

There are available today solutions to these pertinent questions, solutions which make it possible for a medical staff to get a view in depth of patterns of practice without its members having to dissipate their time and skills in the clerical, time-consuming task of endless chart review.

Medical Information System

Forward looking administrators and record librarians now recognize that the hospital's medical record department can no longer function simply as a storage center for charts. The medical record department is gradually coming to be regarded as a data retrieval center with its record librarians functioning as data retrieval experts and performing clerical and non-clinical tasks previously carried out by members of many audit and other quality control committees. With the use of a computerized medical information system the medical record librarian is now able to furnish the members of the audit committee with a wealth of clinical data not heretofore practical or possible for her to obtain, and without her entering the field of medical judgment. Her efforts thus contribute to the elimination of much of the time-consuming chart review so long regarded as indispensable to medical audit.

The Commission on Professional and Hospital Activities makes available to hospital staffs through the Professional Activity Study (PAS) and its extension the Medical Audit Program (MAP) a medical information system which literally permits the medical record librarian to function as the physicians' aide to medical care appraisal.* Suffice it to say, PAS-MAP returns to the participating hospital a clinical abstract of the medical record of each patient discharged from hospital. These abstracts, along with other regularly furnished reports, provide a readily accessible source of data without having to routinely call for, pull, review, and refile patients' medical records.

TECHNIQUES

With a properly organized medical audit committee and a medical records department prepared to function as a data retrieval center, we can now consider the techniques to be used by the departmental audit

---

* Information on PAS-MAP may be obtained by contacting the Commission on Professional and Hospital Activities, Ann Arbor, Michigan.

subcommittees. Each departmental audit subcommittee first decides upon the disease entity it will audit. A review of the routine monthly PAS-MAP analyses often provides the clue as to what disease and operative categories should be audited. They then determine the data to be retrieved from the PAS abstracts. This amounts to the audit subcommittees agreeing upon the parameters which, in their opinion, will reflect the degree of excellence with which a specific disease or operative category was handled in their particular hospital. To illustrate: The department of medicine audit subcommittee decides to audit the medical care given to 100 patients in the 14 to 64 age group who have been discharged from the hospital with the diagnosis of cerebral hemorrhage, nontraumatic (*ICDA* 331.0).* They then determine the data they want on the last 100 cases discharged with this diagnosis. To assist in listing the parameters it can be helpful if they preface their discussion with the statement, "If the treatment of patients with the diagnosis of cerebral hemorrhage in our hospital approaches excellence we should find that:" all patients had a urinalysis, CBC, chest x-ray, a blood pressure recorded; a high percentage of patients had EKG's, skull x-rays, blood sugar determinations, consultations; a small percentage of patients had pneumonia, received antibiotics or blood transfusions, etc. The list of parameters for this diagnostic category might be listed in the following manner:

Number of Patients With	*Should Approximate*
CBC	100%
Urinalysis	100%
Blood pressure recorded	100%
Chest x-ray	100%
Blood sugar	100%
Blood urea nitrogen	100%
Lumbar puncture	High
EKG	High
Consultations	High
Skull x-ray	Fairly high
Angiograms	Fairly high
Albuminuria and no repeat urinalysis	0
Glycosuria and no blood sugar	0
Deaths	?
Autopsies	?
Transfusions	Low
Antibiotics	Low
Physiotherapy	High
Urinary tract infection	Low
Pneumonia	Low
Decubitus ulcer	Low

* *International Classification of Disease Adapted for Indexing Hospital Records by Disease and Operations,* U.S.P.H.S., Publication No. 719, revised 1962.

Undoubtedly the reader can think of items to add to the foregoing. The expected findings as shown might also be debated. But let us look at the rationale behind this approach and note some of the advantages in this technique.

1. Here is a group of parameters which collectively—or some of them individually—may show areas of practice that fall short of the ideal. If a large number of these 100 patients were receiving antibiotics or transfusions, or if very few were receiving physiotherapy, or if nitrogen derivative determinations were not being ascertained on many patients, or if patients with glycosuria or albuminuria were not being followed up, certainly these then are indicators pointing out areas of practice deserving attention by the staff.

2. Up to this point the audit subcommittee has not had to search laboriously through these 100 charts to obtain this information. They have only had to sit down and list the items that singly or collectively might serve as indicators to show how close to the level of excellence they are practicing. This is a task that can be done in a very short time.

3. The record librarian, using the PAS medical information system, then compiles a statistical report for the audit subcommittee. In furnishing this report the record librarian has not had to go to the charts. The required data in the illustration is all obtainable from the routine PAS listings.

4. On receipt of this report, and depending on the findings, the members of the audit subcommittee render the value judgment as to the quality of care being afforded patients with this diagnosis. They may feel they have to go further. If for example they found what they regarded as an undue number of patients with urinary tract infections or very few patients with lumbar punctures, they might decide to call for those charts and review them in detail.

5. The anticipated findings as shown in the example given are not intended as hard-and-fast standards. This is a question of the members of the particular audit subcommittee agreeing among themselves as to the standards they feel their confreres in the hospital should be striving to attain. It is quite conceivable that some of the intended indicators may pose additional questions to the audit subcommittee for which they do not have a ready answer. For example, what is a reasonable or acceptable incidence of urinary tract infections in this diagnostic category and particular age group? The answer may be readily available in the literature. Or the audit subcommittee may wish to take advantage of the huge wealth of data available in the PAS-MAP library in Ann Arbor and request PAS to advise it of the incidence of urinary tract infection in this diagnostic category among a group of 10 or 20 hospitals. To illustrate further, the audit subcommittee may wonder what the death rate is

for this diagnosis in other hospitals? By referring to one of the PAS-MAP publications, the medical record librarian would be able to report that among 254 PAS hospitals the death rate for this diagnosis was 45.5 per cent and the autopsy rate was 21 per cent.*

6. The audit subcommittee then submits its findings, along with its comments, to the main audit committee. This latter group, which coordinates all the audit subcommittees, may have noticed that certain patterns of practice prevail in other departments. For example, they may find that in each department there are a few patients with glycosuria not being followed up with blood sugars, or that the number of blood pressures being recorded falls far short of 100 per cent, and so on. They may decide this is sufficient reason to get out a message to the entire staff. Reports in one or two different diagnostic categories may suggest that antibiotics are perhaps being used to excess; but to get a broad view of practice before beaming a message to the staff, they may request the record librarian to determine the antibiotic utilization rate in several disease and operative categories. By the same token, their observations may lead them to conclude that certain therapeutic and investigative procedures reflect standards of care superior to those reported in the literature—this too, of course, should be communicated to the staff.

7. Although this technique takes advantage of the statistical approach, it must be made abundantly clear there is no intent to imply that statistical descriptions are a substitute for medical judgment. The use of this method *does not mean* that members of a staff have to practice identical medicine or conform to norms. Those physicians who are critical of the statistical approach because they think it is being offered as an alternative to medical judgment are missing the point. It is simply that the use of statistics—properly applied and interpreted—is an extremely useful and time-saving *aid* in our attempts to get a detailed and overall view of patterns of practice.

Additional Examples

The following lists of parameters, or possible indicators, further illustrate what can be done with a large number of disease and operative categories. Additional items could be added to these lists; however, the data to be retrieved by the record department personnel for the following are routinely provided on the PAS abstracts and are hence easily obtainable without having to have recourse to the patients' charts. Selecting the diagnostic grouping (*ICDA* 780–795.9) of Symptoms, Senility and

* Death and Autopsy Rates for 50 Leading Causes of Admission, 1963, *The Record* (C.P.H.A.), 3:12 (Feb.) 1966.

Ill-Defined Conditions, the department of medicine's audit subcommittee would agree upon the items likely to indicate, singly or collectively, the standard of care afforded patients in this grouping. This particular category, which cuts across departmental lines, can oftentimes be quite helpful in gaining a measure of the staff's diagnostic acuity. In listing the parameters for which the record librarian is to supply the data, the audit subcommittee would commence with the approach that if the patients with diagnoses falling into this category only are being treated at the level of excellence we should expect, the findings should be:

Number of Patients With

CBC
Urinalysis
Blood pressure recorded
Serology
EKG
Chest film
Blood sugar
Nitrogen derivatives determined
Sedimentation rate
Consultations
Albuminuria and no repeat urinalysis
Glycosuria and no blood sugar
Elevated blood pressure (140/100 or greater)
   and no diagnosis of hypertension recorded.
Elevated blood pressure and no EKG
Hormones
I.V. fluids
Transfusions
Antibiotics
Deaths
Autopsies
Vague diagnoses such as:
   Pain in back
   Pain in chest
   Pylorospasm
   Pyrexia of unknown origin
Proportion of all admissions (excluding
   maternity and newborn) constituted by
   this diagnostic grouping.

Should Approximate

(The audit subcommittee lists what it feels each of these parameters should show.)

Using the same approach for the operation of Tonsillectomy and Adenoidectomy (*ICDA* 27.2) in the age group under 14 years, the surgical or pediatric audit subcommittee can obtain an excellent view of how this operation is being handled. Notwithstanding the fact that T&A histories and physicals are usually very brief, there is a great deal of information that can be gleaned from the PAS abstracts as the following example illustrates.

Number of Patients With	Should Approximate
Blood pressure recorded	(The audit subcommittee lists
Urinalysis	what it feels each of these
WBC	parameters should show.)
CBC	
Hemoglobin or hematocrit	
Pre-op hemoglobin of 9 Gm or less	
Pre-op hematocrit of 28 or less	
Albuminuria and no repeat urinalysis	
Glycosuria and no blood sugar	
Pre-op temperature over 100°	
Elevated blood pressure (140/100 or greater) and no diagnosis of hypertension recorded.	
Pre-op WBC of 4,000 or less	
Pre-op WBC of 14,000 or more	
Antibiotics	
Post-op hemorrhage	
Blood transfusions	
Myringotomies	
Chest complications	
Deaths	
Proportion of patients 3 years or younger	
Proportion of all admissions of age group under 14 years (excluding maternity and newborn) constituted by this category.	

Here, and with any diagnostic, therapeutic or investigative category, the significance to be attached to these parameters must be determined by the members of the audit committees. The mere listing of a particular item does not in itself necessarily indicate or imply excellent nor less than ideal practice. For example, the fact that "myringotomies" are listed in the foregoing example does *not* infer that this is an indication of good or poor practice. For that matter, it is quite conceivable that in a sample of 500 T&A's there will be some myringotomies. It is in the extent to which they are done that we are interested. The "acceptable extent" has to be determined by the members of the committee. This might even necessitate particular charts being pulled and reviewed. The approach illustrated by the foregoing three examples can be carried out with practically any diagnostic or operative category.

The Monthly Statistical Report

The statistical report of clinical work, produced for the medical staff by the medical records department each month, frequently follows very much of a stereotyped pattern in many hospitals. It usually shows the number of patients discharged and the deaths and autopsies for each clinical department and the subspecialties—and it often shows very little else.

With the use of the PAS-MAP medical information system the monthly statistical report can be structured in such a way as to give the executive and audit committees, as well as the staff, a much broader picture of professional activities in the hospital. The routine PAS-MAP reports now make it possible for the records department to provide average and median lengths of stay of a wide range of diagnostic and operative categories for each clinical department. In addition, the record librarian can, at the request of the staff, furnish numerous clinical items of interest indicating the extent to which certain standards are being met. In other words, the old familiar, stereotyped, so-called statistical analysis can now be replaced by a much more meaningful report.

In discussing some of the clinical items—possible indicators—that might be included in this report, I would like again to stress one or two points. By themselves such items may provide the starting point for an interesting look into related areas of practice. The listing of an item does not infer that something should or should not be. For example, in reporting the percentage of coronaries with anticoagulant therapy, some physicians might be quick with the reply, "So what, you can't fault us because we don't use anticoagulants." Of course not, nor is it the intent to fault anyone! The point in this example is that if a staff is using anticoagulants in 100 per cent or in a high percentage of coronaries it might then wish to study its care of patients with coronary occlusions further and compare it with a group of hospitals in which anticoagulants are used very little. Considering another example, in the following list, the incidence of newborns with conjunctivitis, the question might well be posed, "What is the significance? What is the standard here?" It would be difficult, as with any infection rate, to come up with a specific figure because of the wide differences in recording and reporting; but nonetheless, the routine reporting of such items can be of considerable help to a staff in indicating trends. The following list of clinical items illustrates some of the data which the record libarian can easily retrieve from the PAS-MAP reports and include in the monthly statistical report.

Per cent of acute inflammatory disease in primary appendectomies
Per cent of appendices with acute inflammatory disease that are ruptured
Newborns with conjunctivitis
Newborns with infected cords
Discharged patients not having met Joint Commission requirements of
    hemoglobin and urinalysis
Death rate for coronary occlusions
Coronary occlusions in hospital less than 10 days (excluding death)

Per cent of coronary occlusions with anticoagulant therapy
Per cent of congestive heart failure patients receiving I.V.'s
Per cent of cesarean sections which are classical
Per cent of hysterectomies which are subtotal
Pneumonias without chest x-rays
Antibiotic utilization rate in newborns, deliveries, hernias, etc.
Hemorrhoidectomies with blood transfusions
Varicose veins with blood transfusions
Newborn deaths associated with induction
Newborn deaths associated with breech delivery
Autopsy rates of same
Wound dehiscences
Per cent of eneuresis cases with cystoscopy, etc.
Other

Any audit committee with a little thought and with attention to the scope of this medical information system can add a great many items to the foregoing list. The value of such items might be questioned by some members of the staff, e.g., "What is the point in reporting the per cent of cesarean sections that are classical? We seldom ever have any classical sections." The fact of the matter is that a staff—particularly a large staff and even in medical centers—does not know what it has unless it actually takes a look. This is one way of looking and ascertaining those areas which might be worthy of a second look. If a staff does not have a volume of cases sufficient to make monthly reporting worthwhile, it can easily set up a mechanism whereby the record librarian reports on these possible indicators at quarterly intervals. With the main audit committee receiving a copy of the routine statistical analysis, these data can often be the stimulus to initiate audit studies in areas of practice which might otherwise not be considered.

There has been no attempt, and for very good reasons, to apply specific figures to the foregoing and to regard them as standards. There is a tendency to cling to a specific figure once it is attached to a particular facet of practice. Unfortunately, one still sees the printed word lending support to time-honored but misleading statistical yardsticks, such as the infection rates should not exceed 1 per cent; unnecessary surgery should not exceed 10 per cent; a hospital's death rate should not exceed 4 per cent; etc. These are *not* meaningful figures. The significance of the statistics obtained for the parameters listed above must be determined by consideration. Often comparative data from other hospitals may be obtained from PAS. Their main value lies in the fact that they form part of a very useful screening mechanism.

SUMMARY

An effectively organized medical staff, knowledgeable in the technique of medical audit, taking advantage of a computerized medical information, and using the medical record librarians as data retrieval experts, can obtain a view of medical practice without dissipating the skills and time of its members in time-consuming, tedious, and often futile chart review. In certain circumstances there is no substitute for actual review of the medical record. However, the audit committee which confines its efforts solely to reviewing charts of specific disease entities even though it has well-established criteria to match against the care reflected in the record is not getting a broad view of medical practice in that hospital. The use of a computerized medical information system, coupled with the statistical approach outlined in this chapter, not only tremendously reduces the amount of chart review but also serves as a valuable screening mechanism. It makes it possible, and practical, to look at medical practice on diagnosis, operation, therapy, and investigative bases.

25

The Tissue Committee

I.

By Frank P. Lloyd, M.D.

Frank P. Lloyd was in the private practice of obstetrics and gynecology in Indianapolis, Indiana,
for 10 years before becoming the director of
medical research of the Methodist Hospital in
1963. He received the M.D. degree from Howard
University and had residency training at Freed-
man's Hospital in Washington and at the Columbia Presbyterian Medical Center in New York.
He is a diplomate of the American Board of
Obstetrics and Gynecology, a Fellow of the American College of Surgeons, and a Fellow of the
American College of Obstetricians and Gynecologists. He is chairman of the Research Committee of Methodist Hospital and chairman of the
Education Committee of the department of obstetrics and gynecology.

The Guide Issue of Hospitals, JAHA, August 1,
1965 gives the following data on the Methodist
Hospital of Indiana: Beds, 870; Admissions, 28,
625; Census, 760; Bassinets, 108; Births, 3,691;
Newborn census, 47; Total expenses, $12,300,-
000; Payroll, $7,716,000; Personnel, 2,030.

Quality control is a far-reaching phrase in our present society. The
demand for this control exists in every field of science, engineering, industrial research, manufacturing, and marketing. The product, the millions
of dollars expended, and the integrity of the organization may be contingent upon this control.

Service to humanity is the principal objective—the "product"—of the medical profession.[1] No excuse need be offered for the provision of quality control in the practice of medicine. While governmental control now exists on the periphery of medicine, and may encroach further, the regulating bodies in the art and science of medicine are its own organizations, founded by and composed of practicing physicians. The concern of our nation for the health of its people is second only to its concern for the defense of the country. If our "product" is good health for our citizens, then we must search for ways to provide quality control in their care.

A technique used in hospitals to ensure quality control of surgery is the tissue committee.[2] The committee may range from a large and formal group in a large teaching center to a loosely knit group in a small community hospital.[3,4,5,6] Nowhere is quality control more important than in the small community hospital, for it provides medical care for the surrounding area and hospital facilities for all physicians in the area. The entire reputation of a small medical community may rest upon the work of the surgeons who practice there.

Despite great achievements on many fronts of medicine, the long-standing inequalities in the quality of medical care practiced in our communities remains to be solved. To contend that there are no differences when medicine is practiced without controls is to disregard the changes found after the introduction of control committees into the hospital organization.[7,8,9,10,11] When substandard medical practice exists or when deterioration of medical care develops, it is usually because of a lack of self-discipline of the medical staff. If a staff is to be successful, this self-discipline is vital.

The lack of general standards for tissue committees makes it difficult to compare their work in different settings; however it gives the freedom of adaptability to the various localities, the freedom that is absolutely necessary for the successful function of these committees.

Most physicians who accept staff privileges at a hospital want to practice medicine according to acceptable standards, and they believe that the medical staff should control the activities of its own members. Far from resisting the introduction of a tissue committee, they encourage its establishment. No longer is the tissue committee looked upon as the "surgical police force" and the special nemesis of the gynecological surgeon, but rather as the regulating body of the surgical specialties. Its influence has extended beyond the confines of the operating room to include the evaluation of the total care of the surgical patient.

In most hospitals, the establishment of a functioning tissue committee has brought about a reduction in unnecessary surgery. The clinical records at these hospitals have shown a great improvement in legibility, context, and coherence. There has been no increase in mortality and necessary surgery has not been postponed or left undone.[12]

There should be considerable freedom in setting up the tissue committee. In some areas, one committee may function for several small hospitals in the community. If possible, a pathologist, a general surgeon, a representative of a surgical specialty, an internist, and a general practioner should form the basic group.

The tissue committee should report to the executive committee or the professional standards committee of the staff, who then make any necessary punitive recommendations to the governing board of the hospital.

ESTABLISHED CRITERIA

A most important aspect of the tissue committee is its commitment to govern by previously established criteria. If the medical staff is large enough to be divided into specialty sections, each section should develop criteria for their procedures to be reviewed by the tissue committee. This in itself is an educational experience, and it is most unlikely that a section would set criteria for itself that are not up to the standard practice of its specialty. The standards selected usually will be ones of excellence. This procedure is especially important when men of varying degrees of ability and training practice in a hospital because established criteria tend to bring the standards of practice up to recognized levels.

JUSTIFICATION OF SURGERY

The criteria established by the various departments and sections become the vehicle to determine the justification of the surgery performed. Established criteria tend to remove the reluctance to judge surgery and largely reduce the temptation to render inconsistent judgments that may favor certain members of the staff.

After the criteria have been established, an abstract is prepared by medical record room personnel who are trained to complete this form. All cases that conflict in some way with established criteria are reviewed by the tissue committee. This technique saves much time and allows a review of all types of surgery for which criteria have been established. A similar method may also be useful in hospitals using the Professional Activity Study (PAS).[13]

Criteria cannot be established to reflect all facets of clinical judgement. Cases which are not found to be justified by criteria may have justification based on clinical judgment, and these cases, of course, will be easily justified by an alert committee if the patient's record is complete. This then leaves only those charts for review that do not fit the criteria and for which there is inadequate documentation for the justification of surgery.

When a case is criticized as lacking justification, the surgeon is notified of the action of the committee. Usually there is no resentment against the tissue committee for this criticism since the criteria used in judging the case were proposed by the physician's own section. No action is taken against the staff member unless there is continued or flagrant disregard of the criteria for surgery.

Members of a section may suggest changes in the criteria from time to time; if the section agrees, the changes are transmitted to the tissue committee for incorporation into the established criteria. This allows new techniques and procedures to be introduced into a hospital with the official support of the staff; and by circulating these changes in criteria, the medical staff is kept abreast of new developments.

As statistics from the tissue committee accumulate, comparisons with other hospitals in the community and other communities may point up defects as well as strong points of the criteria and standards of practice used in the hospital. These findings, reported to the various specialty sections, provide material for discussions, continuing reevaluation, and education of the staff.

Initially, an outside consultant may suggest criteria and review procedures, but for the full benefit of the staff, definition and refinements of criteria must be their own continuing effort.

SOME EXPERIENCES OF A TISSUE COMMITTEE

A tissue committee was established at a midwestern hospital in 1953, with the late Paul A. Lembcke, M.P.H., M.D., serving as a consultant in

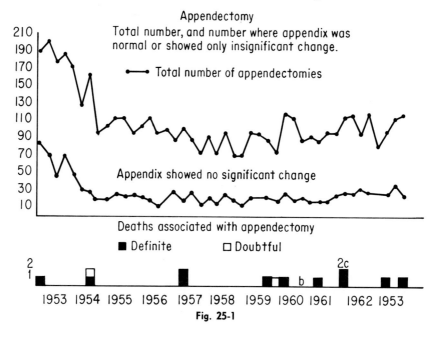

Fig. 25-1

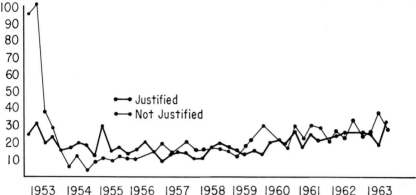

Number of Hysterectomies With Removal of Both Ovaries or of only Remaining Ovary.

Fig. 25-2

establishing criteria for some surgical procedures.[14] Refinements of criteria have been a continuing function of the various surgical sections of the hospital. Several examples illustrate the impact that the tissue committee has had on surgical practices.

1. The justification for appendectomy was stated as "acute inflammation of the appendix at the time of operation being verified by pathological report." The surgical condition and the pathology report on which justification is based are (a) drainage of appendical abscess; (b) acute gangrenous or acute supperative appendicitis; (c) removal of appendix where abscess was previously drained; (d) carcinoid, mucocele, oxyuriasis of appendix; (e) acute fibrinous or acute hemolytic appendicitis; and (f) acute appendicitis.

The incidence of appendectomies and the trends in the classification of cases for 11 years are shown in Fig. 25-1. Besides the reduction in the number of cases reported as not justified, there has been a definite improvement in medical records, to the point where a definite preoperative diagnosis is now made on all cases. There is also a sharp increase in the consultation notes when findings are indefinite.

2. Hysterectomy with removal of both ovaries was justified in the original criteria only if the patient was over 45 years of age or if there was disease of the ovary requiring removal. Figure 25-2 shows the trend in justified hysterectomies with removal of both ovaries.

3. Subtotal hysterectomy was not justified unless some unusual condition was found at the time of surgery and it was fully documented in the record. Figure 25-3 shows the trend in the number and per cent of subtotal hysterectomies performed.

4. Primary uterine suspension was justified only in cases of documented severe displacements of the uterus and in some cases of sterility. Figure 25-4 shows the trend in the number of primary uterine suspensions.

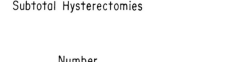

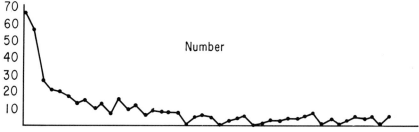

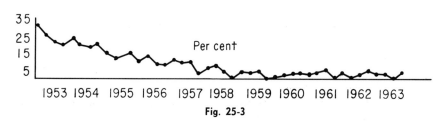

Fig. 25-3

Although there has been definite decrease in unjustified surgery, no instance has been found where necessary surgery was not done.

SUMMARY

The function of the tissue committee is best described in the statement of the Board of Commissioners of the Joint Commission on Accreditation of Hospitals, at its meeting on April 4, 1959:

The *tissue committee* "should be more than a negative or inhibiting influence. It should not be solely content to abolish outmoded or dis-

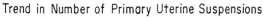

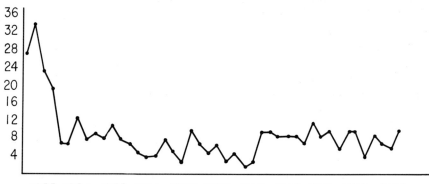

Fig. 25-4

credited techniques and procedures. It should strive for the adoption of better methods of treating patients and of curing disease. It attains these objectives by continuing analysis, review, and education." [2]

BIBLIOGRAPHY

1. Editorial: The Newer Research, *Calif. Med.*, 95:251–252 (Oct.) 1961.
2. Tissue Committee of a Hospital Medical Staff, *Bull. of the Joint Comm. on Accreditation of Hospitals*, No. 21 (Aug.) 1959.
3. Fox, L. P.: Hospital Departments and Tissue Committees, *Obstet. Gynec.*, 7:576–581 (May) 1956.
4. DeCamp, L.: The Tissue Committee in a General Hospital, *N. Carolina Med. J.*, 21:53–54 (Feb.) 1960.
5. Henley, P. G. *et al.*: Uses and Abuses of the Tissue Committee, *JAMA*, 168:2243–2245, 1958.
6. Editorial: Progressive Care, *Mod. Hosp.*, 91:66 (Sept.) 1958.
7. Myers, R. S.: The Tissue Committee Proves Its Worth, *Bull. Am. Coll. Surgeons*, 44:189–191 (July–Aug.) 1959.
8. Verda, D. J., and Platt, W. R.: The Tissue Committee Really Gets Results, *Mod. Hosp.*, 91:74–76 (Sept.) 1958.
9. Monardo, G. D.: The Tissue Committee—An Educational Tool, *Hospitals*, 29:81–84 (Feb.) 1955.
10. Verda, D. J., and Platt, W. R.: The Effectiveness of the Tissue Committee at the Missouri Baptist Hospital, *Bull. Am. Coll. Surgeons*, 43:449–451 (Nov.–Dec.) 1958.
11. Daseler, E. H.: . . . For the Triumph of Evil, *Bull. Am. Coll. Surgeons*, 40:22 (Jan.–Feb.) 1955.
12. Williams, J. W.: The First Duty of the Tissue Committee, *Mod. Hosp.*, 84:100–106 (June) 1955.
13. Slee, V. N.: How to Make the Tissue Committee's Work More Effective, *Mod. Hosp.*, 92:96–98 (June) 1959.
14. Lembcke, P. A.: Medical Auditing by Scientific Methods, *JAMA*, 162:646–655 (Oct. 13) 1956.

II.

By John McGee, M.D.

John McGee is Chief of Surgery of the Marin General Hospital in San Rafael, California, and he has been a member of the tissue committee.

He received the M.D. degree from Johns Hopkins University, and he was a resident in surgery at the University of California School of Medicine, where he is now a Clinical Instructor in Surgery. He is a diplomate of the American Board of Surgery.

The Guide Issue of *Hospitals, JAHA,* August 1, 1965, gives the following data on Marin General Hospital: Beds, 220; Admissions, 9,651; Census, 147; Bassinets, 40; Births, 1,737; Newborn census, 18; Total expenses, $3,755,000; Payroll, $2,515,000; Personnel, 450. There are three other short-term general hospitals in the community of 100, 59, and 30 beds. The population in the 1960 census was 147,000.

THE PAST

In 1918, Standards of Patient Care were formulated by the American College of Surgeons; these were adopted by the Regents of the College on December 20, 1918. The most effective requirement for ACS approval was that the medical staff review and analyze at regular intervals the clinical experience in the various departments of the hospital.

The ACS expanded this requirement in 1929 and recommended that particular attention be paid to the results of surgery and to the pathological findings in relation to the clinical history.

After unofficially suggesting it for several years, in 1951 the ACS established the provision that a tissue committee be required of a hospital seeking approval. The tissue committee would review all surgery and report to the medical staff upon the justification for surgery.

In 1952, The American College of Surgeons relinquished the accreditation program to the Joint Commission on Accreditation of Hospitals, which has continued to emphasize the importance of the tissue committee.

The primary goal of the ACS was the elimination of unnecessary surgery, and this has been achieved in many hospitals which have had the necessary staff organization and cooperation. In these hospitals, the tissue committee has been very effective in reducing the incidence of unnecessary surgery. The elements essential for propr functioning of a tissue committee are:

A medical staff which is willing to have its work audited and which is willing to do the work.
A pathologist who has the courage to "call them as he sees them!"

All tissues removed must be sent to Pathology for examination.

A staff organization which can and will discipline surgeons who perform unnecessary surgery.

THE PRESENT

The ten year experience of a hospital with the right combination of these essential ingredients has been notable in several respects.

Appendectomy. The number of normal appendices removed has been reduced. At one of our first meetings, one surgeon was found to have a 60 per cent normal tissue rate; another, 100 per cent. When they were confronted with these figures, the first surgeon became more particular about the indications for the procedure, and the second surgeon stopped doing abdominal surgery. For the last three years, our normal tissue rate has been from 16 per cent to 19 per cent. No surgeon has been out of step, and it is rare that an appendectomy is judged unnecessary.

Hysterectomy. The same results have been obtained in the pelvis. One of the early reviews uncovered a surgeon who had removed three normal uteri in a brief period; his gynecologic privileges were withdrawn. Another surgeon inappropriately removed a gravid uterus, and his privileges were decreased.

Our tissue committee still keeps a close check on pelvic surgery, but it now rarely comes up with the verdict: unjustified surgery.

The number of subtotal hysterectomies has been reduced. For several years, our committee has asked each surgeon to explain why he did a subtotal operation when we felt that a total hysterectomy was indicated. The percentages of hysterectomies that are subtotal has consequently dropped from 10 per cent to 2.5 per cent. There is a good reason for nearly all of them now.

Exploratory Laparotomy without Removal of Tissue. There has been a marked decrease in the number of these procedures since the tissue committee began to audit them. In recent years, every one of these has been judged justified.

Specialty Surgery. In the surgical subspecialties, it is extremely difficult to evaluate the indications for and the techniques of surgery since many procedures have become so far removed from general surgical training. Only a surgical subspecialist can appropriately evaluate the work.

In our hospital, the department of surgery is now organized into sections corresponding to the surgical specialties. Each section is charged with reviewing the clinical work done in the field of its specialty. The justification for surgery is one facet of their audit.

Other Procedures. All tissues are coded by the pathologist in the following manner:

Code 1. Tissue disease generally requiring surgical removal.
Code 2. Tissue diseased, but surgical removal is not clearly required from the pathological finds alone.
Code 3. No disease.

In a recent year, 322 cases with tissue codes 2 and 3 were reviewed. Twenty-nine cases were referred to the surgeon for additions to the medical record that would justify the procedure. Only seven cases were referred to the appropriate executive committee for more extensive review of possibly inadequate management or unjustified surgery.

Over the ten years that this tissue committee has been working well, the amount of unjustified surgery has been reduced to such a low level that the committee has turned to examination of other facets of care of surgical patients.

THE FUTURE

Many participants in the seminar on the tissue committee at The Hospital Medical Staff Conference at Estes Park, Colorado, in October of 1965 expressed the same progression of committee activities in their hospitals. The tissue committees are looking for additional work to do.

This tendency has been decried by leading proponents of the tissue committee, who feel that any attempt to broaden the activities of the committee will detract from its fundamental purpose, to establish the justification for surgery.

SUMMARY

Everyone will agree that the tissue committee has been a very potent instrument in the reduction of unnecessary surgery across the nation. In many hospitals, this reduction has been the initial medical audit activity. Justification for surgery will always be an important feature of the medical audit of every hospital. However, with the development of audit activities, other features of patient care are coming under careful scrutiny, and certainly each facet of patient care cannot have its separate medical staff committee. It seems likely that there will be some consolidation in medical audit activities. The tissue committee may well be assigned additional duties, or the justification for surgery may become an essential responsibility of the surgical department audit committee.

26

The Utilization Committee

By Vergil N. Slee, M.D.

Vergil N. Slee has been the director of the Commission on Professional and Hospital Activities since its inception more than ten years ago, and he also was the originator and director of the pilot study in the 15 hospitals of the Southwestern Michigan Hospital Council, which was the forerunner of the Commission's Professional Activity Study (PAS). The phenomenal growth of the programs of the Commission can be largely attributed to his vision and energy. He received the M.D. degree from Washington University and the M.P.H. degree from the University of Michigan. He is a Fellow of the American College of Physicians and a diplomate of the American Board of Preventive Medicine. Before becoming the director of the Commission, he was administrator of Pennock Hospital in Hastings, Michigan, and concurrently the health officer for Barry County, Michigan.

(ED. NOTE: *An earlier version of this paper was published in* The Modern Hospital *in December, 1965, and is reprinted by permission.*)

In recent months, the prime subject of discussion in hospitals throughout the country has been the implications of the Medicare legislation for the future of medical practice and American hospitals. While much of the impact is entirely a matter of conjecture, one specific requirement has caused consternation and dismay for many hospitals and their medical staffs. This is the requirement for a utilization review plan, a requirement which is seen as placing yet another burden of committee work on the medical staff.

The purpose of this paper is to develop the thesis that *those hospitals conducting an internal medical audit are already performing retrospective utilization review,* which covers certain points prescribed by the Act. Several aspects in which the medical audit is superior to simple utilization review will be elaborated, and the prediction is made that most hospitals will adopt the comprehensive medical audit in preference to adding one more limited and overlapping committee.

MEDICARE REQUIREMENTS FOR UTILIZATION REVIEW

The Medicare Act requires that every hospital and extended care facility that wishes to qualify as a provider of services must have a utilization review plan. (ED. NOTE: *These requirements are discussed in detail in Chap. 33, "The Impact of Medicare on the Hospital Staff" by Roberta Fenlon, M.D.*) Analysis of the Act indicates that the utilization review plan must have two mechanisms:

1. One mechanism is for live or on-the-spot review of the medical necessity for inpatient services during a continuous period of extended duration. This review must be done in terms of days as specified by regulations. It is similar to the functions of the admission and discharge committee already operating in a few hospitals. I suggest that this be called *medical necessity determination.*

2. The second mechanism is for retrospective review of admissions, duration of stay, and professional services furnished, including drugs and biologicals, with regard to their medical necessity and the efficient use of facilities and services. I suggest that this be called *utilization evaluation.*

Probably the administration and medical staff of the hospital will find it expedient to handle these two problems by two separate methods.

Medical Necessity Determination

Medical necessity determination will require:

1. Defining the "extended care case." This definition must be part of the hospital's utilization review plan.
2. Tagging each admission to the hospital as a member of a class requiring review if the case becomes an extended stay case as defined in the utilization review plan.
3. Establishing a tickler or reminder system for days on which review is required for each case.
4. Notifying a "flying squad" of physicians each day of cases due for review within the subsequent seven days.
5. Developing a pattern for studying individual cases which are referred to the flying squad. This will include consultation with the attending physician.
6. Recording the flying squad's evaluation and determination as to medical necessity for hospitalization.

7. Notifying the patient, his physician, and the hospital when evaluation indicates that further stay is *not* medically necessary. (Benefits cease three days after this notice is received by the facility.)

Medical necessity determination as here described is new to most hospitals although some admission and discharge committees and a few utilization committees have worked on this problem. Innovation and experimentation will be required to develop simple and efficient procedures for this function. Perhaps here, for this single function, the committee will be called a Utilization Committee.

Utilization Evaluation

Utilization evaluation, retrospective study of the use of the hospital, on the other hand, is *not* new. It is this segment of the utilization review plan that is related to the internal medical audit.

Appropriate use of hospital and medical resources and facilities has always been of concern to conscientious and thoughtful physicians and hospital administrators. The medical audit has always pointed out excessive use of drugs, unnecessary hospital stays, and other wasteful practices. The medical audit did not have its origin, however, in attention to the conservation of resources; it sprang from one of the most basic drives in medicine—the drive to provide the best care. Leadership in developing a methodical approach to monitoring the quality of care and maintaining the highest standards came not only from the American College of Surgeons and the American College of Physicians but also from hospitals and particularly from their medical staffs. Special recognition should be given to those hospitals which in 1949 spurred the establishment of the Professional Activity Study and then went on with the American College of Surgeons to develop the Medical Audit Program.

The medical audit movement had barely achieved a good foothold when, in the early and mid fifties, third parties began to demand tighter control of the use of hospital resources. Hospitals were asked and even ordered to establish utilization committees, not primarily to improve the quality of care but to reduce the amount of care. A number of utilization committees with this origin are in operation. To cite only two of the developments, the California Medical Association considers a hospital utilization committee essential, and the Tenth Councilor District of the Pennsylvania Medical Society has been nationally acclaimed for its pioneering in this area. J. Everett McClenahan, M.D.,[1] of Pittsburgh, describes the scope of utilization evaluation in several questions:

1. Was the patient's admission to the hospital necessary?
2. Has the treatment of the patient, while under medical care, been car-

ried out as expeditiously as possible with a minimum of delay in the prescribed treatment?

3. Was the patient discharged as soon as he was medically ready? [1]

Each of the questions obviously reflects the fact that there are criteria or standards for propriety of admission, speed of delivery of diagnostic and treatment procedures, and medical readiness for discharge. Utilization evaluation requires comparison of the care given individuals or groups of patients against these criteria. Since it is retrospective, this evaluation depends on the normal documentation of the medical care provided, the documentation which is found in the clinical records of every discharged patient.

SIMILARITIES AND DIFFERENCES BETWEEN MEDICAL·AUDIT AND UTILIZATION REVIEW

The similarity of utilization evaluation to the medical audit is apparent. *Both depend upon comparing medical care as reflected in medical records against standards representing the desired care.* But there are significant differences between what utilization evaluation usually means to utilization committees and what medical auditing means to American medicine and hospitals. Furthermore, important lessons about effective methodology learned in the medical audit have not been applied in the utilization committee approach.

A medical audit is defined as the evaluation of the quality of medical care as reflected in medical records. In order to see the difference between utilization evaluation and a medical audit, the definition of a medical audit must be dissected. The simple word "quality" holds the key. There is a difference in scope between utilization evaluation and the medical audit.

In a medical audit, quality is defined as the degree of conformity with standards, with accepted principles and practices. These desired standards of excellence demand that certain fundamental things be done for every patient; that an absolute minimum battery of steps and procedures be taken for specific types of patients; and finally that in all instances investigation, diagnosis, and therapy be tailored to the individual patient. The goal is to achieve standards which each physician would like to have met when he or a member of his family is the patient and which he sincerely tries to maintain in his own practice. Note that the scope of a medical audit is comprehensive. A medical audit is just as concerned about conservation of our medical and hospital resources as is a utilization committee. But equal attention is given to the question of whether every patient gets what he needs for his particular problems.

Thus it should be clear that *a medical audit is utilization evaluation and considerably more.* The medical staff which is conducting an internal medical audit is, by definition, carrying out a utilization evaluation although this aspect is only a portion of the medical audit's total function.

The second major difference between the medical audit and utilization evaluation is in the *purpose.* The medical audit exists in today's hospitals as medicine's most potent weapon against professional obsolescence. It was introduced a number of years ago to reinforce the educational arm of medicine by which the fruits of research are transmitted to the clinician and translated into practice. It has been so designed and structured that it is a medical staff's best mechanism for keeping up to date, adopting the new, discarding the old, and making the best use of available resources whether they be hospital beds, tests, drugs, or personnel. As noted earlier, utilization evaluation has *its origin* in the effort to control use of facilities and resources.

METHODOLOGY

The educational nature of the medical audit is reflected in and enhanced by the methodology which has developed over the past several years, methodology which has not been generally adopted in utilization evaluation.

The medical audit is carried out by committees within the medical staff. Note that I have used the plural rather than referring to a single committee. It is quite true that in many institutions there is only one such committee, even as many hospitals have a single utilization committee. This approach has serious drawbacks.

Obviously, if there is a single medical audit committee, it must represent the various medical disciplines and specialties. It is equally obvious that there is work to be done. One of the advantages of rank in the medical staff is that tasks which may prove onerous can be delegated to juniors. The typical committee, then, is made up of younger members of the staff, one each from medicine, surgery, pediatrics, obstetrics, and other disciplines. When the committee faces the task of reviewing care, however, the surgical cases are placed in the lap of the young surgeon, the medical cases with the young internist, and so on; and we have a group of one-man junior subcommittees attempting to function. This produces an almost impossible situation and one which is not likely to be productive.

In contrast, a two- or three-man subcommittee on each of the major clinical services takes advantage of the existing departmental structure of the medical staff, giving each clinical chief a tool with which he can carry out his obligations for review and maintenance of the quality of care. Furthermore, this approach takes advantage of specialty training and interests, and a group is formed which can intelligently and productively discuss the topics falling within its jurisdiction. Not only is this process practical, but it is interesting. General practitioners as well as specialists participate because the goal is education, not judgment of the general practitioner by the specialist. The review is of practice, not of practitioners.

Departmental Audit Committee. Each committee regularly and systematically analyzes *all* of the work of its department in an orderly fashion. It starts with an overall view of the department and moves down to various clinical segments. This can be visualized as a progressive process which goes through two screening steps and is followed by the examination of selected individual case records:

1. First there is a *review of descriptive statistics* which shows the kinds of patients, their diagnosis, the operations performed, use of blood, length of stay, complications, consultations, death rates, and the like.

2. Then follows the *review of detailed statistics of groups of patients* to see if any specific aspects of care are not in accord with the committee's expectations as to what the best care would look like.

3. Finally there is the *examination of the individual cases* contributing to a statistical total which was found to be at variance with the standards expected.

Requisites for a Medical Audit

In this rapid description of the process by which *all* the care can be audited, certain vital requisites should be mentioned.

1. The hospital must provide *a medical record information system* which gives the essential statistical views by department. It must also give progressive detail so that each statistic may be converted into the case histories of individual patients. Such a system involves adequate original clinical records, the use of modern methods of tabulation, presentation and analysis of data, and skilled information retrieval personnel in the medical record department.

2. The second requisite is that *the medical staff be trained in the techniques of medical audit,* a process not taught in medical schools or in residencies. Yet here, as with every skill, there exists a body of technical knowledge which can make the task simpler, more efficient, and more effective. Training concerns two aspects: first, the development of criteria against which the care will be matched; and second, working with information in statistical and coded form in order to screen large numbers of cases rapidly for possible problem areas.

3. The medical staff organization must be streamlined. Such reorganization is now encouraged by the Joint Commission on Accreditation of Hospitals. Its Bulletin No. 40, issued in December, 1965, describes the required functions, leaving committee structure to the hospital. The Social Security Administration's pronouncements on utilization review under

Medicare are also consonant with this advice. A new pattern of medical staff organization is already being set by the gradual disappearance of separate tissue committees, transfusion committees, and other committees covering narrow areas of concern. These are being embraced within the more inclusive approach offered by the medical audit. Retrospective utilization evaluation will not call for an additional committee in the hospital which already has an active internal medical audit. The requirement for evaluation of this segment of medical care, patterns of utilization, is satisfied by the medical audit.

Examples of a Surgical Audit

In order to take this process from the general to the specific, let me describe one audit done by a surgery audit committee.

It is noted that 10 per cent of all patients, except newborns and deliveries, are admitted for *tonsillectomy and adenoidectomy* (T&A). This seems high to the committee, and they find that it is 40 per cent higher than the national average. The decision is made to look into tonsillectomy and adenoidectomy in detail.

A meeting is devoted to *setting up a list of criteria*. These are derived from the committee's own knowledge of what constitutes good practice, supplemented by a search of the current literature and consultation with specialists when doubt arises. The result is a statement something like this: If our T&A practice approaches excellence, we will find:

1. Very few patients below 2 or 3 years of age.
2. Few or no postoperative hemorrhages.
3. Few or no transfusions.
4. Prophylactic antibiotics used only for selected cases.
5. All patients had minimum laboratory work-up of urinalysis and CBC.
6. All patients had blood pressure taken.
7. History taken as to bleeding diathesis.
8. No patients operated while febrile.
9. Very few patients staying longer than the hospital's custom for T&A.
10. No deaths.

Other statements may be added. Note that some, but not all, of these aspects of care would be of concern in utilization evaluation.

This list is reviewed with the *retrieval specialist*, usually the medical record librarian, who is asked to provide the statistics with which the committee will decide if the care measures up to their standards of excellence.

Note that the statements also can initiate *the most fundamental level of investigation of patient care*. For example, the committee may want detail on each individual case operated while febrile. A long stay may be accounted for by a complication recorded only in the progress notes. And the case-by-case study will sometimes uncover further problems. Laboratory work may be most frequently missed on admissions on a particular day of the week because of hospital staffing patterns, or the wholesale use of prophylactic antibiotics may be the habit of only one or two surgeons.

Channels of Follow-up

The medical audit as an educational process does not end here. The *committee's findings* for each topic audited must be documented and summarized. The reports are then forwarded through medical staff channels where they can form the basis for staff education. When there is clear evidence that direct communication with an individual staff member is indicated, this is a task which must not be shirked by the department chief or executive committee. Finally, from the medical staff level, an accounting must be made to the governing board describing the method of audit used, giving specific findings in impersonal terms, and reporting actions which have resulted from the findings.

A NEW PATTERN OF MEDICAL STAFF ORGANIZATION

A new pattern of medical staff organization is being set by the gradual disappearance of separate tissue committees, transfusion committees, and other committees of narrow concern. These are being embraced within the more inclusive approach offered by the medical audit committees. Utilization evaluation will *not* call for an additional committee in the hospital which already has an active internal medical audit. The requirement for evaluation of this restricted segment of medical care—utilization—is satisfied by the medical audit.

SUMMARY

Clearly, the medical audit goes much further than utilization evaluation since it emphasizes the importance of insuring that *all* patients receive *all* that they need in contrast to merely curbing excessive use of facilities or services. The medical audit springs from medicine's own drive to insure for the next patient better care than was given to the last. The evaluation process itself is highly motivated, continuous education for the physicians on the committees, and the findings of the audits are springboards for the staff's formal and informal education programs.

BIBLIOGRAPHY

1. McClenahan, J. E.: Utilization Review under Medicare, *Hospitals, JAHA,* 39:55–58 (Sept. 1) 1965.

27

The Patient Care Committee

By Robert L. Hawley, M.D.

Robert L. Hawley is pathologist at Mercy Hospital in Denver, where he served as chairman of the hospital's Education Committee for many years and where he is now chairman of the Patient Care Committee. Dr. Hawley received the M.D. degree from the University of Colorado, where he is now assistant clinical professor of pathology. He is a diplomate of the American Board of Pathology.

The Guide Issue of *Hospitals, JAHA,* August 1, 1965, gives the following data for New Mercy Hospital: Beds, 250; Admissions, 10,929; Census, 217; Bassinets, 17; Births, 964; Newborn census, 13; Total expenses, $3,470,000; Payroll, $2,253,000.

The bedlam of Times Square is not a desirable atmosphere for the patient who is being prepared for surgery. During a recent study by a patient care committee, just such a frenetic scene was put together from the testimony of hospital personnel representing several departments. It was learned that technicians, orderlies, nurses, visitors, interns, and attending physicians frequently intersected each other in uncoordinated traffic in the patient's room on the evening before surgery. The apprehensive patient surrounded by a milling crowd is not infrequently found in hospitals everywhere, and this is but one example of the lack of coordination between departments caring for the patient in the modern hospital. The quality of care rendered to the patient by several individuals may be seriously compromised if it is not skillfully organized and coordinated, and the technical excellence of finest service may be impaired by multiple conflicts. A history and physical examination will be of lesser quality if it is interrupted by a harassed medical technologist, a surgical aide, or nursing personnel under pressure. It is an inferior blood count that is finally performed at 11:00 P.M. on the evening before surgery by the harried technologist who has made numerous trips to the patient's room only to find other hospital personnel with the patient each time. Such conflicts cause irritation and decrease the level of care the patient receives.

It requires but little imagination to visualize the patient's state of mind when he becomes aware of these conflicts or senses the lack of smooth coordination in his care. He may have just begun to receive intermittent positive pressure therapy, for example, when his lunch tray arrives or the orderly comes to take him to radiology. To the patient it appears that the left hand does not know what the right hand is doing. He may ask himself, "Are these the capable hands in which I have placed myself?" Already sensitized by his fear of oncoming events, he is acutely aware of any disquietude or confusion. While the outcome of his treatment is positively supported by smoothly coordinated and reassuring care, it is adversely affected by discernible conflicts and a hectic atmosphere.

In recent times, hospitals have grown in magnitude and complexity so rapidly that the patient may be dwarfed in the mind's eye of the hospital personnel. Increasingly complicated modes of diagnosis and treatment require a growing number of highly specialized technicians, who individually care for only a limited facet of the patient's problem. This has led to fragmentation of patient care, which in turn has led to depersonalization and dehumanization. Hence, we tend to treat the organ, or a part of the patient, but not him—certainly not all of him. It is not rare for the patient to overhear the x-ray technician say, "We'll take that chest on number 722 next and the skull on 932 after him." The complexity of each hospital employee's job discourages him from being primarily concerned with the total needs of the patient. The more complex the responsibility, the more concerned the physician or technician becomes over *his* technical responsibilities, the more absorbed in *his* problems, and the less preoccupied with the *patient's* welfare.

The concept of total service to the patient is difficult to obtain in the modern hospital. In lieu of one individual caring for all of the patient's needs, the many individuals charged with his care must be welded into a "wrap-around" care, simulating as nearly as possible the tender loving care by one person.

Whether or not there exists a need for the improvement in the care of the sick patient in one's own hospital, it is necessary to know just *what* care is rendered to him. In the modern hospital, we actually may not know what happens to a patient. Who in today's hospital really sees the total picture of the patient from the time he pushes open the front door until he finally awakens back in his room minus his appendix? It is necessary to fit together the successive events that befall the patient in his odyssey to health.

To obtain this *insight into the total picture* of the patient's experience, a study in depth is necessary. This can be accomplished in part by permitting each hospital department to learn what it is that every other department does to and for the patient. In this way, the various departments gain insight into the experience of a patient and at the same time discover conflicts that may have gone unrecognized.

THE PATIENT CARE COMMITTEE

To produce an educational experience of this type requires the assemblage of a pertinent group of department heads. The number should be small enough to encourage informality and relaxed discussion. This group, known as the patient care committee, should include the head of the nursing service, a staff physician, a representative of administration, the chief of radiology, the chief of pathology, and heads of the outpatient, dietary, and admission departments. Head nurses and other departmental heads may be invited to attend the meetings in turn to discuss aspects of their services to the patient. Formal organization is best kept at a minimum to encourage free discussion.

Strong department heads to whom the administration has delegated authority are the key to a successful patient care committee. Many interdepartmental problems may be solved rapidly and directly, without the need of going to the top and down again. The following example demonstrates how problems can be resolved by direct interdepartmental action.

It was learned that as many as 75 patients each morning were receiving a cold and unacceptable breakfast when nurses described this occurrence to the patient care committee. It was found that this was the result of poor coordination between the medical technologist who was obtaining fasting blood specimens and the dietary department which was delivering breakfast trays that had been held. The heads of the dietary, nursing, and pathology departments quickly solved this problem by coordinating departmental schedules. Numerous daily telephone calls between nurses and dietary personnel were eliminated, and many bothersome communications between technologists and nurses were decreased. Above all, patients who previously received cold bacon and eggs now receive a good hot breakfast. This happy solution also strengthened rapport between the departments.

Complete minutes of each committee meeting are kept, and a list of problems is maintained for follow-up. The major portion of time at each meeting is reserved for presentation by one department, and the remainder is used for discussion of any other current problems. It is rewarding to discover that many problems and conflicts can be resolved forthwith.

A necessary ingredient to this format is *placing the patient and his concerns above the prerogatives of any department head.* The sick individual's welfare is on the table, so to speak, in front of all the members of the patient care committee, and as his care is discussed, the consciousness of him pervades the atmosphere.

The Patient Relations Committee

The personal reaction of the patient to his hospital experience is a necessary adjunct to the presentations by head nurses and departmental heads. Many mechanisms may be used to determine these reactions. We have found an interviewing system to be one of the best approaches, and it is best accomplished by hospital personnel who are interested, sympathetic, and objective. The interviewers should wear lay apparel and should introduce themselves as *patient relations representatives.* Certain essential questions should be used, but the interview must be informal and must encourage the patient to pursue whatever subject he may care to discuss. This group of interviewers operates as the patient relations committee, and it reports regularly to the patient care committee. This source of information about patient care brings many problems to light, most of which can be remedied by interdepartmental action. Problems of a minor nature, such as the patient who continues to be served coffee despite repeated requests for tea, are taken care of by direct communication between the interviewer and the appropriate department head.

The Satellite Program

Another project, entitled the Satellite Program, has been launched from the patient care committee. On a year-round basis it is designed to encourage hospital staff at all levels to become involved in the patient's problems and to promote an atmosphere of general concern. In this program, small groups meet to discuss a particular patient and his problems during his hospitalization. Participants in the group are rotated for each meeting. Thus a nurse, x-ray technician, dietician, and admission clerk may meet to discuss a patient recently discharged from the hospital. The nurse describes the details of her care of the patient, the problems encountered, and his reactions. Each department representative in turn relates his services and the special aspects of his care. A staff physician or a house physician should also participate in the discussion. The objective of this program is to allow personnel at various levels in the hospital staff to understand patients' problems more fully and to gain a depth of insight into interdepartmental dynamics. Such group discussions have been found to lead to remarkable insight by hospital personnel, revealing to them how much more they could do for the patient—individually and as a team.

SUMMARY

Experience has shown that a remarkable number of patient care problems, large and small, can be solved or remedied by an objective patient care committee. Discussion at the level of department heads, interviews by patient relations representatives, and in-depth education for all hospital personnel through satellite groups—all are effective techniques. Vastly more important than merely remedying current problems is the progressively improved attitude of hospital personnel toward the human needs of the patient, surrounding him with an atmosphere of reassurance that speeds him back to health and productivity.

THE PATIENT CARE COUNCIL

(ED. NOTE: *The following paragraphs are reprinted from an article by William W. Jack, M.D., "Duties of the Chief of Staff" which was published in* Hospital Progress, *46:77–81, January 1965. This material was presented at the Chiefs of Staff Conference in Denver, October 22–24, 1964.*)

There is a group of committees whose essential interest lies within the area of patient care. These include the patient care committee itself, the infection control committee, the cancer and isotope committee, the pharmacy and therapeutics committee, the diet committee, the intensive care committee, the disaster committee, and now a committee on adverse effects and another on the use of blood transfusions.

This is a worrisome group. Each has an essential function, yet for some it is not a very large function. Each is independent, yet there is over-lap for some. Most of them need representation from administration and nursing, and this means that their recommendations must be spread three different ways. This troika authority can be confusing and frustrating, yet it is necessary. May I suggest a different way, and, in so doing, I wish I could assure you that this different way is practical and effective. Unfortunately, I cannot.

Nonetheless, my suggestion is this. Appoint one or at most two physicians instead of committees to be primarily interested in each of the functions that I have outlined above. Call it the council on patient care. Have it chaired by the vice-chief of staff. Have it include a senior member of administration, not the director; a senior nurse, not the director of nursing. Permit each member of this council to have his own advisory committee, or permit each member to appoint an ad hoc committee for specific projects. Channel the minutes and recommendations of the council to the meeting of the hospital director, of nursing, and chief of staff that I have already referred to. Permit this group to act upon these minutes and recommendations and effect implementation, if approved. This would not deny the director the opportunity of referring any questions to his staff or department heads. This would not deny further study by nursing. This would not deny reference to the staff executive committee if the chief so chose. I can visualize that this council would be most important and could obviate many of the difficulties that these committees have existing alone.

28

The Blood Transfusion Committee

By James J. Bergin, Lieut. Col., MC

Lieutenant Colonel James J. Bergin is assistant chief of the department of medicine of Fitzsimons General Hospital. He was formerly assistant chief of the hematology service at Walter Reed General Hospital; prior to that he was chief of the department of medicine of Rodriquez Army Hospital in San Juan, Puerto Rico. He has been closely associated with the activities of the transfusion committees in these hospitals.

Dr. Bergin received the B.S. and M.D. degrees from Tufts University and is certified by the American Board of Internal Medicine.

"The transfusion of blood when indicated is acknowledged to be life-prolonging therapy of the highest order. To know when to administer, and how much to administer, requires consummate clinical skill. To discuss when transfusion is unnecessary or contraindicated is equally imperative. The reasons against are as important as the justification for it." [1] This editorial comment from *The Journal of the American Medical Association* differs from the recommendation of the earliest pharmacopoeias when blood was favored for the amelioration of lunacy and palsy and for the rejuvenation of the geriatric patient. After Harvey's discovery of the circulation, transfusions of calves' blood into humans was recorded in 1667 in the *Philosophical Proceedings of the Royal Society*.[2]

The centuries passed, and the transfusion of blood was alternately condemned and acclaimed. It was not until the last few decades that the remarkable scientific advances in blood procurement, processing, distribution, and administration have resulted in the ready and needed accessibility of blood. However, availability tempts the nondiscerning user and may catalyze excessive and inappropriate administration of blood.

The issue at hand lies in the answers to the following questions: (1) Is there sufficient knowledge regarding the positive indications for blood transfusion? (2) Is there awareness of the hazards involved? (3) Is there full cognizance of the legal implications? (4) Is there an appropriate response to adverse transfusion reactions? If the answers to these questions are negative, there is a need for supervision and leadership which may readily be supplied at the local hospital level by a blood transfusion committee.

Concern of several national organizations and supervisory bodies about the practices of blood transfusion is reflected in their recommendations. In March of 1961, the Joint Commission on Accreditation of Hospitals remarked on the importance of an educational program to review blood transfusion practices.[3] In October of 1961, the Joint Blood Council recommended a study of the use of blood in all phases of the medical services.[4] In the same year, a committee on transfusion problems of the National Academy of Sciences and the National Research Council began to compile the authoritative book, *General Principles of Blood Transfusion*.[23] In the Department of the Army Technical Bulletin, *The Surgeon General*, the importance and function of a hospital transfusion board were stressed.[5] Let us explore some of the considerations leading to these recommendations.

TRANSFUSION RISK

It has been estimated that between 3,500,000 and 5,000,000 units of blood are administered annually in the United States.[6,7] The number of untoward reactions can readily be determined by considering that the transfusion reaction rate is consistently 3 to 4 per cent. The majority of the 100,000 or more transfusion complications are not mortal; however, of

TABLE 28-1. Immediate Reactions

Type	Manifestation	Cause
Allergic	Urticaria, asthma	Donor antigen
Pyrogenic	Fever, chills, headache	Protein, bacterial pyrogen, leuko-agglutinin
Hemolytic	Chills, fever, myalgia, anuria, shock, death, bleeding	Antigen-antibody reaction, hemolyzed blood
Circulatory overload	Pulmonary edema	Over-transfusion
Toxic	Fever, shock, hemolysis	Bacterial endotoxin
Citrate intoxication	Tetany, cardiac arrhythmia	Hypocalcemia
Potassium intoxication	Paralysis, cardiac arrhythmia	Aged blood
Coagulation defect	Bleeding	Dilution of coagulation factors, fibrinolysis
Air embolism	Dyspnea, death	Air administered

this remarkable number, about 3,000 people die each year.[8] Thus, the risk of infusing a unit of blood is equivalent to that of an appendectomy. How many physicians deliberate at length before recommending an appendectomy, but ponder only briefly before a blood transfusion? The immediate transfusion problems are categorized in Table 28-1. Details of these complications are readily available in the current literature and will not be discussed here.

Other problems may confront the unwary, and delayed reactions supervene after an apparently successful completion of the transfusion.

TABLE 28-2. Delayed Reactions

Hepatitis	Serum sickness
Malaria	Hemosiderosis
Syphilis	Isoagglutination

The incidence of recognized *homologous serum hepatitis* varies from 0.3 to 1.0 per cent of all individuals receiving blood. One of every 200 transfusions is involved.[9] Data from the University of Chicago tabulated the risk of serum hepatitis to be 1.06 per cent from one unit of blood; 2.78 per cent from two units; and 4.82 per cent from five units. The mortality from the disease was 10 per cent.[10] The total number of patients concerned at a national level is sobering.

Since all blood administered is compatible but not identical blood, the danger of *isoagglutinin formation* is apparent; but the subsequent impact on the population cannot be estimated or measured. The other delayed reactions are self-explanatory.

Transfusion reactions occur even in the framework of excellent blood banking. The *reaction rate* has not been lessened during the last decade, so the total number of adverse reactions is proportional to the number of units of blood given. If technique remains stable, then reduction in the amount of blood administered is followed by a decrease in complications. Until there is improved technology, this circumstance will prevail.

THE LEGAL ISSUE

It is appropriate to consider the legal issue. The guilt of negligence rests upon an action taken counter to that which a reasonable and prudent physician would do in the same circumstances. It is well known that action has been taken by the recipient for negligence in the administration of blood. However, Cantor has stated, "It would only seem to normally follow that a person would be liable for damages following and caused by a transfusion that was not indicated by the facts of the case. Even if no negligence could be proved in the collecting, storage, testing, and administration of blood, an action for damages would lie if the plaintiff could prove that the transfusion was not indicated medically." [11] As with other therapeutic endeavors, careful planning must precede the decision to transfuse. Historically, the pathologist in charge of the blood bank has borne this legal burden. However, the judgment of the user also has been defined as subject to legal challenge.

INDICATIONS FOR BLOOD TRANSFUSION

Exchange transfusions excepted, there are two valid indications for the transfusion of blood, according to Crosby: "(1) to improve the stability of the circulatory system when the blood volume has been reduced in such a way as to imperil the patient; (2) to improve the oxygen-carrying capacity of the blood to prevent acute hypoxia or invalidism." [12] Other reasons are less cogent. Consider these indications for transfusion: (1) to provide a tonic; (2) to promote healing; (3) to combat infection; (4) to supply a source of iron; (5) to reverse the trend of a difficult case; and (6) to attain a preoperative hemoglobin level required by an anesthesiologist.

The first three reasons have no basis in scientific fact. Regarding the question of iron, the amount of iron available in a unit of blood is meager compared to that in the readily administered pharmaceutical preparations. The anesthesiologist's requirement demands further consideration. The normal hemoglobin level needed for full physical effort is in excess of the requirement for sedentary activity. Chronically anemic patients and immobilized patients may be asymptomatic at the 6 Gm per 100 ml level. The anesthetized patient is better compared to the bedridden than to the competing athlete, and the needed hemoglobin level is better viewed in this setting. In blood dilution experiments, the oxygen-carrying capacity of blood is not impaired if blood volume is maintained until the hemoglobin level is less than 7 Gm per 100 ml. Higher levels act merely as a reserve and not as a necessity.[12] I am not advocating a lesser number to replace the rigid, anesthetic requirement of 10 Gm, merely a critical analysis of the specific blood replacement requirement in the context of the individual patient. Finally, the hemoglobin result may be in error. Restandardization of instruments resulted in 50 per cent reduction in daily transfusion in one hospital. This amounted to 1,000 transfusions a year,[13] again a reflection of arbitrary blood replacement as contrasted with clinical need.

MONITORING TRANSFUSION PRACTICE

In 1953, the medical staff of Providence Hospital, Washington, D.C., instituted a program of physician education regarding the hazards of blood transfusions and adopted specific indications for blood transfusions to establish uniform criteria for ordering blood replacement. Their results were compiled and analyzed according to the "use factor" proposed by Crosby, which is determined by dividing the units of blood transfused by the number of patients hospitalized.[12] The data obtained by McCoy[14] deserve careful analysis and are depicted in Table 28-3.

TABLE 28-3. Analysis of Blood Transfusion Statistics at Providence Hospital, Washington, D. C.

Year	Hospital Patients	Units of Blood Used	Use Factor
1953	12,786	3,024	0.237
1954	12,500	2,390	0.194
1955	12,866	2,229	0.173
1956	15,011	1,950	0.131
1957	19,817	2,353	0.119
1958	20,535	2,438	0.119
1959	20,907	2,505	0.120
1960	21,045	2,317	0.110

It can be seen that in spite of an increasing patient population the total number of units of blood administered decreased, and there was a dramatic reduction in the *use factor.* The author states that in no instance was a patient denied needed blood.

The experience of a small, nonteaching community hospital was described by Walz.[15] (ED. NOTE: *Mercy Hospital in Mount Vernon, Ohio, has 140 beds and had 6,849 admissions in 1964, according to the Guide Issue,* Hospitals, JAHA, *Aug. 1, 1965.*) A transfusion committee was established and charged with the responsibility of education, delineation of acceptable uses of blood, and monitoring of all administered transfusions as to justification. The results were compiled as shown in Table 28-4.

TABLE 28-4. Analysis of Blood Transfusion Statistics at Mercy Hospital, Mount Vernon, Ohio

Year	Hospital Patients	Units of Blood Used	Use Factor
1958	5,007	894	0.180
1959	5,427	881	0.160
1960	5,850	976	0.165
1961*	6,176	709	0.114
1962	6,954	629	0.090
1963	7,052	479	0.070

* Transfusion committee organized in May, 1961.

The experience in this hospital is comparable to that of the Providence Hospital in Washington, D.C. During a three-year period, the amount of blood used decreased by one-third although hospital admissions increased, and the "use factor" was halved. The greatest reduction in blood use was in the surgical and obstetrical services.

The decline in blood utilization as reflected in the "use factor" has been experienced throughout the country wherever transfusion committees have promulgated physician education and carefully monitored transfusion practices.[1]

THE ONE–UNIT TRANSFUSION

The one-unit transfusion has come under the particular scrutiny of transfusion committees. The incidence of its employment has been well documented. Allen et al.[16] reported a 37 per cent incidence in Chicago. Morton from the University of Rochester noted a 44 per cent incidence which dropped to 36 per cent during the four-month period when an investigation of blood transfusion practice was carried out.[17] From the Cleveland Clinic, King remarked on a 30 per cent incidence.[18] From Ann Arbor, Michigan, Diethrich[19] also reported 30 per cent. There is common agreement that from 40 to 70 per cent of all single-unit transfusions are unjustified. Powell reported a level of 80 per cent unjustified single-unit transfusions, dropping to 52 per cent as the practice of this therapeutic modality was scrutinized.[20] An interesting observation was made by Walz[15] who noted a rise in single-unit transfusions from 18 per cent in 1961 to 29 per cent in 1963 as the "use factor" dropped from 0.114 to 0.070.

The use of the single-unit transfusion often clearly reflects the ability of the physician. As Crosby states, "Sometimes it demonstrates an unusual skill in the use of transfusion as a therapeutic tool. At other times it is an act of thoughtlessness or incompetence." [21] Consider the patient referred for hemorrhoidectomy for the purpose of extirpating the site of blood loss which was causing a severe iron deficiency. Appropriate specific iron replacement had raised the hemoglobin from 3 to 9.8 Gm per 100 ml during the three weeks prior to surgery, but, at the insistence of the anesthesiologist, the surgeon reluctantly gave 500 cc of blood so that the magic number of 10 Gm of hemoglobin could permit anesthesia to be given. It is needless to comment on the defects in this type of inflexible thinking. MacDonald has remarked that a patient with a hemoglobin of 11 Gm would be safer *donating* a pint of blood preoperatively than receiving one.[22]

Justified One-unit Transfusions. The patient with an acquired hemolytic anemia who receives one unit of blood every five days is an example of valid usage. The surgeon, inserting an aortic graft, notes a brisk loss of blood with an otherwise unexplained change in vital signs. He orders a unit of blood infused concomitant to control of the bleeding site, and subsequent physiologic homeostasis follows. Such a surgeon is to be complimented for his therapeutic capability. An additional transfusion would only double the transfusion reaction risk. Thus, there is an essential place in medicine for the single-unit transfusion. Monitoring this aspect of medical care sharply reduces the unwarranted practice. The effect is one of increasing the incidence but obviating the tragedy of death due to a needless transfusion. As Crosby stated, "There is some concern lest shotgun condemnation of the single unit transfusion impede the wise physician or pervert the foolish." [21]

THE NEED FOR A BLOOD TRANSFUSION COMMITTEE

The blood transfusion committee acts in an advisory capacity, usually working as a subcommittee under a medical audit committee. In military hospitals, the blood transfusion subcommittee reports to the medical audit committee, which in turn reports to the commanding officer. It occupies a comparable position to the tissue committee. Similar areas of administrative responsibility exist in the civilian hospital structure.

The Composition of the Committee. The composition varies with the needs of the hospital. It is recommended that the committee represent the specialties of pathology, medicine, obstetrics, surgery, and anesthesiology.

The pathologist who directs the blood bank, investigates transfusion reactions, and supervises hemoglobinometry often serves as the chairman. Ideally the representative from medicine is a hematologist and consults on complicated hematologic problems. The members from obstetrics and surgery are well acquainted with the problems inherent in hemorrhagic emergencies and operative management, and they represent the users of 80 to 90 per cent of all blood transfused in the hospital. The direct and intimate guidance they exert with their colleagues is invaluable to the functioning of the committee. Generally speaking, the anesthesiologist applies more numerical demands on quantitative hemoglobin levels than his confreres, and blood replacement often follows his dictates. He is more amenable to monitoring by working within the committee structure than without, and he is an essential contributor to the success of the committee.

The Functions of the Committee. The functions are as follows: (1) education in the vagaries of blood transfusion therapy; (2) constant vigilance of applicable laboratory procedures, such as hemoglobinometry, cross-matching, and blood processing; (3) investigation of transfusion reactions; (4) setting standards for blood replacement; and (5) review of records for indications of transfusion and proper recording of transfusion reactions. Particular attention is directed to records of transfusion reactions, of single-unit transfusions, and of more-than-three-unit replacements. The demands of the hospital dictate the extent and depth of the review, but the above would serve as a guide as to the minimum duties.

The failure to diagnose accurately and to treat effectively a patient who has had a transfusion reaction has special medicolegal import. All hospitals and laboratory supervisors appreciate the difficulty in obtaining precise clinical information and laboratory measurement in a suspected transfusion reaction. Diethrich[19] noted that although the procedure to be followed for a possible reaction was readily available to all physicians and on every hospital ward, 20 per cent of blood transfusion reactions were not even reported to the blood bank. The legal implications are obvious. This deficit of action and recording quickly lessens under the dynamic monitoring, education, and consultation of the committee.

SUMMARY

The mere presence of a blood transfusion committee is beneficial, and the reporting of data on a monthly basis to the hospital staff generates improved transfusion practices. The vast majority of physicians react constructively to the leadership offered.

Experience has shown that appropriate committee action is followed by a reduction in the total number of tranfusions administered, and the number of transfusion reactions necessarily parallels this change. Committee action also fosters prompt recognition, thorough evaluation, complete recording, and appropriate therapy of transfusion reactions.

DISCUSSION

(ED. NOTE: *The following is an edited transcript from the Discussion Seminar on the Transfusion Committee led by Dr. Bergin at The Hospital Medical Staff Conference held in Estes Park, Colorado, October 11–13, 1965. It is appended to amplify some of the material presented in his chapter.*)

Pathologist: I believe the risk of serum hepatitis is less if one draws blood from the upper-class population.

Comment: There have been contradictory data regarding the incidence of hepatitis from the upper-, middle-, and lower-class population. However, one thing can be said: the risk of hepatitis cannot be eliminated as long as blood which is less than six months old is used. Of course, we are discussing the use of whole blood, and, therefore, the risk of serum hepatitis is always present.

Anesthesiologist: You made the comment that the anesthesiologist is the one who makes the greatest numerical requirement for level of hemoglobin before surgery. In my hospital, it is just the reverse. My greatest difficulty is in stopping surgeons from using blood when the hemoglobin is below 10 Gm per 100 ml.

Comment: This is a very refreshing attitude.

Pathologist: In my hospital, the biggest problem is the general practitioner, internist, or pediatrician who gives a unit of blood to a patient who is chronically anemic but asymptomatic. I am thinking of patients with terminal cancer or uremia—sometimes, they give two units. It would be very difficult to pick them up by surveying records.

Comment: The most important means of stopping this practice is by education of the medical staff on a recurrent monthly basis. Present sample cases and discuss the problem in general terms. Eventually, the total physician population will become aware of the inappropriateness of transfusing a chronically anemic but asymtomatic patient. Second, the transfusion committee will periodically review charts of patients with various diagnoses such as cancer or uremia, and then it is easy to detect this practice.

Pathologist: You have described a decline in the "use factor" in two hospitals. I am always suspicious of this kind of data because a new team of doctors who use more blood, such as thoracic surgeons, could be added to the staff, or a team could move to another hospital and less blood would be used.

Comment: These data were analyzed in this regard, and there was no essential change in the patient population or the doctor population in the institutions concerned.

Pathologist: If the bylaws of the hospital specify which patients should be transfused, how is the problem of the transfusion of asymptomatic, chronically anemic patients controlled?

Comment: Again, by the education of the medical staff and by the review of charts. However, physicians who transgress recurrently are invited to come before the committee. The committee is never punitive because it has no authority. It gathers and forwards data to an executive committee wherein lies the authority to do something about privileges, etc. However, it is salutary for the doctor to come before the committee and he is always warned in regard to the specific problem at least a week ahead of the meeting. When he comes, he usually answers in one of three ways. He may acknowledge an obvious error, and this is personal education of the highest order. He may supply data that are not in the chart and clearly justify the transfusion. In this case the physician is guilty of poor recording, and again he is educated. Or he may decide to buck the system. In this case the committee merely forwards the data to the executive committee. But it should not end there. The case should be brought to the medical staff to exploit this opportunity for education.

Pathologist: Are there any recommedations about a physician justifying the use of blood before it is given?

Comment: Yes, this is one of the areas to be implemented in the immediate future. The request for blood will be subject to audit in a manner quite similar to that of the tissue committee with its preoperative, postoperative, and tissue diagnoses. Even more important, especially in smaller hospitals, information will be given to the pathologist which will help him place an order of priority on the blood to be administered.

Pathologist: I have the nurses do the immediate investigation of transfusion reactions because the doctors are almost never in the hospital at the time it happens. They are in their car going to another case which may be 60 miles away.

Comment: I believe the physician should be in attendance for a blood transfusion, at least for the first 15 minutes. The majority of hemolytic transfusion reactions will become apparent by that time.

Pathologist: That is all right if you have an intramural staff, but we do not.

Internist: In our hospital, the staff is entirely extramural, and we do not have resident physicians. It is mandatory according to the bylaws of the hospital for the physician to be present at the time the transfusion is started and for 15 or 20 minutes afterwards.

Comment: Legally, I see no alternative to this practice.

Internist: It is unfortunate that the clinicians involved in giving transfusions cannot be here for this discussion. The greatest interest is always shown by those who are already fully aware of the problem and have to deal with it on a daily basis.

BIBLIOGRAPHY

1. The Transfusion of Blood, *JAMA*, 189:690 (Aug. 31) 1964.

2. Cannan, R. K.: Foreword in "General Principles of Bood Transfusion," National Academy of Sciences, J. B. Lippincott Company, Philadelphia, 1963.

3. Blood Transfusion Services, *Bull. Joint Commission Accreditation Hospitals*, No. 26 (Mar.) 1961.

4. Joint Blood Council Transfusion Review Program, *JAMA*, 180:230 (Apr. 21) 1962.

5. General Principles of Blood Transfusion, Department of the Army Technical Bulletin 8–15, *Office Surgeon General*, (1 Oct.) 1963.

6. Pirofsky, B.: The Use and Abuse of Blood Transfusion and Blood Derivatives, *GP*, 22:127–137 (Sept.) 1960.

7. Santer, D. G.: The Use and Abuse of Blood, *Am. Assoc. Blood Banks Bull.*, 12:7–11 (Jan.) 1959.

8. Hirsh, B. D.: Responsibilities in Blood Transfusion, *Medicolegal Digest*, 1:21–26 (Jan.) 1959.

9. DeGowin, E. L.: Transfusion Reactions, *Med. Sci.*, 6:99–114 (July 25) 1959.

10. Sayman, W. A., Gauld, R. L., Star, S. A., and Allen, J. G.: Safety of Liquid Plasma—A Statistical Appraisal, *JAMA*, 168:1735–1739 (Nov. 29) 1958.

11. Cantor, P. D.: A Legal Look at Blood Transfusions, *GP*, 16:82–84 (Aug.) 1957.

12. Crosby, W. H.: Misuse of Blood Transfusion, *Blood*, 13:1198–1200 (Dec.) 1958.

13. Waid, M. E., and Hoffman, R. G.: The Quality Control of Laboratory Precision, *Am. J. Clin. Path.*, 25:585–594 (May) 1955.

14. McCoy, K. L.: The Providence Hospital Blood Conservation Program, *Transfusion*, 2:3–6 (Jan.–Feb.) 1962.

15. Walz, D. V.: An Effective Hospital Transfusion Committee, *JAMA*, 189:660–662 (Aug. 31) 1964.

16. Allen, J. G. *et al.*: Blood Transfusions and Serum Hepatitis: Use of Monochloroacetate as Antibacterial Agent in Plasma, *Ann. Surg.*, 150:455–468 (Sept.) 1959.

17. Morton, J. H.: An Evaluation of Blood Transfusion Practices on a Surgical Service, *New England J. Med.*, 263:1285–1287 (Dec. 22) 1960.

18. King, J. W., and Senhauser, D. O.: Trends in Blood Utilization, *Transfusion*, 2:344–348 (Sept.–Oct.) 1962.

19. Diethrich, E. B.: Evaluation of Blood Transfusion Therapy, *Transfusion*, 5:82–88 (Jan.–Feb.) 1965.

20. Powell, N. A., and Johnston, D. G.: Criteria for Blood Transfusion, *Calif. Med.*, 97:12–15 (July) 1962.

21. Crosby, W. H.: Editorial Review: The Single Unit Transfusion, *Transfusion*, 4:329–330 (Sept.–Oct.) 1964.

22. MacDonald, I.: Editorial, *Bulletin, L.A. Co. Med. Assn.*, 91:57–58 (Mar. 16) 1961.

23. National Academy of Sciences, "General Principles of Blood Transfusion," J. B. Lippincott Company, Philadelphia, 1963.

Part IV

Perplexing Situations for the Medical Staff

29

Special Problems of Large Hospitals

By Donald C. Carner and Ronald D. Yaw

Donald C. Carner is the executive vice president of the Memorial Hospital of Long Beach, California. He received the A.B. and M.B.A. degrees from the University of Chicago, and he serves as a preceptor for their graduate program in hospital administration. He is active in hospital consulting and committees and boards of many national organizations. He has contributed to the hospital literature frequently, and he also writes articles on hospital affairs for lay magazines.

The Guide Issue of *Hospitals, JAHA*, August 1, 1965, gives the following data on the Memorial Hospital of Long Beach: Beds, 444; Admissions, 20,481; Census, 359; Bassinets, 46; Births, 2,539; Newborn census, 30; Total expenses, $7,660,000; Payroll, $4,716,000; Personnel, 869. There are three other voluntary non-profit, short-term general hospitals in Long Beach. The capacities of these are 188, 239, and 349 beds.

Ronald D. Yaw is the executive vice president of the Blodgett Memorial Hospital in Grand Rapids, Michigan, a post he has held for many years. He is the immediate past president of the American College of Hospital Administrators and a past president of the Michigan Hospital Association.

The Guide Issue of *Hospitals, JAHA*, August 1, 1965, gives the following data on Blodgett Memorial Hospital: Beds, 420; Admissions 16,-251; Census, 330; Bassinets, 66; Births, 2,475;

Newborn census, 35; Total expenses, $5,721,-000; Payroll, $3,597,000; Personnel, 988. There are two other general short-term hospitals in Grand Rapids, Butterworth Hospital with 467 beds and St. Mary's Hospital with 370 beds. The population of Grand Rapids in the 1960 census was 202,379.

In August of 1965, the chief administrative officers of 24 hospitals, ranging in size from 275 to 800 beds and located across the nation, were asked to outline the two biggest problems their respective hospitals faced. The problems mentioned most frequently were:

1. Communication.
2. Need for better management.
3. Need for leadership within the staff.
4. Pressure of outside forces.
5. Outpatient services.
6. Need for more full-time physicians.
7. Financial factors.
8. Better coordination within communities to achieve more effective use of facilities and manpower.
9. Current unrealistic government attitude toward cost reimbursement.
10. Comparison of cost in high-quality large institutions with low-quality small hospitals.

Each problem is defined and considered in the following 10 sections. (ED. NOTE: *Mr. Carner is responsible for the first five sections and Mr. Yaw for the second five.*)

COMMUNICATION

Perhaps a brief review of the reasons why communication within the hospital is difficult will give us an understanding of the reason many hospitals list this as a major problem.

The hospital is a complex organization subject to many diverse forces. Everyone connected with the hospital has his own special interests, and they often pull in divergent directions. Some physicians see the hospital as an adjunct to their practice and an extension of their office; others visualize the hospital as a threat to the private practice of medicine. The vendor sees the hospital as a source of income and profit. The fire marshal looks upon the hospital as a hazard with potential danger to hundreds of lives. Health insurance companies see hospitals eating up their premium income. The Internal Revenue Service wonders if the not-for-profit corporation is really that and whether it should really be tax free. Employees look to the hospital as a source of livelihood. To students, the hospital is a source of clinical material. Volunteers work at the hospital to gain the satisfaction of helping others. Unions would like to capture workers as dues-paying members. Patients seek to regain their health. Visitors discharge long-standing social obligations. Research workers look for answers to their problems.

The ultimate objectives of the hospital have long been considered to be patient care, education, and research. However, patient care and research can easily work at cross purposes, as can patient care and education. Even education and research can run counter to one another. Furthermore, none of these objectives is clearly measurable, in contrast to the goal of a profit-seeking organization. General Motors, for example, is a relatively simple organization which can readily determine whether a unit of its organization is profitable and worth retaining. Is it possible to determine whether a patient recovered as rapidly and completely as he could, or whether a student really learned all he should, or whether a research project was fully productive? Even the question of whether a hospital employee is proficient is difficult to measure, but a worker at General Motors either meets set job standards or he is not proficient. Further, General Motors has no one comparable to the physician in his level of interest, his responsibility as agent in directing the expenditure of patient-customer funds, his almost unquestioned authority to issue orders directing employees, and yet with no direct responsibility to "management."

How can communications be really effective in an organization such as the large hospital that involves so many different groups of people with diverse interests and goals, none of which are easily expressed, completely understood, or readily measured?

NEED FOR BETTER MANAGEMENT

Why is better management needed? It may be helpful to draw again a comparison with a large profit-seeking corporation. General Motors has developed one of the most competent management teams in the world, and this is the primary reason for the company's success. Keep in mind, that the term being used is "management," not "administration." The direction of the affairs of the medical staff is included in management. The chief of staff may practice medicine at the patient's bedside, but at the executive committee he is practicing management.

Management in the hospital must be especially skillful because it must lead by persuasion rather than by exercise of authority as at General Motors. It is *not* suggested that hospital employees manage the staff physicians. Hospital administrators have their own problems with which to cope; contrary to what some might believe, hospital administrators do not want to have their hospitals take over the practice of medicine. Any thinking hospital official realizes that to be effective the physician must preserve his individuality and his independence. Each patient presents an individual set of problems, and the solution can only be determined on an individual basis by an individual physician thinking independent thoughts. I certainly do not want my physician to diagnose my problems and to prescribe therapy on a group basis by using page 297 of the procedure manual. We are constantly striving to have hospital employees develop the depth of personal interest and individual identification that is so characteristic of the physician.

Strong, competent management *is* essential in the modern hospital. But some physicians are fearful of strong, competent management. Although they want all the benefits, they are fearful that management will want to take over medicine; hence, they may try to circumscribe management and retain the maximum degree of control of the hospital. Think what happens without effective management. The plant and equipment become obsolete in spite of the fact that physicians demand the costly new tools that are pouring out of research laboratories. Patients of physicians must be hospitalized; but they are frustrated in their desire for a safe, comfortable environment, for excellent nursing, air conditioning, electrically operated beds, television, good food, and clean rooms. With poor management, personnel become sloppy and lax; physician's orders are not carried out; errors mount; costs rise; newspapers criticize; grand juries investigate.

Today a hospital may employ people in as many as 145 different job skills. Turnover is very high in many job categories; in some, half the work force is replaced each year. This calls for recruiting, screening, testing, checking references (25 per cent of the male applicants have police records), orienting, training, and supervising. Most employees need supervision to do the job the way it must be done when lives are in the balance. The days of dedicated, religiously motivated workers are over.

Hospitals must stock as many as 10,000 different items. These must be purchased, at the best price, stored, distributed, accounted for, charged to the appropriate cost account, and paid for. Ultimately, there is income from many thousands of patients and hundreds of insurance carriers. It is not unusual for a large hospital to work with 10 million dollars each year. This money must be safeguarded, accounted for, invested, and disbursed. Buildings must be anticipated and designed; specifications must be developed; contracts awarded; construction carried out. If you have recently built a home or an office and struggled with the architect, building codes, inspectors, suppliers, and unions, you have a first-hand feeling for the problems connected with hospital expansion.

There was a day when a cigar box was actually used to transact hospital business. They put the money in and took the money out, and if they ran short, a philanthropist made up the difference. Now computers are essential to keep track of the fiscal and business matters; while full-time fund-development officers work to secure bequests, life income, and annuity gifts. Appraisers, actuaries, CPA's, tax men, and attorneys are called in as needed.

Research, which is now common in large hospitals, requires coordination and financing. Teaching grows more complex by the year, involving not only the program content, faculty, recruiting, and affiliations, but also apartments, playgrounds, large stipends, service beds, and expansion of outpatient clinics. Direction of a full-fledged program in medical education requires first-class management by physicians.

Negotiations with various levels of government recur constantly, and the "beginning has just begun," as the fellow said. To make the day more interesting, there may be a law suit filed.

Attention to these daily details is essential, but highly important is the need for hospital management to plan ahead, to anticipate problems, and to have an effective solution on hand before a crisis develops.

Where do you find qualified management people, and how do you pull them into the hospital field or into medical staff management? How do you keep them if they are good and yet keep them from appearing as a threat to the medical staff?

Do you have an answer? Consider this. If medicine and hospitals are "one" as seen by the courts and the public and the government, why do we not recognize this development and revise the hospital corporation structure to accommodate the change? Representatives of the medical staff and management should be brought into the governing board as full-fledged voting members, yet a majority of civic leaders should be retained to assure that the public interest is paramount. Would this not strengthen the board by emphasis upon (1) motivation, (2) expertise, and (3) responsibility?•

NEED FOR LEADERSHIP WITHIN THE STAFF

The majority of all medical staffs need better leadership. Why? All elements of the hospital are growing in size and strength and organization. Unless the medical staff keeps pace, the other elements will outdistance them, not because of a particular desire to do so but because of a void in medical leadership. To illustrate, compare staff leadership with that of the governing board. The governing board usually has a high proportion of successful businessmen skilled in leadership. The turnover of board members takes place at a very slow rate. Now look at the contrast with the medical staff. The chief is usually elected by the staff, then officially appointed to office for a year or possibly two. In only a small number of hospitals is the period significantly longer. Seldom does this leadership compare favorably to that of the governing board. What about administrators? Many are the product of years of learning, testing, and hard experience as they rise to top level management positions. Not only do they have training and experience but also the time to carry out the job.

The process most staffs use to select their leaders places the chief of staff at a very serious disadvantage and does not help the hospital either. Every competent administrator would prefer to work alongside top quality, consistent medical staff leadership with a physician heading a strong, cohesive, aggressive staff, rather than see a series of very good doctors with insufficient leadership experience and little time thrust into a position in which they must cope with a multitude of hospital problems and keep up their practice at the same time.

What is the outcome in this rather typical situation? The chief of staff is placed in a poor position in the power structure, and he spends most of his time in a defensive capacity trying to protect the medical staff from a gradual erosion of the doctor's position. Often he is limited to fighting a rearguard action, and he may have a great deal of difficulty in marshaling the strength and support essential to achieve constructive and positive new objectives. This may be why many medical staffs are organizationally proficient at blocking action and poor in terms of forward progress.

Medicine is beginning to recognize that the chief of staff is a *key* figure. Heretofore, the channel of communication was usually restricted to national, state, and county medical association leaders. Today, more and more matters are flowing directly to the attention of the chief of staff.

How can we get physicians to accept the fact that to have effective staff leadership, they must be willing to stop the annual game of musical chairs. They must be willing to place strong leaders in the position of chief of staff and keep them there long enough for them to become truly proficient.

Someone must have found an answer to the dilemma of how to attract strong, ethical, competent physicians and make it possible for them to function long enough to give the staff the quality of representation and leadership so sorely needed today. At the same time, it is essential to keep out of office the cheap medical politician who would use the power to his personal advantage.

PRESSURE OF OUTSIDE FORCES

Because the so-called health market has become a 30 billion dollar business, doctors and hospitals are subjected to a constant stream of slanted information from many national, state, regional, and county organizations. Much of the information that flows into your office and into mine and that reaches the employees may be generated by people who are engaged in one dispute or another at a national level and who are determined to direct people in a particular way. Some of it may serve a useful purpose, but most of it is self-serving. The current drive by labor leaders to unionize hospital workers is an example. If they could pick up annual dues of $50 from 2 million hospital workers, this would add up to quite a tidy sum per year. The insurance industry is very concerned about utilization committees, in an effort to protect their premium income and profits. Hospital and medical organizations are not above sending inflammatory letters couched in emotional terms. Because the letters are written by people who are deeply concerned with a problem, even though *they* see it on a somewhat remote level, they are not likely to weigh the concern and the new problems which may be created in local communities where none existed but where the potential for misunderstanding is always present. For example, there is the recent hot dispute between the American Medical Association and the American Hospital Association regarding the question of whether contract specialists belong to one sector or another of the Medicare legislation. I recall receiving temper-stirring letters from both organizations for no useful purpose. I find it difficult to think that contractual doctor-hospital arrangements, worked out over a period of time and tested through years of experience, are suddenly going to be tossed aside because of a political struggle between two great organizations.

But how should we cope with the flow of propaganda which, if followed, would split doctors and hospitals, hospitals and employees, patients and doctors, and destroy the time-honored relationships that seem to be doing the job quite well?

OUTPATIENT SERVICES

The remarkable increase in the use of hospital emergency rooms and outpatient services is well documented. The emergency room question is discussed in another chapter; here we shall discuss the expanding demand for hospital outpatient services. It is not unusual to see large hospitals which offer not only outpatient laboratory and x-ray facilities but also isotope service, therapeutic x-ray, physical therapy, occupational therapy, speech therapy, and other diagnostic and therapeutic services which individually compete with private practitioners. These are usually outpatient units that offer service which the physician himself does not want to provide but which some of his patients must have.

How can hospitals meet the doctor's need for highly specialized, supplementary diagnostic and therapeutic service without getting into the realm of competition with the medical staff?

NEED FOR MORE FULL-TIME PHYSICIANS

Several years ago, Beetle Bailey was discussing the food in the unit mess hall. "It's so terrible no one can eat it and besides, the servings are too small." This has a familiar sound. From some medical circles we seem to hear, "We must put a stop to the increasing trend towards salaried physicians in hospitals, but why can't we have more of them." Some of the reasons for the increasing use of physicians on a salary basis are obvious; others are less so.

One reason is the expensive, rapidly obsolescing equipment which must be concentrated in one place with the inevitable tendency to similarly concentrate the highly specialized medical personnel. X-ray and laboratory services are examples.

Another reason is the scarcity of paramedical personnel who are too few to scatter throughout the community. Medical technologists, physical therapists, occupational therapist—these scarce people and the equally scarce physician supervisors tend to clump around hospitals.

A little understood reason is that medicine develops needs before the public develops the understanding and the willingness to pay. Physiologists, research workers, hematologists, endocrinologists—these are but a few who, from a medical point of view, are essential; but from a sales point of view they are unprofitable. The answer is often subsidy.

There is an increased used of physicians on a salary basis as a direct response to the demands of the medical staff for more time-consuming tasks such as conferences, review committees, and teaching programs. Result—directors of medical education and medical directors.

The final reason is hardest to spell out. Society has made of the doctor a one-man grand jury without his consent. He is expected to ration scarce items in wartime, to decide whether this sick day is or is not paid for, to judge whether his colleagues keep patients in the hospital too long, to determine a person's ability to drive a car safely. Each item requires a physician's judgment. No payment accompanies the burgeoning demands on a physician's time and personal strength, and resentment and rebellion is the inevitable and understandable reaction of the overburdened man in practice. The resentment spills over into other areas including service in the emergency room, service on utilization panels and tissue committees, service in clinics, and care of student personnel; and this could potentially increase the number of hospital-paid physicians. The matter is further complicated by distrust or concern. Some physicians regard salaried practice as an unfair control by hospitals, while most administrators are concerned about having to dig up the money to pay the salaries of this enlarging group.

Dr. T. Stewart Hamilton raised an interesting question several years ago when he wrote, "We must ask ourselves if salaried practice is really a hazard to good medical care or if it is only a paper dragon." [1] Personally, I lean to the paper dragon concept. It is high time we identified the public's needs and set about meeting them rather than wrangling about how many and whose slips of paper we use to finance our lives. I suspect there may be contrary views.

FINANCIAL FACTORS

Controlling costs in a hospital today is largely a problem of moral issues. A moratorium on rising costs can be achieved by imposing a moratorium on progress.

Hospitals are not insensitive to the public's clamor about rising costs, and, in general, they have tried to control costs in areas where this can be done. While group purchasing, use of methods engineers, and group operation of service facilities such as laundry are far from universal, these techniques are widely used.

It does little good to defensively wail that cars, food, and clothing have increased in cost. It does little good to make inexact comparisons with expenditures for liquor, cigarettes, and cosmetics. There is only one substantial question. Are we overtreating our patients? If so, who determines this?

At this minute, in the coffee corner of some hospital a doctor who is a little gray at the temples is saying, "When I was an intern I got a lousy 20 bucks a month, a pair of white shoes, and a carton of Chesterfields for Christmas; and I worked day and night seven days a week." And he will be interrupted by the doctor next to him who points out that he did not even get the Chesterfields. The latest version of this story is that the intern and resident years are "no loss—no gain" years. The stipend should be sufficient to allow the house officer and his family to live a normal life and to enjoy the good things in moderation as a junior member of the professional community. To do this the hospital has added about 2 dollars per day to the cost of care. I think it is probably the best 2 dollars the patient spends, but many disagree. House staff salaries now make up $2\frac{1}{2}$ to 4 per cent of the hospital's expenses, roughly the cost of laundry and linen service.

Two decades ago, the most expensive item in our laboratory was an $875 autotechnicon. Today our routine chemistry examinations are done on a $14,000 autoanalyzer—but this is out of date; a newer one, costing $35,000, does 12 chemistries at once. Twenty years ago we had seven people in our laboratory; today, over ten times that number.

Is this cost justified? Yes.

The electronic computer that is used today to calculate the decay rate of our cobalt bomb costs one-third as much as we had invested in all of our deep x-ray equipment 25 years ago. Would we want to turn back all this progress and return to lower cost days? Morally we could not. Does the public want us to undo all this and return to lower cost days? They not only want but demand the newest. Those who are so quick to be critical of increased costs appear to forget who it was that brought the increases about and why.

COMMUNITY COORDINATION OF FACILITIES AND MANPOWER

I have no basic quarrel with proper planning, and I think facilities should be effectively used; but I have serious misgivings about the source and direction of some of the planning now under way in our hospitals. Many who espouse the planning cause are, in fact, more interested in cost reduction than in planning for progress. I find no fault with truly effective planning groups which are representative of and knowledgeable about that which is being planned. Physicians, hospital administrators, and truly community-minded civic leaders can render an effective service.

What I do not like is the planning by companies with newly gained knowledge which equates competence in building automobiles, for example, with competence in the health professions. I find it hard to accept the notion that x-ray therapy device A is to be preferred over x-ray unit B, and under no circumstances should x-ray unit C be found within 100 miles of another such unit. Especially do I find it hard to accept this from a company which proudly announces that their lowest priced car is available in 188 models and which produces three complete families of cars that are essentially identical.

I wonder about those who would keep our laboratories open 168 hours a week, further diluting our already thin staff, and at the same time press for elimination of all costs of education from our payment formulas.

It is unrealistic to overlook the fact that, in any multi-hospital community, there are bound to be allegiances and traditions which cannot be wiped away in a meeting or two. A little friendly competition is as good for hospitals as it is for auto companies. I would not, however, like to see us reach their heights of absurdity in duplication of services.

I have intentionally been a little negative in this planning business. I see us going too far too fast and doing too much "wide blue yonder" thinking and not enough plain old spade work. Good planning should start at the intrahospital level and proceed to the interhospital level, with all competent, interested groups participating. The real need in our hospital structure today is not so much for bureaucratic planning from above as for the recognition that there is much to be done with what we have. Group purchasing, centralized services, the use of management consultants, all are available now and not widely enough used.

They may not have the glamour, but they contain the ingredients for more effective use of our facilities.

UNREALISTIC GOVERNMENT ATTITUDES
TOWARD COST REIMBURSEMENT

This topic needs a definition of terms. Big government generally can do a better job than little government in this area. The federal government has strived for many years to pay hospitals their costs. Joint form #1, developed by the American Hospital Association and Washington, while not perfect, has been something that hospitals can live with. It is in the area of state, county, and city government that reimbursement problems arise. Their own programs are often poorly put together, and it is here that federal programs get tampered with. As an illustration, the intent of the Children's Bureau is to pay realistic costs, but this intent is altered in most crippled and afflicted children's programs at the state level. We have all seen the sabotage of the Kerr-Mills program by county and state officials. That bill never had a ghost of a chance of meeting the need in the majority of states, and large numbers of people were denied the help intended by the federal government. The alacrity with which four out of five hospitals signed up for Blue Cross as their fiscal intermediary may be an indication of the desire not to have the federal intent subverted by other elements of our governmental structure.

It is interesting to speculate on the reasons for this differing attitude at different levels of government. The federal government appears to accept responsibility for caring for segments of the population and seems to view itself as a purchaser of this care. States and counties on the other hand seem to consider themselves as benefactors who make grants to supplicant hospitals and doctors.

Big government is quick to use existing mechanisms; small government rarely does, preferring to handle all details itself. An example of this is Medicare. I believe that a sincere effort is being made to pay hospitals reasonable costs and to delegate as many functions as possible down to the hospital level. It will be interesting to see what efforts will be made at county, city, and state levels to alter this program.

In general, whenever tax health dollars go through the filter of local social welfare departments, our troubles are multiplied—patients become clients, health dollars become a bounty, and the intent of the legislative branch of government undergoes a change.

COST COMPARISONS OF HIGH-QUALITY LARGE HOSPITALS
WITH LOW-QUALITY SMALL HOSPITALS

Obviously, large size does not guarantee quality; neither does small size mean mediocrity. But perhaps we might agree that there is a synergistic action between people and things in a larger hospital that makes quality care more probable there.

One of the problems is, of course, identifying what is quality care. Often we find ourselves judged on nonessentials. I cringe when I hear my hospital described as a good hospital because we serve good coffee or hear a hospital termed a poor hospital because of the parking facilities. A patient who receives a careful diagnostic study by a well-supervised fourth-year resident and has his case discussed in rounds frequently resents this intrusion and considers himself the recipient of poor care. Unfortunately, the reverse may often be true.

Complexity begets complexity. The introduction of an open heart surgery program, for example, requires increases of equipment and personnel in several other fields. The increases in these fields lead to ages in the areas of education and research. A small hospital cannot operate a nursing school or a costly residency program.

Although efforts are being made to gear facilities and staffing to patient needs, it is an unfortunate fact that many patients do not need a complex hospital for any part of their stay and many more do not need these facilities for all of their stay. And since to the sick or injured person nothing involving him is minor, he will continue to go to the complete hospital. The large hospital of the future will need to offer care at four levels—intensive care, general care, extended care, and a "no care" section for diagnostic and evaluation admissions. Even this will not be a panacea.

An equalizing trend in hospital costs is the definite upgrading of the smaller hospitals. Better trained physicians moving into rural areas, standardization of nursing and other professional salaries, and the desire to meet higher standards for accreditation are all factors that tend to close the cost gap.

Another helpful trend is the concentration of foundation and federal grant funds in the larger, more complex hospitals. The trend is slight but definite in the direction of lifting the expenses of research and education from the back of the hospitalized patient.

Finally the larger hospital, simply because it is large enough to be engaged in educational ventures, is vulnerable to the spiraling demands of more and more accrediting groups. The smaller hospital has only to meet the modest demands of the Joint Commission on Accreditation of Hospitals. The larger hospital must cope with the requirements of the National League for Nursing, which specifies nurses with master's degrees for teaching, and the specialty boards, which set definite work load points at which additional medical personnel are required for continued approval of training programs.

There is no end in sight. It is difficult to identify a single area where costs will not increase, partly because of legislation and partly because of progress.

BIBLIOGRAPHY

1. Hamilton, T. S.: Physicians and Hospitals—The Challenge to Cooperate, *Hospitals, JAHA,* 37:13 (July 1) 1963.

30

Special Problems of Small Hospitals

I.

By Jo E. Anderson, M.D.

Jo E. Anderson is a general practitioner in a small group practicing in Le Sueur, Minnesota. This agricultural community of 3,310 (1960) is located 60 miles southwest of Minneapolis. The Minnesota Valley Memorial Hospital, the only hospital in the community, is relatively new, having been established in 1960. It has 39 beds, and in 1964 there were 870 admissions, 135 births, an average daily census of 17, and 34 personnel (Guide Issue, *Hospitals*, JAHA, August 1, 1965). The *American Medical Directory*, 23rd edition, 1965, lists three general practitioners in the town, one of whom has a secondary specialty of pediatrics, and a general surgeon. Dr. Anderson received the M.D. degree from the University of Kansas School of Medicine in 1954; following a rotating internship, he served a two-year general practice residency at the University of Colorado School of Medicine.

(ED. NOTE: *This chapter is in two parts, presenting the viewpoints of two authors and their experiences in two different settings—one in a recently-established small hospital, the other in a long-established small hospital.*)

When considering the special problems of the small hospital, one should start by asking several pertinent questions which can be applied to his own hospital:

1. Why does the hospital exist? Was it built because of a real need? Was it built as a convenience for the physicians, the patients, or the community? Do the original reason for building it still exist?

2. What is the purpose of the hospital? Has it been content to exist as a place where the sick become well? Should the hospital feel a responsibility for leadership in the area of public health and preventive medicine? Does the hospital and its board have specific goals in mind? What plans has it made to change its existing service to meet new conditions and new demands?

THE SMALL COMMUNITY

The problems of living in a small community often become the problems of the small hospital. All too often, everything that is done becomes common knowledge and the subject of the town gossip at the bridge club and the checker game. This places the hospital, its board, administration, and staff under great strain to yield to the pressure of small influential groups. In our hospital we have found that a good administrator who is at the same time a "foreigner" to the community and an ardent supporter of the hospital is a very effective way of dealing with many of these pressures. A good administrator will be an effective one because he realizes his primary obligation is to run the hospital in a businesslike manner. A second and very important element of smooth community relations is a widely representative hospital auxiliary. In our community of 3,500, there are 190 active auxiliary members.

THE ADMINISTRATOR

In the small hospital the administrator must assume an increased vigilance over areas which are outside the usual direct supervision of the administration. He must ask himself, "What are my responsibilities toward quality of care and utilization in my hospital?" This may bring him into conflict with the medical staff who feel this is none of his business. It is at this point that a well-trained administrator who does not yield to pressures is very helpful, and such a sense of responsibility will do much to help the hospital work toward high goals. To make this working arrangement with the medical staff smoother, we have found it helpful to have the administrator present and participating in each medical staff meeting.

PERSONNEL

Staffing and personnel problems plague many small hospitals. Curiously enough we find that our *custodial employees* are among the most loyal.

They are not unionized. Many boast of the title Department Head; and most are more than willing to return for extra hours when called and even return without being called "just to check something."

Geographical location, local industry, and size of the community play large roles in the availability of *nursing personnel.* Like other communities, we have many trained nurses in town, but very few wish to work full time. The hospital has found that a few regular full-time registered nurses can carry the load quite adequately if supplemented by part-time nurses. When a patient needs more nursing care than this arrangement provides, private duty nurses are utilized. This permits women who desire to keep up their nursing skills to work in the hospital under supervision; it also provides a fairly large group of nurses who are familiar with our hospital upon whom we can call for general duty in an emergency. Refresher training is available to these nurses through our affiliation with a larger teaching hospital. A local training program for nurses' aides has also proved helpful. During this past year a teen-age Candy-Striper program was begun.

MEDICAL STAFF ORGANIZATION

The organization of the medical staff of a small hospital often poses problems. Many times there are few staff physicians, and often they represent even fewer offices. Lucky is the hospital where all the staff work together to improve their hospital!

At our hospital, a formal organization of the medical staff according to the recommendations of the Joint Commission on Accreditation of Hospitals seems to work best. Meetings, while informal, usually proceed along parliamentary rules, and reports from the various committees are given. Committee appointments are kept fairly permanent so that physicians come to feel a greater sense of responsibility.

A question regarding the *physician's responsibility to the hospital* sometimes arises. Should procedures which can be done in the office be done in the hospital? If both are equally available, should the doctor see patients at night in his office or the hospital? We have felt the availability of assistants and the laboratory makes it possible to practice better medicine by seeing the patient at the hospital. In addition, it helps increase the hospital's clinical load and thereby its finances. This question ultimately involves the doctor in a reappraisal of his responsibility for making the hospital a financial success. Without his patients the hospital could not operate; with his patients he may lose money for procedures which could be done in the office, although perhaps not as well.

ACCREDITATION

Should the small hospital seek accreditation by the Joint Commission on Accreditation of Hospitals? I would submit that working to achieve accreditation or to maintain it is a very desirable goal for every eligible hospital. The standards set by the Joint Commission for medical care are *minimum*, not maximum, standards. They serve as a goal and a stimulus for the administration and the medical staff.

The maintenance of charts is an important part of the accreditation standards. One solution we have found helpful is to make the dictation of records extremely easy. The busy physician is much more likely to dictate complete records than he is to write them longhand. We are able to have a typed history and physical examination on the chart within two days. Discharge summaries are likewise typed, with carbon copies for the physician's office records.

ANCILLARY FACILITIES

The ancillary facilities of the small hospital deserve special consideration. Most hospitals depend heavily on income from these services to balance the financial budget. If laboratory procedures are available, they will be used by the staff, but only if they are dependable. Good x-ray and laboratory technicians are difficult to find, but they are very important to the success of a small hospital's operation. Given the facilities, the services of a visiting radiologist makes possible many diagnostic studies equal to those of larger centers.

AFFILIATION WTH A TEACHING HOSPITAL

In 1960, when the Minnesota Valley Memorial Hospital was established, the health planners for our community envisioned a rural health center with the acute hospital as its nucleus. As an aid in achieving this, a formal affiliation was established with a metropolitan teaching hospital 60 miles away. (ED. NOTE: *Mount Sinai Hospital, Minneapolis, Minnesota, is affiliated with the University of Minnesota School of Medicine. It has 305 beds, and in 1964 there were 9,662 patients discharged and 712 births.[1] The hospital is approved for 14 rotating internship positions and 18 residency positions in medicine, surgery, and pathology.[2] This affiliation is discussed further in Chap. 42 on Continuing Education in the Non-teaching Hospital.*) This affiliation, has helped to provide an atmosphere to encourage medical practice of a high quality. At the administrative level there has been close consultation over problems which have developed. Financial savings are realized by both hospitals through bulk purchasing of supplies. Department heads from the smaller hospital spend training periods with their counterpart at the affiliate hospital. Consultation visits by the larger hospital's personnel—operating room nurse, librarian, medical records librarian, pharmacist, dietician, and others—have helped to solve problems and develop procedures for our hospital. All pathological specimens are reviewed by the affiliated hospital pathologist who periodically visits us and discusses tissues from our own cases with the staff.

Over the past three years, postgraduate seminars have been presented at our hospital by specialists from the affiliate hospital staff. We have become better acquainted with these consultants, and they have a better idea of the type of cases which can be handled in our hospital. A telephone call about a problem will often be enough to solve it because the consultant is acquainted with the staff physician and his facilities. The potentials of the affiliation have not yet been fully explored.

THE FUTURE

What does the future hold for the small hospital? Will it be squeezed out of existence by regional centers? Will Medicare make of it a geriatric care center? Can small hospitals still attract physicians? These are questions which deserve serious consideration by the board, administration, and staff of small hospitals. I believe that the small hospital which survives in the future will be the one which clearly sees its purpose and reason for existence. The physicians who make up the medical staffs of these hospitals must take their responsibility for leadership seriously, or we may find our practice of medicine severely restricted by rules not of our making.

DISCUSSION

The questions raised during our discussion seminars center around two major problem areas—those related to the emergency room and those related to the role of the physician as a member of the hospital staff.

Emergency Room Questions

Patients are using the Emergency Room more and more as an Outpatient Department. How does a small hospital get *staff coverage* for this?

There is a trend toward greater use of the hospital for all medical services. Many factors are involved such as insurance, unavailability of the patient's own doctor, and a growing philosophy that a hospital is a service institution and that "this is a service which is part of my rights." Physicians and hospital administrators must recognize these attitudes and either accept or reject the concept of extended hospital services. If an active outpatient service is encouraged, the first problem to be faced is coverage by staff doctors.

Some hospitals pay stipends to members of their staff for regularly being "on call" for emergency service. Many others depend on volunteer coverage recruited from the medical staff. A few hospitals attempt to preserve the emergency room and at the same time offer outpatient service by providing office space for doctors within or adjacent to the hospital. One traditional medical arts type of building in the Pacific Northwest has incorporated in it a hospital floor for emergencies. In another area, an attempt to avoid overtaxing the hospital emergency room resulted in the building of a condominium office across the street by 20 physicians who take turns staffing it at night. This preserves the private practice aspect while meeting the problem of availability at all hours.

What can be done about the *increasing use of the emergency room?* One hospital gives each outpatient an informational brochure instructing him in ways of getting his doctor after office hours. This includes information about answering service, doctors taking calls for colleagues, and so on. It also emphasizes that the doctor can often better attend to the patient's problem in the office during office hours where complete records and assistants are available.

Some physicians, particularly in small hospitals, encourage patients to meet him in the emergency room after office hours. This solves the problem of seeing the patient in the office without adequate help or in the home without available diagnostic services. The hospital may also be used as an answering service for the doctor who remains available by checking in with the hospital switchboard from time to time.

Hospital Staff Questions

How does a small hospital staff *restrict previously granted privileges?* Provisions should be made in the medical staff bylaws specifying the manner in which privileges are granted or restricted. An annual review of the privileges of every staff member is a good policy, with recommendations being sent to the board whose ultimate responsibility it is to grant privileges. Should the staff feel the need to restrict or remove a man's previously granted privilege, the doctor involved should be notified personally, not by mail, and given a chance to be heard in a formal fashion. This is often a very difficult and delicate problem, but it should be considered in the light of the best interest of the hospital and its patients.

How does the staff get the physicians to *complete their patient charts?* The importance of taking a good history is rightly emphasized in medical school, but the importance of recording it in usable form is often neglected. Accurate and complete records are necessary for good medical care; still, incomplete charts are a problem for nearly all hospitals. The medical records librarian is the key to complete charts by providing easily accessible facilities for dictating records and by persistent, good-natured nagging. Taking a few charts each day to the doctor for completion is preferable to presenting him with a large batch all at once. But the medical staff itself bears full responsibility for this work. Emphasize recording histories and physical examinations on the chart early and make dictation available.

Good records become contagious. Other staff members begin to dictate more complete records, then summaries, and soon a friendly professional rivalry is producing complete charts promptly. Also important is the idea of working toward a common goal—to achieve or maintain accreditation.

If a doctor gets behind on his charts and does them all retrospectively, the question of quality of care may be raised. Retrospective physicians' notes which disagree with current nursing notes may be most embarrassing in the court room.

But what do you do about the *doctor who will not complete his charts?* Good staff bylaws should provide specific measures, such as automatic suspension of a delinquent physician's privileges. This may range all the way from complete suspension with no privileges to suspension of privilege to admit certain categories of patients. Usually, the length of the suspension is limited to a period sufficient to complete the unfinished charts and also is limited to non-emergency admissions. Some hospitals even go so far as to inform other hospitals in the region of the suspension. In some cases there is mutual respect for such suspensions, and the recalcitrant staff doctor finds himself unable to admit patients to any hospital. These are the extreme measures. The mechanisms for all disciplinary measures should be clearly defined in the bylaws. Usually the enforcement is delegated to the administrator, and this should be done in an impartial manner.

How does a small hospital *attract doctors?* Hospitals in rural areas are finding this increasingly difficult. With only 18 per cent of the medical graduates in the United States going into general practice, the odds are against the small hospital. It is encouraging to find that the problem is less acute in states where preceptorship programs are a part of the medical school curriculum.

In rural areas where staffing has become a problem, the hospital should reassess its function and its role in providing an atmosphere attractive to new physicians. This might include providing clinical or office facilities in or adjacent to the hospital, continuing education opportunities, and affiliations with larger metropolitan hospitals. Obvious, uniformly high-quality medical care is probably the greatest magnet, and this is best demonstrated by a systematic internal medical audit program.

How is it possible for the staff of a small hospital to carry out *all the committee functions* we have heard about here? Small numbers of doctors on the staff means that everyone must wear several hats. It also means that one or two who fail to carry their load will hamper the whole staff. It is quite acceptable for the entire staff to sit as a committee for tissue, records, utilization, and credentials, but separate minutes should be kept.

The use of the Professional Activity Study and the Medical Audit Program of the Commission on Professional and Hospital Activities will help to assess the type, amount, and quality of medical care being given in the hospital. To assure the best use of the data, it is strongly advised that hospitals planning to use these services send representatives to Ann Arbor for tutorial sessions.

BIBLIOGRAPHY

1. Guide Issue, *Hospitals, JAHA*, (Aug. 1) 1965.

2. "Directory of Approved Internships and Residencies," American Medical Association, Chicago, 1965.

II.

By James G. Price, M.D.

James G. Price is a general practitioner in Brush, Colorado, a community of 3,621 population (1960), located 90 miles east of Denver. The Brush Hospital has 34 beds, 1,260 annual admissions, 142 births, an average census of 17, and 32 hospital personnel (Guide Issue, *Hospitals, JAHA*, August 1, 1965). The active medical staff consists of four general practitioners. Dr. Price received the M.D. degree from the University of Colorado School of Medicine in 1951. He practices in partnership with two other physicians, and he is the immediate past president of the Colorado Academy of General Practice. He was born in the hospital in which he practices.

The term "small hospital" is ambiguous. My own point of reference is colored by my experience in a 34 bed hospital, and for this discussion we shall consider a hypothetical small hospital of less than 50 beds. It is likely to be the only medical facility in a rural community. The staff consists of not more than 10 physicians and perhaps as few as 2. All of the physicians are general practitioners, and most of them do major surgery. The nearest fully equipped and fully staffed major hospital is at least 75 miles away. More than likely, the hospital is lucky to break even at the end of the year, and it may need some annual financial support from the community.

What sorts of things go on in this hypothetical small hospital? A good share of its cases involve acute trauma, especially that caused by automobile wrecks and farm accidents. It handles most of the medical problems of the area including acute emergencies such as coronary occlusions, strokes, and severe croups. Practically all of the babies of the area are born here. Elective referral of the pregnant woman to a major center for some specific cause is a rare exception, and the obstetrical emergencies which arise usually do not lend themselves to being transferred elsewhere. A considerable amount of closed orthopedic work is handled as well as most kinds of minor surgery. The amount and type of major surgery depends upon the capabilities and desires of the various staff members, but it is not unusual to find hysterectomies and other pelvic surgery, appendectomies, hernias, and cholecystectomies being done routinely. Open chest work and intestinal resection may be done by necessity in extreme emergency.

The typical small hospital handles up to 90 per cent of the medical and surgical problems of the community. Basically, it functions in providing the same kind of care to its people that the city hospital provides to its people. It offers care to people who are so sick or injured that they cannot be moved. It allows patients to be close to their families and businesses, with a physician who knows their idiosyncracies and histories. In essence, it is just another hospital, somewhat diminished in size and scope of activities from the city hospital, but giving the same basic services.

The need for this hospital varies with the geographical area and generally seems to be decreasing. The number of such hospitals decreased from 44 per cent of all short-term general hospitals and special hospitals in 1953 to 36.8 per cent in 1964. During this same period, the percentage of hospital beds in smaller hospitals decreased from 11.5 to 9 per cent.[1] In Colorado, 53 per cent of the general hospitals have less than 50 beds, but these hospitals account for only 12 per cent of the total beds in the state.

Population increases and shifts have made it possible for some areas to support larger hospitals, while in other areas population decreases have closed small hospitals. Without question, modern transportation makes it easier and faster to move a patient long distances. Until some sort of all-weather rapid transportation is developed, there will continue to be serious emergencies which demand immediate treatment on the spot; and we have yet to find a good substitute for the convenience of "being sick at home." It appears that the small hospital is here to stay.

COMMUNITY-HOSPITAL RELATIONSHIP

Since the small hospital is located in a small town, it is subject to all the hazards and advantages that are part of small-town living. It must deal with a degree of "togetherness" with the community that is unknown in metropolitan areas. Almost everyone in the town knows almost everyone else, their families, their illnesses, and their problems. Genuine concern and simple curiosity on the part of the townspeople attend the hospitalization of anyone; and if John Doe goes to the hospital, his doctor can expect to be asked what is wrong with him. The doctor preference of each person is a matter of casual public knowledge; and should anyone collapse on the street, his own family doctor would most likely be called.

The administrator and the hospital trustee are probably patients of a member of the medical staff, and their opinions about the hospital and its operation are influenced, consciously or unconsciously, by their physician's comments. The selection of a family physician by one of the laboratory or nursing personnel may give rise to the question of preferential treatment to that physician and his patients.

It is customary in some areas for the local radio station to broadcast the name of every patient admitted to the hospital. The weekly newspaper also publishes this list and may categorize each patient as surgical or medical. It is quite customary and acceptable for a patient to publish in the newspaper an all-inclusive thank you note to friends, his preacher (by name), and his doctor (by name).

The fact that a person may have donated $5.00 to the annual hospital drive gives him a proprietary interest in the overall financial situation of the hospital, and he feels free to give the board members advice on all administrative decisions.

All of these situations are not necessarily bad—they are simply facts. Since illness and hospitalization involve a great deal of personal contact, the personal knowledge about each patient can be of great value in providing prompt care tailored to his specific quirks and needs. It is obvious that the small hospital has glass walls, and the administrator, the board, and the medical staff must take this into account in making decisions. The real problem arises when a controversial decision must be made, or when a long-time employee must be fired, or, worse yet, when surgical privileges are revoked or other disciplinary action involves a staff member.

The magnitude of the potential and probable public reaction may be enough to cause a faint heart in the decisionmakers, for the marginally operating hospital cannot afford a major public split which costs it a segment of its clientele. It is not implied that shoddy performance by any person—staff or janitor—is therefore permanently tolerated, but delicacy and tactfulness may take the place of more straightforward solutions.

ADMINISTRATION

The administration of a small hospital may be by the community itself, a church organization, a hospital management corporation, or in some cases by a private corporation. The type of administrative body which is best will vary from hospital to hospital.

The large *hospital management corporation* has some real advantages —it supplies an experienced administrator; it can save money by central purchasing; it can help nurses and technicians; it may provide a financial backing to tide the hospital over lean days. Most important, the administrator may be responsible primarily to the parent organization and secondarily to the hospital board, according to clearly defined contractual terms. This may be good or bad. On the other hand, the community may not be able to change administrators should this be desired. Hospital services and personnel may be unduly curtailed in a false economy drive; and in the unlikely event that the hospital operation becomes profitable, part of this profit will leave the community. Church management may offer a similar picture, with the possible additional difficulty of conflict due to patient-administration difference in religious belief. Anything less than wholehearted enthusiasm and cooperation of the public can easily spell disaster for the small hospital.

The administration has certain responsibilities for maintaining quality of care. These responsibilities may be exercised through ex officio membership committees of the medical staff, and the administration can insist upon the maintenance of generally recognized standards of medical and surgical care, whether or not the hospital is accredited. Often it may apply leverage toward this end through the pathologist serving the hospital and also by flatly stating that their organization cannot be associated with mediocre medical care. If the same administrative organization is used by other nearby hospitals, a realistic baseline for utilization and length of stay can be developed for the area. It is not inferred that the administration should assume the duties and responsibilities of the medical staff, but it can offer great help and stimulation should there be any faltering in maintaining high standards.

The financial obligation of the administration is to operate the hospital on a sound financial basis, meet obligations to local merchants, purchase wisely, and constantly try to keep costs of hospitalization down to the lowest level consistent with good care, adequate help, and suitable equipment and supplies. Even a small hospital is a valuable industry to its community, and the community has the right to expect efficient management.

STAFFING

A shortage of *nurses* is common to hospitals of all sizes, but the problem may be compounded in the small hospital by an almost absolute lack of career nurses. In our hospital, every working nurse would gladly return to her family if an adequate replacement could be found. Community pressure and her own conscience rather than a desire to work often are the major motivating forces. This situation results in nurses working split shifts or one shift per week or in a complete lack of registered nurses for night coverage. Vacations and illness are a nightmare to the nursing supervisor. Many of the nurses have not worked for 10 or 15 years, and they are unsure of their own abilities and unfamiliar with current methods. In a hospital where one nurse must cover all services except major surgery, the fear of bungling a delivery may be enough to keep a nurse from working at all. The usual small town and small hospital present very little enticement to the new graduate who, perhaps having enjoyed the help of an intern or resident staff during training, feels quite inadequate to undertake all the never-before-performed duties of a small hospital nurse. The only solution to this problem, and at best it is a long-term one, is to encourage local girls to go into nursing by providing inspiration and subsidy with the hope that some will return. Licensed practical nurses and nurse's aides are somewhat easier to find, and a well-trained, experienced LPN may often be given increased responsibility.

Qualified *laboratory technicians* are relatively scarce but usually can be found. Not infrequently the laboratory technician also serves as x-ray technician since the volume of work does not warrant two full salaries.

The services of a *physical therapist* may be available through a state agency or often not at all, in which case the burden falls upon the physician. His interest in this field and his available time will determine how much or how little of this therapy the patient receives.

THE MEDICAL STAFF

The complexity of organization will vary with the number of doctors on the staff, the simplest organization being merely a president and a secretary. Local dentists who might be called to do work in the hospital commonly receive courtesy staff privileges. This is also true in the case of out-of-town specialists who come to the hospital occasionally. The hospital cardiologist, radiologist, and pathologist usually are not residents of the community, but they have staff privileges in order to have their reports appear on the records.

The usual *committees*—tissue, death, and record—often consist of the entire staff acting as each committee. The hazards of this arrangement are apparent. A physician may be called upon to justify some portion of his treatment to another physician, his competitor, who until this admission considered himself the family doctor for this patient. A similar situation is the absurdity of one staff member presenting a death review to his partner who knew the patient very well and even helped take care of him!

The quality of the functions of a small staff is directly dependent upon the personalities of the members. If there is persistent serious conflict of opinion, the staff organization will likely cease to function altogether.

Utilizing the services of the hospital pathologist may be a great aid in *settling staff disputes*. His actual presence, which may involve considerable travel on his part, is essential; unless he is present he may make judgments without full clinical knowledge of the patient. Many pathologists are willing to make an outright condemnation of only gross and obvious surgical fiascos, and these usually constitute only a minor fraction of the judgment errors which may exist. Indications for operations such as tonsillectomy and adenoidectomy, hysterectomy and other pelvic surgery, and cholecystectomy will vary widely, according to the opinions of different surgeons. The pathologist cannot be expected to evaluate blindly the patient's pain, disability, or symptomatology.

When questions of professional competency arise, supervision by a senior staff member may be enough to solve the problem. Such an easy solution is rarely the case in the small hospital, and an obvious need for *discipline* presents a serious quandary. Rarely can matters be settled in anything resembling an impersonal fashion. Revocation of surgical privileges is quickly construed as sour grapes, and sadly enough, this may not be entirely untrue. Airing of dirty linen is always distasteful. At times a committee from a neighboring hospital or the state medical society may be able to provide a disinterested appraisal with recommendations for discipline. This helps to remove a major burden from the staff.

Do not conclude from this discussion that the staff of every small hospital is an ugly little volcano ready to erupt; the majority of them are quite the opposite.

Privilege delineation is usually handled in the small hospital simply by applying for and receiving surgical privileges for any procedure of which the surgeon is deemed capable by training or experience. As the size of the staff increases, the procedures for privilege allocation more nearly parallel those of large hospitals.

One can hardly be a staff member without being exceedingly aware of *hospital finances*. The administrator is usually much happier if he has no beds for patients than if he has no patients for beds, and one may not hear much in the way of over-utilization complaints from that quarter. The admission and discharge committee (the entire staff) often functions as a model of unstated reciprocity—based upon the fear of having one's own patients rejected. An honest rejection may lose an entire family as patients and gain only a frosty smile from the administrator. It is unquestionably the duty of every staff member to reduce overhead and hospital costs in any way that does not conflict with the best care of the patient. This includes a realistic attitude in demands for new and expensive equipment.

LICENSURE AND ACCREDITATION

Accreditation by the Joint Commission on Accreditation of Hospitals is a desirable goal for even the smallest eligible hospital. Achieving this goal means that the hospital has met certain minimal standards designed for better care of the patient. Achieving accreditation is neither simple nor permanent, but once done, its major value is that it keeps all personnel from the board to the janitor alert and on their toes. To maintain accreditation, attention is continually directed to all facets, including some which might otherwise be neglected such as disaster planning, record quality, and staff organization. All is for the benefit of the patient.

State licensure may or may not be a problem, depending upon the specific regulations of the particular state. Unfortunately, some state regulations for licensure are written with only the large hospital in mind, and at best with only vague ideas of the problems of the smaller hospitals. Some requirements, if met to the letter, would cause the operating expenses of the small hospital to rise so high that the hospital would simply be out of existence. Ignoring the failure of the small hospital to meet existing regulations is a poor substitute for regulations which are adequately demanding to assure good patient care and yet realistic enough to be within the reach of all.

HOSPITAL FACILITIES

The *laboratory* of a small hospital is usually under the direction of part-time, non-resident pathologists who may seldom visit the laboratory. The scope of work performed depends upon the desires of the staff, the training and supervision of the technician, and the equipment. The more complicated tests are usually sent to the pathologist's office. Facilities of the state laboratory may also be available.

An *electrocardiograph* is standard equipment, and most members of the medical staff have at least a rudimentary familiarity with reading electrocardiograms. The tracings may then be mailed to a cardiologist who reports by telephone. At times this may lead to an unneeded overnight stay in the hospital. Direct transmission of electrocardiograms by telephone lines is becoming available in some areas.

Modest *x-ray and fluoroscopy facilities* are available in most small hospitals. One-day teletype reporting of routine x-ray interpretations and telephone reporting of urgent findings are services that are now commonly provided by the radiologist. Fluoroscopic examinations are scheduled for the regular visits of the radiologist.

A *walking blood bank* can be very effective if the services of the technician are completely reliable. In many areas, several small hospitals become affiliated with a central blood bank organization and are thereby able to exchange blood between the hospitals as well as obtain unusual types from the central blood bank, often by air transportation.

CONTINUING EDUCATION

Every conscientious physician finds it necessary to continue his medical education on a regular, systematic basis. This can be done in a variety of ways, and it may be through his own hospital. It is not difficult for the staff of a small hospital to organize *refresher seminars* with members of a medical school faculty or other teachers who come to the hospital for clinics and formal presentations.

Equally important is the physician's responsibility for the *education and training of other hospital personnel* who render patient care. He should insist that some time be devoted to this function regularly, perhaps each month or each quarter.

Small hospitals rarely have interns or residents, but it is not unusual for a medical student to be about, assigned either to the hospital or to a member of the staff during a required or elective preceptorship supervised by the medical school. The instruction of these students is one of the more pleasurable duties of a physician. The benefits from this association are not unilateral, for the students have much to offer— enthusiasm, friendly but candid criticism, and often some of the latest information, theoretical though it might be.

In the small hospital, where regulations are likely to be somewhat more lax than in the city, stagnation is easy and may eventually become disastrous. Lack of stimulating associations can produce serious mental lethargy which ultimately causes patient care to suffer. The necessity of some form of systematic continuing education is absolute.

THE FUTURE

If the welfare of the public were the sole factor in determining the destiny of the small community hospital, its future would be assured. However, many critical problems of operating a small hospital may make its very existence precarious. It is therefore quite possible that relatively small shifts in the medico-economic structure could destroy the narrow margin of successful operation. The demise of the small community hospital could conceivably be brought about by some measure designed to improve the public health, perhaps some future measure similar in concept to the regional hospital complexes for the care of heart disease, cancer, and stroke as proposed by the President's Commission. (ED. NOTE: *This concept is in contrast to the provisions of Public Law 89–239 establishing regional medical cooperative programs, not complexes, for education, research, training, and demonstrations in the fields of heart disease, cancer, stroke, and related diseases. The emphasis of this legislation is definitely on educational opportunities for the practicing physician and on cooperative arrangements.*) If some measure should drain off to treatment centers a significant segment of the patients well cared for in the community hospital, it could represent the margin of an adequate daily patient census needed for the successful operation of the hospital. Conceivably, community facilities could be reduced to something resembling a military triage area where little or no definitive treatment is attempted. The shortcomings of this dismal picture are obvious—the extreme emergency when time is critical or when weather conditions make transportation impossible requires immediate, adequate treatment.

An additional hazard of downgrading the small community hospital to the level of a community clearing station is the decreased attractiveness in recruiting physicians for practice in small communities. Where there are no hospitals, likely there are few physicians.

On the other side of the scale is Medicare which may greatly increase the demand for hospital beds in hospitals large and small. Experience with current governmental insurance programs demonstrates that the insured segment of the population insists upon more and longer hospitalization.

The dwindling number of physicians seeking staff appointment in the small community hospital is a growing concern in many areas. Most members of the small hospital staff are general practitioners. With an ever decreasing number of medical graduates entering general practice, serious physician shortages already exist in many rural areas.

CONCLUSION

The small hospital has many problems that are either non-existent or of minimal importance in the larger hospitals. This is not to say that the small hospital does not provide a needed service, but, as with all good things, much effort is required to make it work.

BIBLIOGRAPHY

1.   Guide Issue, *Hospitals, JAHA*, (Aug. 1), 1965.

31

The Emergency Service

I. THE ORGANIZATION OF AN EMERGENCY SERVICE

By Roswell K. Brown, M.D.

Roswell K. Brown is the associate director of the Field Program of the Committee on Trauma of the American College of Surgeons. He received the M.D. degree from Cornell University. For many years he was a member of the faculty of the University of Buffalo School of Medicine where he was clinical professor of surgery and Assistant Dean. He has served on the National Board of Medical Examiners. He is a diplomate of the American Board of Surgery and a Fellow of the American College of Surgeons.

We hear a great deal about changes in patterns of medical care these days, one of which is the tremendous increase of patients attending hospital emergency departments.* Doctors are no longer available in their offices at all hours of the day or night, nor do they make house calls as frequently as they used to. In previous generations, an emergency situation was handled by calling the doctor. Nowadays the patient is taken to the hospital, or an ambulance is called.

The great increase in patient load in the emergency room is largely due to patients who have non-urgent complaints. This tends to obscure the fact that there has also been an important increase in the number of seriously injured patients.

* Emergency service problems are also discussed in the chapter "Problems of Small Hospitals."

(ED. NOTE: *The annual number of emergency room visits in the United States has tripled in the past decade. Many factors have been cited as causes of this onslaught. One of the more intriguing ones proposed is the sharp decline in the number of general practitioners, their number having decreased from 95,000 fifteen years ago to 68,000. Of these, only 45,000 are treating patients full time. From one-third to one-half of all emergency room visits are estimated to be for non-emergency conditions.*)

THE ACCIDENT TOLL

Each year there are over 10 million disabling injuries and 100,000 accidental deaths in the United States. Serious injuries are happening at about the same rate as breathing—20 breaths a minute, 20 injuries a minute. If the amount of life lost by accidental deaths in the United States is computed by adding up the life expectancy of each person killed, we find that 1,400,000 years of human life are lost each year in the United States.

The emergency unit of the hospital has greater potential in terms of years of human salvage than all of our work in heart disease, cancer, and stroke. Let us face the question, "Is the hospital best serving today's needs of the community or is it preoccupied with the problems of the past?"

The American College of Surgeons Committee on Trauma

The American College of Surgeons is dedicated to improvement of patient care. Its Committee on Trauma is presently carrying out a program designed to improve emergency services through invitational surveys. The survey is not an inspection, and emergency departments are not accredited nor given any rating. Surveys are arranged through the state chairman of the Committee on Trauma of the American College of Surgeons who appoints a survey team, usually made up of one or more surgeons, administrators, and emergency department nurses, all from other hospitals. A preliminary questionnaire is completed in advance of the survey by those responsible for the emergency department. Members of the visiting team make systematic on-the-spot studies with the corresponding members of the local staff. An evaluation report is then submitted.

THE EMERGENCY SERVICE COMMITTEE

An emergency service committee is essential because the department needs careful supervision and guided growth to meet the increasing and changing demands of modern times. The physician who serves as director of the emergency department is responsible for day-to-day functions. The committee is responsible for policy decisions. It should include:

1. The administrator
2. The director of the emergency department
3. Representatives of the major clinical services: medicine, surgery, obstetrics-gynecology, pediatrics and psychiatry
4. Nurses who are in charge of emergency service nursing
5. Sometimes representatives of the ambulance services

To place responsibility for the emergency service directly in the hands of the executive committee of the medical staff is not enough. The solution of many problems requires the intelligent cooperation of other professional sectors of the hospital.

STAFFING

Physicians. Prompt, competent medical attention must be available in the emergency department at all times. It has been said that all patients should be seen within 15 minutes. This, of course, is too long a delay for a patient with respiratory obstruction, severe bleeding, or cardiac arrest. Certainly the nurses should be qualified to administer life-saving measures in dire emergencies in the absence of doctors, but they should not undertake treatment in ordinary circumstances. The waiting room in the emergency department is for relatives and friends, not for the emergency patient.

There are now many different organizational plans for emergency service staffing. Some seem to be only temporary expedients, but others offer good professional patterns for the future.

The Hospital with Interns and Residents. Some of the most valuable educational experiences for interns and residents are to be had on the emergency service. Of course, it is never justifiable to exploit these young doctors by giving them responsibilities without proper medical and surgical supervision. This is unfair to the interns and residents as well as to the patients; and it may create incidents which result in poor public relations for the hospital, to say nothing of the liability suits. The so-called "ladder of learning" plan affords an ideal organization for the best possible patient care. Each member of the staff delegates supervised responsibilities to those below and at the same time accepts responsibilities and advice from those above. This is certainly the best plan for the continuing education of the entire staff. A hospital with a good educational program will have excellent emergency service coverage; and it may well be the most important aspect of professional training.

The Hospital without House Staff. In the hospital without house staff, the emergency service is staffed in many different patterns by physicians in practice. Cooperative planning is needed to provide competent care with reasonable promptness and without conflicts of interest.

A common practice is for members of the staff to cover the emergency service in rotation. The frequency and duration of duty depends upon the size of the staff, their ways of life, the distances of their offices and homes from the hospital, and other considerations. Some physicians serve emergency department duty for 24 hours once every month or so. Others have duties at specified hours of a certain day every week. The schedule should be worked out carefully and fairly. Some practitioners who vigorously opposed being regimented have later found the emergency duty to be both interesting and rewarding. Duty rosters should be made up several months in advance and always be prominently posted on the emergency room bulletin board as well as mailed to each doctor concerned.

Some hospitals have met the problem by hiring physicians for either full-time or part-time work. Emergency department employment may be quite desirable for young practitioners who need the financial support, and it may also be a good method of becoming known in the community. Some institutions hire physicians only for the hours when members of the staff are not routinely at the hospital. For others, all that is needed is a fair system of rotation of calls to bring in doctors who live nearby.

The methods of staffing the emergency service are countless, but the success of any method depends upon mutual agreement and understanding. Almost any pattern of service may be successful if the staff understands the philosophy and backs the program. No staffing pattern can be satisfactory unless the physicians are well paid, either by fee or by salary.

The physicians on duty should have access at any hour to consultation and professional help from their colleagues. It is well to set up duty on the basis of first, second, and third call. A roster of available specialists should be on the bulletin board. The x-ray department and laboratories must provide 24-hour service.

In the future, it seems likely that more and more groups of physicians will practice together with their offices in or near the hospitals, thus furnishing rather complete emergency care.

(ED. NOTE: *A recent innovation in several parts of the country is a contractual arrangement with a group of physicians to provide emergency services for the hospital. This may be with or without the direct billing of the patient for services by the physicians.*)

Nurses. On the emergency service, a special type of nurse is needed who, in my opinion, is the best nurse that exists. She has wide qualifications, both technical and personal. She has the ability to get along with the demanding public, the suffering, the dying, the drunk, the disorderly the hysterical relatives, the stupid helpers, and the difficult fellow nurses and surgeons who are sometimes quite unreasonable. The good emergency service nurse takes all of these difficulties in stride without interruption in efficient emergency patient care.

The inevitable wide fluctuations in the work load are the nature of emergency services. If the staffing of nurses follows the dictum that "too many nurses may be worse than too few," the emergency department should then be able to mobilize extra nursing help rapidly and on short notice.[4] Inexperienced nurses and highly specialized nurses do not belong in emergency departments except as observers or for training.

Auxiliary Personnel. That nursing and administrative functions can be combined is admirably illustrated by the many competent nurses in small hospitals and especially by some of the very efficient nuns. In small institutions, all the functions—nursing, secretarial, bookkeeping, and record librarian—may have to be vested in one person. In most hospitals, however, this work should be supervised by nurses.

Surgical technicians, first-aid experts, qualified ambulance attendants, male nurses, and orderlies may be useful in the emergency department. Practical nurses and nurses aides may also be of great service, but they should work under careful supervision.

Nurses often need the services of male attendants, sometimes very quickly; if they are not assigned to the emergency room, they should be available nearby on call. There seems to be a dearth of intelligent, dependable male paramedical workers. An established paramedical profession of male first-aid workers, with adequate pay and public recognition, I believe, would attract young men to a lifetime career. The young man who is now interested in a health career has a wide variety of professions and vocations from which to choose, but unfortunately the nursing profession goes by a name that implies femininity. We have great admiration for male nurses and for first-aid specialists, but we do not like to call them "nurse," though they be as well qualified as their female colleagues. This group of paramedics needs respect and a new professional name.

The emergency department also needs maid and janitorial services. The workers assigned should be able to act as nurses aides at times when all hands must help with patient care. On the other hand there should be no secretaries or nurses or doctors who are unwilling to do cleaning duty when necessary.

Ambulance Personnel. It is beneficial for ambulance personnel to be assigned to emergency department duties either as a permanent arrangement or for training purposes.

Ideally, the immediate care at the site of the injury and care in transportation should be a responsibility of the emergency service charge nurse in that she records a critical evaluation of the first-aid performance of every ambulance case. These records should be reviewed by the emergency department committee with appropriate corrective measures instituted when indicated. At the Hurley Hospital in Flint, Michigan, meetings are held for critical discussion of performance with the ambulance personnel, the emergency department nurse, and the surgeons, with resulting improvements in patient care.[1] Ambulance Councils have been organized in some areas of New Jersey. These councils, made up of the volunteer squads that serve a given hospital, are for education and critical self-evaluation. They obtain the help and guidance from the nursing and medical profession through honorary membership and by inviting key persons to participate in their meetings.

POLICIES, RULES, AND REGULATIONS

Policy matters and rules and regulations are determined by the hospital staff through the emergency department committee and the executive committee. The following usually should be included:

1. The emergency department should be open at all times. Every patient must be seen by a physician; otherwise a clerk or an orderly may inadvertently send away a patient who is in desperate need of care.

2. The policies concerning physician fees and hospital charges should be clearly understood.

3. The type of treatment undertaken in the emergency room should be only that which can be done better there than anywhere else in the hospital. General anesthesia is usually not feasible.

4. There should be no revisits in the emergency department. Removal of stitches should be done in the physician's office or in the outpatient department.

5. Elective minor surgery, such as sebaceous cystectomy, generally should not be allowed in the emergency department; but if it is permitted, there must be a clear understanding that emergency patients always take precedence and elective operations may have to be interrupted at any time.

6. Careful records of history, physical findings, treatment, and disposition are a necessity for optimal patient care. Teaching programs cannot exist without good records. Research programs are dependent on accurate records. Legal considerations require records, especially accurate notes as to the disposition of the patient.

7. A poison control chart and manual, standard textbooks, and the hospital's own book of Standard Procedures should be readily available.

8. The emergency department instruments must be of the same high quality as those in the rest of the hospital. Worn-out, outdated, cast-off instruments should not be used for this most important work of the hospital.

9. Stretchers should be x-ray permeable and constructed so they may serve as examining table and observation bed if necessary.

BUILDINGS

Why are standards about the facilities and buildings necessary? One hospital built a new wing in such a way that it closed the entrance to the emergency department, leaving the only access through the front door of the hospital, one floor below the emergency department. We know that this hospital was not really interested in the problems of the community—it was content to have accident work taken elsewhere. In another hospital, the emergency department entrance is more easily accessible to the general public than the main entrance. The resulting constant flow of traffic interferes with proper emergency service function.

The emergency service entrance should be well marked and easily accessible but away from the main entrance of the hospital. The ambulance drive should be smooth and even, with minimal turns, without curb, and without an unloading platform. Everything possible should be done to avoid jarring the ambulance patient. The unloading area should be covered, and in rigorous climates it should be enclosed. Stretchers and wheel chairs should have storage space near the entrance.

The construction of the emergency room should provide a large area for immediate care, without partitions but with curtained cubicles so that the staff may take care of several seriously injured patients at the same time and so that the treatment area for any one patient may be either small or large, according to the needs.

Special purpose rooms, such as the following, should be provided:

Small treatment rooms for special types of cases, such as eye injuries.
A quiet room for disturbed or drunken patients.
A doctor's call room.
A waiting room, separated from the working area and equipped with toilets, drinking fountain, and telephone. Relatives and friends and the curious public must not be allowed to crowd into the treatment area.
A room for ambulance attendants, police, and press, also with a telephone.
An observation area. Some patients seen in an emergency department can be properly evaluated only by observation over a period of several hours. It may be wise to have a strict rule that any patient remaining in the emergency department for 8 hours, or some other appropriate period of time, must be admitted or transferred.
The x-ray department should be nearby, or there should be an x-ray unit within the emergency service area. The same considerations apply to the laboratories.

Each emergency department needs careful supervision for the problems of current operation and also for future developments. This requires inter-professional cooperation of administrators, doctors, nurses, and ambulance personnel.

Several publications which are useful guides for improving emergency services and facilities are given in the references.[2,5,6,7,8]

BIBLIOGRAPHY

1. Curry, G. J.: The Ambulance Attendant: His Qualifications and Training, *Bull. A.C.S.*, 41:465–467 (Nov.–Dec.) 1956.

2. Kennedy, R. H.: Guidelines for an Effective Emergency Department, *Hospitals*, 37:101–116 (June) 1963.

3. Knowles, J. H.: The Medical Center and the Community Health Center, *Bull. N. Y. Acad. Med.*, 40:731–742 (Sept.) 1964.

4. New, P. K., Nite, G., Callahan, J.: Too Many Nurses May Be Worse Than Too Few, *Mod. Hosp.*, 93:104–108 (Oct.) 1959.

5. Spencer, J. H.: Emergency Room in General Hospital, *No. Carolina Med. J.*, 25:325–330 (Aug.) 1964.

6. "The Emergency Department in the Hospital—A Guide to Organization and Management," American Hospital Association, Chicago, 1962.

7. A Model of a Hospital Emergency Department, Committee on Trauma, The American College of Surgeons, Chicago, 1964. (Brochure)

8. The Emergency Department: Organization and Operation, The American College of Surgeons, Chicago, 1965. (Motion picture)

II. COMMUNITY EMERGENCY MEDICAL SERVICES

By J. C. Owens, M.D.

J. Cuthbert Owens is professor of surgery at the University of Colorado School of Medicine. He is a member of the Colorado section of the Committee on Trauma of the American College of Surgeons and the coordinator for medical education for national defense. He received the M.D. degree from Marquette University School of Medicine and is a diplomate of the American Board of Surgery. He has been very active in the emergency service field, serving as chairman of the Health and Medical Care Workshop of the Governor's Traffic Safety Conference in 1963 and as a member of the Governor's Medical Advisory Board for Traffic Safety Council. He was involved in Task Force Disaster Planning of the National Academy of Sciences and the National Research Council, and he currently serves as chairman of the ad hoc committee on Voice Communication for Medical Emergency Service of the National Academy of Sciences and the National Research Council.

The organizational structure for community emergency medical services must meet the demands and changing concepts which have been noted in data gathered from recent surveys. While these reports initially centered on hospital emergency departments in large institutions, improvement of emergency medical services is vital at all levels of care and in all communities, regardless of size.

The greatest weakness in emergency medical care is the lack of coordination and cooperation among the facets of emergency medical services—emergency departments, ambulance services, first-aid and rescue units, and accident prevention units. The lay press has stated that emergency medical service in the United States is an "unorganized crazy quilt of bits and pieces that just don't fit together." All the required facilities, techniques, and systems are available; what is needed is to put them all together and make them work. Each community should study and develop means for staffing and equipping its emergency medical services.

Although standards for emergency medical services are desirable, some communities cannot make practical use of them; in these areas the standards should remain as guidelines toward effective, high-quality emergency care. However, the size of the institution or community can seldom if ever be a legitimate excuse for not having excellent initial emergency medical care.

Ambulance and Rescue Units

The ways and means of transportation of the sick and injured are important factors in reducing deaths and other serious effects of injury and illness; however, those in the health professions seldom think of the ambulance business as a member of the family of health services. The close contact which once existed between the medical profession, hospital staffs, and ambulance personnel has been lost. We know of only two small hospitals which conduct a critique with the first-aid personnel on every patient the ambulance service brings to the hospital. These two hospitals probably have the best initial emergency care of any community in their two states because of this coordinated effort.

It is uncommon to find a city, county, or state with a model ambulance ordinance. Most ambulances are poorly constructed, equipped, and manned for managing emergencies. Without an ordinance there is no law to regulate them or the people who drive them and attend the patients. Ambulance drivers are the only unlicensed personnel who care for the sick and injured, yet they are dedicated individuals who receive little respect and little financial reward.

The ambulance service should be improved so that emergency care can be administered as close as possible to the site of the emergency. The first purpose of an ambulance service is to reduce mortality and morbidity for emergency patients; the second purpose is transportation. Improvement is impossible if first-aid training is lacking, if equipment is minimal, if standards are nonexistent, and if the community fails to show interest in the service until an obvious mistake is made or there is a threat to discontinue the service.

First Aid

What do hospital emergency department personnel know about first-aid training in their communities? In many hospitals one finds no knowledge whatsoever, and small hospitals give a better report than the large ones. In some communities, the response to calls for volunteers for first-aid training has been so poor that it is left up to a few interested individuals who are usually city or county officials. When there is little interest in first-aid training in a community, the hospital emergency facilities and the ambulance services are usually poor.

Signs

Highway and street signs locating a hospital are seldom adequate to assist the public in case of an emergency. Not only are highway and street signs lacking, but in some instances there is no sign to identify the hospital. Upon arrival at the hospital emergency entrance, several additional problems may face the patient: thoughtlessly parked private cars and delivery trucks may block the driveway to the emergency unit entrance; in multilingual areas, only English may be used for signs; some hospitals seem to make a game of which door to enter for emergency service, for many unmarked possibilities may be noted. Adequate identification of hospital emergency facilities has never been more important than today.

Communication

Prompt and direct voice communication for all community emergency services insures maximum coordination for emergencies of any magnitude. No project is more important than assuring that all emergency medical services have adequate radio communication. Lack of communication has been the greatest bottleneck initially in every disaster encountered in this country. A well-organized communication system that is used daily not only increases the efficiency in managing needs for immediate medical care but also has a tremendous potential for coordination of community emergency medical services.

Emergency Department Census

There has been a sudden and unbelievable increase in the patient load in hospital emergency departments. Both physicians and hospitals have brought strong public awareness of scientific progress and its place in comprehensive medical care. The public expects this progress to be immediately available in the emergency department of every general hospital. This concept has augmented the use and function of the hospital, brought about architectural changes, and forced a re-evaluation of the purpose and perspective of the institution. The modern physician must bring his pattern of medical practice into conformity with the changing concepts. He can afford neither the equipment, the personnel, nor the time necessary for emergency medical care in his office.

Many causes have figured significantly in the increased emergency service load, but public awareness that the hospital is always available with a full complement of staff and equipment seems to be the chief one. Emergency service census figures should be evaluated on the basis of the patient's interpretation of his illness, facilities for medical care in the community, the time of the day and day of the week, the availability of physicians, and whether the patient is a resident or nonresident.

Decreasing the Non-emergency Census. Although each hospital is an individual entity, all experience similar types of emergencies. The problems of decreasing the non-emergency load are discouragingly numerous. There will always be some non-emergency patients because of varying interpretations of "what is an emergency."

There are four units in the organizational planning of a hospital which can relieve the emergency department of non-emergent patients: the admitting desk, the outpatient department, the screening clinic, and the ambulatory laboratory and radiology clinic. An examining room apart from the emergency unit should be available in every hospital. This encourages good public relations since the most emergent patient is given priority; if treatment is not instituted, the patient is not charged.

Separate examining rooms for non-emergencies are noted more frequently at small hospitals than at large institutions. Since the outpatient department is next to the emergency unit in most hospitals, some keep the area open as an OPD until 10:00 P.M. or utilize the space for enlarging the emergency department during the peak load period after 5:00 P.M. when the OPD would be closed.

In large hospitals, screening clinics have become essential to lessen the load and economic burden on the emergency area.

Many hospitals may provide offices for physicians in or adjacent to the building. This apparently follows a national trend.

Trends in Specialty Care

Surgical patients, and especially trauma cases, once monopolized the census of emergency rooms. In recent years, the quantity of non-surgical emergency patients has increased and has necessitated a number of specialists other than surgeons to practice in the emergency unit.

The value of assigning observation beds to the emergency area has been recognized by internists and surgeons; the need for facilities for respiratory and cardiac resuscitation and for the subtle methods of predicting and monitoring shock due to medical conditions are also recognized. Pediatricians have become aware of the potential of the emergency unit in centralizing poison control, in immediate care of acute respiratory obstruction, in the management of accidents which cause high mortality and morbidity in children and adolescents, and in handling the large number of children who need attention after 5:00 P.M. when most physicians' offices are closed. Psychiatrists and psychiatric social workers have also begun to see patients in the emergency unit. Each service recognizes the teaching asset which is available in the area.

Accident prevention investigation is beginning to appear in the emergency department along with instruction in first aid and triage techniques, all of which enhances the team aspect of emergency care.

Assignment of Nurses

The nurse's position in the emergency department has become more prominent with the growth of the department. If she is to keep up with her increased responsibilities, she needs special graduate courses. These courses need to be developed, for few have been offered other than an annual program presented by the American Hospital Association on Emergency Department Organization and Management of Nurses.

Indoctrination of nursing personnel is woefully lacking in a majority of hospital emergency units. Substitute nurses frequently are not aware of emergency unit policies, equipment storage, or even techniques for assisting in emergency procedures.

Emergency procedures instituted by nurses are usually discouraged in the absence of a physician. Nurses should be encouraged to add procedures for direct care of the patient to their duties in assisting the doctor, whether he is present or not. If nurses are not permitted to have greater responsibilities in the direct care of the patient during the absence of a physician, another individual needs to be added to the medical field—the emergency department technician. The common dictum that emergency department coverage should be such that a patient is seen by a physician within 15 minutes after arrival is totally inadequate for the patient who needs vital care within 3 to 5 minutes. A few hospitals utilize men who were former armed forces corpsmen or hospital administrative corps officers. These men also may replace orderlies when required.

Physician's Call Systems

Although many methods for calling physicians have been devised, none has had much success in solving the problem of securing immediate emergency medical care. A physician should be available on second call if unexpected or unusual situations arise, and some mechanism should also be available whereby specialty services can be obtained. No system is really effective unless a doctor is on call in the hospital, an impossible plan for small hospitals.

Short of full-time salaried physicians, good systems that have been observed in several hospitals include the following:

1. In a 350-bed hospital with complete specialty coverage and with only interns on the house staff, 70 general practitioners rotate call in the hospital from 5:00 P.M. to 8:00 A.M.

2. In a 200-bed hospital with complete specialty coverage but with no interns or residents, 50 general practitioners rotate call at the hospital on a 24-hour basis.

3. In a small hospital, all doctors have radio communication with the hospital.

Every physician should be expected to shoulder some part of the responsibilities in the community for emergency medical care. It is unrealistic and impractical for all emergencies to be handled by a few interested physicians; medical schools and internship and residency training programs should continually stress this approach.

Although specialty coverage may be difficult for small communities because of distances involved, the specialty fields should seek methods of improving the present poor situation. Movement of critically ill or injured patients from one hospital to another is a serious hazard which should be eliminated.

Emergency Department Manual

Standard procedures and policies for the emergency department should be written and readily available in all hospitals. A complete lack of standards or routines may involve not only medical care standards, but also administrative standards and procedures. The hospital administrator, physician, or nurse cannot excuse the environment and its lack of predictability when there are no standard procedures.

Standards are usually available from the State Health Department to assist the hospitals in writing their own emergency manual which will properly indoctrinate the personnel. Standards are also available from the American Hospital Association and the American College of Surgeons.

Emergency Department Committee

An emergency department committee should formulate and execute policies. Committee members should represent the major clinical services, hospital administration, and nursing services, as well as the ambulance services and a community coordinator who oversees all emergency medical services in the community. Failure to have this wide representation may lead to disorganization, with the services being merely paralled adjuncts without coordination.

Medical Audit

Current hospital practice demands a systematic medical review of in-patient medical records, but such a review is rarely if ever applied to emergency department medical records. An audit of this type has tremendous educational value and also provides an organized method of determining adherence to policies and standards. Recommendations for changes in hospital practice and emergency department policy procedure may be developed by the emergency department committee from the findings of the audit. The few institutions which have undertaken this program have found it to be invaluable in improving the organization and management of the emergency department.

Disaster Plans

Despite the requirement of the Joint Commission on Accreditation of Hospitals that all hospitals have a disaster plan and have two trial runs each year, less than half the hospitals are able to produce disaster plans. The majority of disaster plans that do exist are incomplete, inadequate or outdated. Some of the best plans have been found in hospitals with less than 50 beds.

Taking a program out of mothballs on rare occasions and expecting it to work efficiently is inconceivable, especially if daily emergency care is not coordinated with the plan.

Equipment

Adequate facilities—including necessary medications, airways, tracheostomy tubes, manual positive pressure breathing apparatus, defibrilators, and suction machines—should be immediately available in the emergency department and should be as simple as possible to meet the needs. Borrowing equipment or having emergency equipment in areas away from the emergency department should never be permitted, even if duplication of equipment is necessary. The stretcher or examining table should be freely movable and should be x-ray permeable to limit needless transferring of the patient. Exchange stretchers should be arranged with ambulance services to further decrease patient movement and eliminate needless waiting by ambulance personnel.

Reference Materials

Reference books on such subjects as toxicology, ambulatory surgery, fractures, public health, and pediatrics should be available. The physician is at a disadvantage when he is required to institute treatment for a condition not related to his specific interests unless he has immediate access to suitable references.

Economics

The public expresses great dissatisfaction over the minimum fee charge when no procedure has been performed and especially when their physician meets them in the emergency room for his convenience. Administrators state that the fees are a many-sided necessity, but they constitute a significant public relations problem.

There is no argument against the hospital receiving a just financial return for emergency services, but there are many instances in which the charge is abused. For example, a "courtesy" space may not be provided for a physician to see a patient whom he has requested to meet him at the emergency department, even though the complaint is not emergent. Hospitals must make reasonable charges, but a profit should not be expected from the emergency department. The costs must be balanced with the service rendered.

Many economic deficiencies may be noted in the emergency unit, such as undercharging and not including x-ray and laboratory procedures on emergency room patients in the cost analysis. A master record must be kept on the number of patients seen, the length of time they were present, the type of complaints, and the treatment given. It is inconceivable that a realistic budget necessary to operate the unit can be accurately determined without this information.

Procedures

As a general principle, surgical procedures in the emergency department should be limited to suture of lacerations, reduction of fractures, and local or regional block anesthesia. Exceptions may be resuscitative emergencies or supportive treatment for acute conditions of a serious nature. There should be specific policies regarding the type of cases to be taken to the operating room, rather than leaving the decision to the discretion of the physician.

Policies should be established on the use of antiseptics, scrubbing before suturing lacerations, and the use of a cap and mask during the procedure, all of which should follow the same practices as in the operating suite.

No procedure needs more attention than the emergency treatment of airway obstruction and other critical respiratory problems. Every physician who practices in the emergency unit should be skilled in the installation of an endotracheal tube, in performing a tracheostomy, in applying positive breathing by means of an ambu bag, in obtaining physiologic proof of adequate tissue oxygen perfusion, and in performing cardiopulmonary resuscitation in cardiac arrest. The care of the open airway is one of the most frequent weaknesses found in emergency units, despite reports that 10,000 deaths from automobile accidents each year result from chest injuries; and respiratory obstruction is probably the most common single cause of sudden death in infants and children.

Methods of monitoring shock—determination of central venous pressure or of arterial and venous oxygen saturation, the tilt test, etc.— should be initiated in the emergency department before the patient is moved. Established hospital policies for tetanus prophylaxis, poison control, burns, and others should be prominently posted.

CONCLUSION

Certification by the State Health Department is the only factor that governs a hospital other than the legal responsibility of the board of trustees. Membership in the state hospital association, which requires certain administrative standards, is not mandatory and has no jurisdiction over the doctors. The state medical society can control its members, but not the hospitals, and not all physicians are members. Other than those few communities that have a model ambulance ordinance, no organization controls the ambulance services, directly or indirectly. Community coordination of all services is essential in local and state-wide medical planning for mass casualties and disasters, as well as for patients who require emergency services daily. Every community should have a coordinator, counselor, or committee to study and advise on the problems of emergency medical services.

Emergency medical care is changing. These services are becoming more important in health care activities of every community. All individuals in the health field should realize that the mortality and morbidity of patients in need of emergency care is high, and they should take a hard look at the emergency medical services really offered.

32

Disaster Planning

By George L. Thorpe, M.D.

George L. Thorpe is the director of outpatient services at St. Joseph Hospital and Rehabilitation Center in Wichita, Kansas, and he is the chairman of the hospital's disaster committee. He received the M.D. degree from Tulane University. He is a member of the American Academy of General Practice.

A disaster may be defined as the arrival, with little or no warning, of many more casualties of all types and degree of severity than our personnel and physical facilities are equipped to handle, at a time of partial to total disruption of normal service in the institution. Hospitals have widely varying patient capacities, supply problems, storage space, community resources and support, and medical, nursing and technical talent with enormous differences in ability, availability, and adaptability. With these variables in mind, each hospital should design a plan adapted to its own specific needs, one that is strong enough to accommodate maximum casualty loads foreseeable for that community.

PLANNING COMMITTEE

It is the rare institution that can depend on a single individual to do all of its planning, although this might be ideal in the smaller hospitals. A disaster planning committee needs the help of all departments and services within its organization for developing its plan and for leadership during a disaster situation.

Membership on the committee may include administrators, clinical (medical) director, business manager, director of nursing service, director of volunteer service, food manager, building engineer, comptroller or chief accountant, supply officer, public relations officer, medical records librarian, chief of laboratory service, and chiefs of clinical departments whose services might be critical.

The *functions* of the disaster committee are:

1. To develop the hospital's disaster plan
2. To coordinate the hospital's plan with a community-wide disaster plan or with community Civil Defense
3. To develop departmental plans in support of the hospital disaster plan
4. To assign staff physicians to specific areas of the hospital, including physicians allocated to the hospital by the county medical society
5. To establish standard emergency medical care procedures for the hospital
6. To conduct and supervise training programs for physicians, nurses, technicians, attendants, and custodial personnel on management and medical aspects of mass casualties
7. To supervise drills to test the hospital disaster plan in various simulated disaster situations
8. To review and revise the disaster plan at regular intervals as indicated by periodic drills
9. To designate subcommittees to assume specific functions of the disaster committee (i.e., emergency food and water storage, etc.)
10. To individually supervise and direct the operation of their own areas in event of an actual disaster
11. To provide education and information for all concerned.

ADAPTABILITY

Planning should be based on facilities, supplies, and manpower that are normally present or available to the hospital. Promises of outside support should not be depended upon to activate the plan. In every division of the disaster plan, a *distinct chain of command* should be established so that the absence of one or several individuals will not delay the activation of any part of the plan. This places responsibility upon those to whom the plan has given authority to act in the name of the planning unit.[1]

In the hectic atmosphere created by disasters there must be *one person to coordinate* all efforts being made to handle casualties as efficiently and quickly as possible. This assignment normally is given to the hospital administrator because of his intimate knowledge of the resources available for immediate use. The adaptability of a disaster plan hinges on the ability, availability, and adaptability of the person in charge. Not all hospital administrators are emotionally and psychologically suited to cope with the uncertainties, responsibilities, and stresses of disaster situations. The plan should designate in numerical order several individuals with known ability to assume direction of the plan in event of a disaster and to provide an unbroken chain of command under all circumstances.

MAJOR AREAS OF RESPONSIBILITY

Medical Care of Casualties. This is the reason for all the planning. Physicians by their training and by the nature of their daily practice are able to cope with emergency problems routinely. A subcommittee of physicians should plan the assignment of medical personnel to the various teams (i.e., surgical, fracture, shock, triage, etc.) to make the maximum use of the talents available.

Nursing Service. Like medical care, this requires a minimum of planning. In disaster situations, the assignment of duty areas is an extension of the normal nursing routine.

The Administrative Area. This requires the greatest amount of pre-disaster planning, for it comprises all the functions of supply, service, communications, publicity, transportation, repair, and maintenance. These areas are most likely to encounter unforeseen interruptions. Administration must cope with the hysterical relatives of casualties, disrupted communications and utilities, damaged or destroyed buildings and supplies, transportation and security troubles, recruitment and direction of volunteer man power, and urgent requests from the medical and nursing areas that seem almost impossible to fulfill.

MEDICAL SERVICE

It is within the medical service division that the direction and treatment of the patient originates. The physician in charge is responsible for the overall supervision of the medical care that patients receive. Upon authority of the doctor, the nursing division will function.

Type Sorting Casualties (Triage). Sorting of the injured by the most mature physician available, usually a general practitioner or a surgeon, is the key to the management of mass casualty patients; it is only by this means that they may be categorized properly and separated so that there is a minimum time lag between injury and onset of therapy. In its application, sorting considers the necessity for overlooking no one and for doing the greatest amount of good for the largest number of casualties.

Priority of Treatment. Patients are categorized by their injuries to determine priority of treatment.

Group I minimal injuries—no priority. Some in this group may be able to assist in the care of patients in the other categories.

Group II immediate—highest priority for surgical treatment. In this group, relatively short procedures may suffice to save life. Definitive surgery can be delayed.

Group III—Next highest priority for surgical treatment. The delay in the surgical treatment of this group may lead to infection, but their lives will not be unduly jeopardized by the delay. The time lag between the injury and surgery will depend upon the number of professional personnel and facilities available.

Group IV—Lowest priority. This group is operative procedures requiring reconstructive measures. These patients need such lengthy and technically complicated procedures that institution of therapy for one of these casualties would theoretically jeopardize the lives of several casualties in higher priority groups. The treatment of this group is not one of masterful neglect but rather consists of emergency measures to maintain the patient until the availability of facilities, supplies, and personnel permit definitive treatment.

Area Sorting Casualties. The experiences reported from disaster situations indicate the advisability of establishing areas for the holding and treatment of categories such as shock, burns, fractures, immediate surgery, medical problems, post-anesthesia, and morgue. The conversion of service areas (dining areas, classrooms, auditoriums, etc.) into wards must be planned and the needed equipment for their use provided. The type of disaster, the available personnel, and the physicial facilities dictate these arrangements.[2,3]

Nursing Service

Disaster planning in the area of nursing is mainly a matter of personnel mobilization and assignment of nurses, orderlies, and volunteer help to medical teams and to areas as the situation indicates. The care of patients who are in the hospital at the time of the disaster and their movement to temporary areas in order to clear wards and rooms for critical casualties are largely nursing service functions.

The establishment of a *nursing manpower pool* (made up of nonworking RN's, LPN's, nurse aides, and technicians) who agree to respond to call for service in a disaster and with a predetermined method of notification is one of the most effective means of supplementing the nursing service.

Administration

The administrative area requires the most detailed planning for disaster situations. So varied are the demands and so critical are the needs in the presence of all sorts of disruption of normal services that the ability to cope with a disaster might be measured by the resourcefulness and ingenuity of the administrative leaders. The following outline gives the major areas of administrative concern:

A. Supplies
    1. Medical: community resources, government agencies with medical stockpiles
        a. Dressings
        b. Drugs
        c. Anesthetics
        d. Oxygen
        e. Emergency cabinets with keys available containing essential supplies prominently labeled "Disaster" or "Emergency"
        f. Prepackaged emergency hospitals
    2. Utilities (when normal sources are disrupted)
        a. Water with alternate sources and purification methods
        b. Fuel for heat and cooking
        c. Electricity for auxiliary circuits to operating rooms, emergency rooms, x-ray, etc.
    3. Food (methods of preparation if normal utilities are disrupted)
        a. Kitchen stores for patients and help
        b. Special foods for nurseries and diets
        c. Alternate sources and emergency stockpiles
B. Communications (usually designated as the Control Center)
    1. Telephone switchboard
        a. Direct phone lines for alternate use
    2. Disaster radio
        a. Local amateur radio "ham" clubs
        b. Special hospital channels with self-contained power service
        c. Civil Defense net with independent power source
    3. Messenger system using community organizations, such as Boy Scouts
C. Traffic (this may be the most difficult problem)
    1. Internal (signs prepared in advance to direct traffic flow)
        a. Routing of casualties
        b. Control of visitors
        c. Supply routes
    2. External (signs prepared in advance)
        a. Roads cleared for incoming casualties
        b. Guarding entrances of hospital to keep out non-essential people
    3. Auxiliary source of transportation
        a. For transport of dismissed hospital patients
        b. Personal vehicles for emergency transport

D. Personnel
1. Regular hospital employees to carry an identification pass: "_____ is a key person in the _____ Hospital disaster plan. This person's services are required at the hospital."

Signed _____

Administrator

2. Establishment of a volunteer manpower pool for all to draw on as needed
3. Establish and activate a system of notification of volunteers in co-operation with the nursing service

E. Records⁴
1. Identification tags
2. Admissions
   a. Personal property security
   b. Master casualty list
3. Disposition
   a. Master discharge list
   b. Morgue

F. Evacuation. If the hospital has an internal disaster or if its plant becomes endangered during a disaster, provision for the evacuation of its patients must be included in all plans.

On this basic framework, each hospital must build a disaster plan suited to its particular needs. No attempt has been made to discuss the enormous amount of detailed planning that is necessary and which must be based on individual hospitals and local situations.

TYPES OF DISASTERS

Community Disasters (Train Wrecks, Plane Crashes, Theatre Fires, and Injuries to Persons in Large Assemblies). This requires mainly expansion of beds, medical manpower, and reserve supplies, all of which should be readily obtainable from nearby sources.

Natural Disasters (Tornadoes, Floods, Earthquakes, and Severe Storms). Such disasters are much like community disasters except for the complications of loss of utilities, transportation difficulties, and communication problems. Even in these instances, additional supplies and help are rapidly obtainable from outside the disaster area. Evacuation of patients to other less crowded facilities usually can be speedily arranged.

Atomic Attack. Disaster planning for atomic attack cannot be on an individual institution basis because the problems are totally different.

If one considers the results of even a small atomic explosion, it is apparent that cooperative planning between adjacent communities is the only logical approach. A few facts will illustrate the problem.

If an eight megaton weapon is exploded in your area (few atomic weapons are now below 20 megaton size), expect the effect of blast and heat to destroy all physical and biological materials within a 4-mile radius of the epicenter. In a 4- to 8-mile radius there is a good possibility for survival of individuals in shelters from the initial effects of blast and heat. In this area, frame houses would be destroyed, flying debris would cause considerable injury, and people in the open would sustain third degree burns. In addition, everyone within this 12-mile radius who reflexly looked at the flash would sustain severe burns of the retina. The effects of radiation released by this weapon is another story which we shall leave to the experts in that field, except to note that a probable lethal dose of radiation would be sustained by all who survived the initial effects of heat and blast within a 9-mile radius.

The above facts indicate that for the first few days following the explosion the casualties treated would consist mainly of walking wounded who were able to travel 20 to 25 miles with little or no help. Other types of casualties would be found only by rescue squads from nearby, nonaffected areas.

SUMMARY

Planning can improve service in times of disaster; dry runs and drills make the plan work. Frequent revision must be accomplished; new personnel must be trained; and every employee must have a thorough understanding of the part he plays in the event of disaster. These measures will produce efficient care of the greatest number of casualties in the shortest time.

The American Hospital Association in Chicago offers several services including a list of aids in disaster planning. If you have a plan and would like to know how well it measures up to the demands of a disaster, get a copy of their "Check List for Hospital Disaster Planning," and check yourself out. The Bacon Library of the American Hospital Association will lend an excellent file of material.

BIBLIOGRAPHY

1. Carlisle, B.: If a Disaster Should Hit . . . Would Your Hospital Be Prepared? *Hosp. Management,* 80:39–41 (Sept.) 1955.

2. Mills, W. J.: Emergency Medical Treatment of Casualties at Providence Hospital, *Alaska Med.,* 6:39–41 (June) 1964.

3. Langston, D. V.: A Hospital in a Disaster Area, *JAMA*, 189:306–307 (July 27) 1964.

4. Siffen, F.: Medical Records for a Disaster, *Hospitals, JAHA,* 38:79–97 (Mar. 16) 1964.

33

The Impact of Medicare on the Hospital Staff

By Roberta Fenlon, M.D.

Roberta Fenlon is an internist in private practice in San Francisco, California. She received the M.D. degree from the Universty of Iowa and is a member of the American College of Physicians. She has been active in organized medicine and has the distinction of being the only woman who has been president of the San Francisco County Medical Society in its history of 98 years. For a number of years, she has been a counselor of the California Medical Association. She is a member of the Mental Health Advisory Board for the city of San Francisco.

Dr. Fenlon is an active member of the staff of Children's Hospital in San Francisco and has served as vice-chief of staff and as a member of the executive committee. She is also associate clinical professor of medicine at the University of California School of Medicine in San Francisco. When the Medicare legislation was implemented in the fall of 1965, Dr. Fenlon left her practice for four months to serve as the Chief Medical Consultant to the Social Security Administration for Medicare. Since returning to her practice, she has continued to serve as a consultant.

The physician's role under Medicare will be the same as it always has been. When he hospitalizes a patient or sends him to a nursing home, he will assume the same responsibility both in the admission process and in the medical care after the patient has been admitted. The significant change is in the hospital environment. Participating hospitals and nursing homes must have a utilization review mechanism which some may not have had in the past. This requirement will have important effects upon the staff physician, and and it is essential that he understands its potential impact upon the hospital medical staff.

UTILIZATION REVIEW

The utilization review plan provides for *continuing reviews by mechanism of the institution's own choice or creation.* It can be a hospital staff committee including two or more physicians, or it can be a group outside the hospital which is similar in composition to the staff committee. The committee or other mechanism set up under the plan will be responsible for undertaking two kinds of reviews.

The first kind of review, which may be on a sample basis, looks into the various elements of *utilization retrospectively*—admission, services provided, and length of stay—from the standpoint of their medical necessity. This review is essentially educational; that is, the committee's activities, by providing a professional scrutiny of practices within the institution, result in the formulation of appropriate professional criteria with regard to the medical necessity for hospitalization and the provision of medical services.

The second kind of review must be of *the individual beneficiary remaining in the institution for a period of "extended duration."* For this review, the period or periods that shall be considered long stays are specified in the law. Each committee will be asked to specify in its plan the number of continous days of hospitalization following which a review would be made to determine whether further inpatient services are medically necessary. This review is to be made within one week following the last day of such a specified period of continuous hospitalization. When the committee's findings with respect to the medical necessity for continued hospitalization disagree with those of the attending physician, the committee is required to notify the attending physician of its findings and also to provide an opportunity for consultation between the committee and the physician. If, after the consultation, the physician members of the utilization review committee decide that continued hospital care is not medically necessary, the attending physician, the patient, and the administrator are so notified. Social Security funds are then relieved of the liability of paying for further care after the third day following the day the institution receives notice of such finding. However, no report will be required from the committee other than that the case has been considered if the committee does not come to a negative conclusion. The judgment of the attending physician in an extended care case must be considered carefully by the review committee.

Underlying Principles. These should be taken into consideration by the hospital staff in effectively and reasonably implementing the utilization review provisions:

1. The plan should have as its overall objective *the maintenance of high-quality patient care and an increase in effective utilization of hospital services.* This is achieved through an educational approach involving a study of the patterns of care and bed utilization.

2. It must always *maintain the right and responsibility of physicians to make the decisions* regarding hospital admission, course of treatment, and length of stay based on the medical needs of the patient.

3. Under its governing body and through its medical staff, *the individual hospital must carry full responsibility for the effectiveness and efficiency of the operation of the utilization review plan.* Since no two hospitals are alike, each must develop its own utilization review procedures within the framework of professionally established criteria and the allowable limits of the law. This provision is based on congressional committee reports which clearly indicate that the intent of Congress was to provide a flexible framework within which hospitals and physicians could develop, in the light of professional considerations, the most appropriate procedure for each individual institution. *Explicit* in these principles is the inviolability of the physician's right and duty to exercse his medical judgment. *Implicit* is the joint hospital-physician responsibility for effective hospital utilization.

The hospital administrator must also be concerned with facets of the hospital's *day-to-day operation which influence efficient use of the hospital facilities.* He can assume his share of the responsibility by assuring that the utilization review functions performed by the medical staff have the support and assistance of the hospital's administrative staff in assembling information, facilitating chart reviews, conducting studies, exploring ways to improve administrative procedures, maintaining committee records, and promoting the most efficient use of available health services and facilities. In addition, he must see that the costs incurred in connection with the implementation of the utilization review plan are included in the definition of reasonable costs, which are reimbursable to the extent that such costs relate to health insurance program beneficiaries.

Although the law states, in describing the utilization review plan, that reviews shall be conducted by a "staff committee" or by a group outside the hospital, *more than one committee may properly be involved in utilization reviews.* Thus, the medical care appraisal and the educational aspects of review need not be conducted by the same committee or group. Also, it is not mandatory that the medical staff create a new committee; *existing staff committees may assume the review responsibility* stipulated in the hospital's review plan.

It is obvious that the staff physician will find himself working closely with hospital administration and with his fellow physicians. This increased interdependence should be beneficial to all parties. Increased knowledge and understanding of one another's problems could give increased strength to the involved individuals.

The public has demanded that advances in medical care be available to all, and it wants evidence of it. When it has not been evident, hospitals and physicians have often been subjected to legal action, and this has placed a great burden particularly upon the physicians. By necessity, he has had to order tests which actually only corroborated his knowledge. X-rays have been taken for "proof" of his physical findings. Specific procedures which were indicated have been modified or dispensed with entirely. It is hoped that utilization review will eliminate much of this vexing problem and strengthen the position of those interested in quality care at decreased cost.

Utilization review should be planned so that all physicians participate on a rotating basis. The knowledge gained should be valuable and stimulating and should encourage even better professional relationships.

Much of the added burden of another hospital committee can be alleviated by *using existing committees* in some instances and by the use of record room or other hospital personnel. Help in post-hospital planning should be made available through the hospital and home health agencies. Families, hospitals, and the community will share what previously has been primarily the physician's burden.

Conceivably, utilization review may *stimulate physicians to take more refresher courses* or to seek opportunities for additional training. Case discussion has traditionally been the stimulus for further study—utilization review conferences should be no exception.

The medical staff must plan together, particularly in the first few months, for the *admission of so-called "elective" cases.* This step is essential if the hospital and staff are not to be overloaded and if beds for the acutely ill are to remain available. Programing for this can be easily achieved if the staff is an organized and actively planning group.

The burden of *resisting the unnecessary use of hospitals and nursing homes,* for such use will be tempting to some of the elderly and their families, will rest primarily on the physicians. It will not differ in kind but it may differ in degree from the responsibility in dealing with subscribers to any hospital insurance plan. The utilization review committee should prove valuable in this respect because the physician will have professional support for his opinions. The family and patient must abide by them or assume full financial responsibility of hospitalization. The legal responsibility of the physician does not change under Medicare, but now he will have both colleague and administrative support for many of his professional decisions.

HOSPITAL-BASED PHYSICIANS

Under PL 89–97, physicians' charges in teaching hospitals, except fees for interns and residents but including those of the hospital-based specialists, are reimbursable under the medical insurance plan (Part B); they cannot be included under the hospital insurance plan (Part A). The benefits under Part B are on an elective basis and are financed by both the enrollee and by matching funds from the general revenue of the government. The hospital benefits (Part A) are financed primarily from contributions of individuals during their working years (Social Security), and the coverage is not voluntary. Hospital costs must therefore be separated from physicians' services.

Each individual hospital and hospital-based physician must reach some agreement wherein the requirements of the law are met. Existing arrangements between hospitals and hospital-based physicians have varied widely, and there may be variation from one department to another. The Medicare program does not require any change in these arrangements, but there must be an analysis to distinguish between the medical and surgical services rendered by a physician and the hospital services.

The hospital and the physician may, if they wish, pool the two payments through assignment of the physician's fee to the hospital and subsequently distributing the proceeds according to their pre-existing agreement. They may, on the other hand, change their previous agreement in any way that is mutually satisfactory as long as the total cost of service to patients is not increased.

The impact of this requirement in the law has occasioned much soul-searching by physicians in general and by the hospital-based physician in particular. The anesthesiologist, psychiatrist, and roentgenologist have in many instances previously clarified their position. The pathologist has not always been able to do so. Now the decision must be made by every individual hospital-based specialist. The following methods are available to him:

1. Being fully compensated by the hospital which bills for all services.
2. Becoming involved with a percentage of income from the department and billing for his position.
3. Making arrangements to undertake the responsibility for employment of personnel, to provide the equipment and supplies needed, and to bill the patient directly for their charges.

While there is a choice, the fact is that the specialty societies involved have recommended that their members make arrangements which will maintain their independence—they should coordinate their services closely with other medical and hospital services, and there should be no control by the administration or any unlicensed person. If these recommendations are ignored, the specialists may become separated from their colleagues, a mutual loss which could undermine hospital staff morale. If the medical staff is organized without benefit of all the physicians concerned or if one group of physicians is primarily responsible to the administration, the consequences could be disastrous to not only the patients but also to the hospital.

OTHER ASPECTS OF PL 89–97

In general, *the conditions of participation for hospitals are the same as those now required by the Joint Commission on Accreditation of Hospitals.* In fact, after Medicare was enacted, the Joint Commission included in its requirements the duties of a utilization committee. For physicians not practicing in an accredited hospital, this may mean an all-out effort to gain its accreditation. Although this may be a burden, the reward should be worth the effort in improving the quality of hospital care.

Certification and recertification for hospitalization may be by a stamp or preprinted form which the physician will sign along with his orders.

Reimbursement procedures are similar to those of private insurance. The physician, if he chooses to accept an assignment of the patient's insurance rights, will receive payment from the designated insurance company in his area, or he may bill his patient directly in whatever amount he deems proper. If he accepts assignment, he completes the lower portion of the official form which asks only for the essentials of the fee, the procedure performed, the date, and where it took place. The insurance company will reimburse him for 80 per cent of the reasonable charge for this procedure. The other 20 per cent may be collected from the patient. If the physician decides to bill the patient directly, he must supply the patient with a receipted bill which itemizes the type of services and where and when rendered.

Congress specified the *three guidelines to be followed by the carriers in making determinations of what constitutes a "reasonable charge."* First, the reasonable charge must be generally in line with the physician's usual and customary charge for the same service. Second, the reasonable charge must conform with the prevailing charges for similar services in the locality. Third, the reasonable charge on which Medicare beneficiary payments are based cannot be higher than the reasonable charge which would be determined by the intermediary carrier for its own policy holders. The actual determination of charges is in the hands of the carriers; but if the physician does not choose to accept payments from them under the assignment, he is not bound by their determination of what is reasonable.

Medicare is designed to help the aged meet their medical bills, not to make changes in either the medical care that is given or the manner in which it is given. The hospital insurance plan could reassure the physician that all procedures necessary for the patient can be obtained, and there need be no consideration of his limited finances or the problem of depleting his savings.

Under both the hospital insurance plan and the voluntary insurance plan, a patient may obtain 20 days of *diagnostic studies at a hospital on an outpatient basis.* He must pay the first 20 dollars of the charges. There has been a growing trend to center medical practice and medical care around the general hospital. The inclusion of these diagnostic studies in the law could accelerate this trend with more and more physicians leaving the central parts of a city to practice near or even in the hospital of their choice. The trend could also give rise to various forms of group practice depending upon the size of the hospital staff. More interdependence among physicians and the allied professions, technicians, and administration will be forthcoming.

CONCLUSION

No one has a crystal ball, but the impact of this legislation could entirely change the practice of medicine. The basic issues underlying this change revolve about whether the costs will increase unreasonably and whether the patient will receive depersonalized care. The answers will depend not only upon the physician but also upon society—governmental agencies, allied health fields, voluntary health agencies, hospitals, insurance companies, and legislators will all contribute to the final outcome. Nevertheless, the responsibility will remain primarily with the physician. The Hippocratic Oath and the basic objective of the medical profession, as stated by the American Medical Association, commit physicians "To promote the art and science of medicine and the betterment of the public health."

Part V

Graduate Medical Education and the Hospital

34

Education for Health and Medical Service— The Long Pull

By Ward Darley, M.D.

Ward Darley is a native of Colorado. After receiving the M.D. degree and his internship and
residency training at the University of Colorado
School of Medicine, he practiced internal medicine in Denver for a number of years and was
active in the staff organizations of several of
the Denver private hospitals. During this period
he was a member of the volunteer faculty of
the medical school and rose from the rank of
instructor to professor of medicine. He is a diplomate of the American Board of Internal Medicine and a Fellow of the American College of
Physicians.

Dr. Darley became Dean of the University of
Colorado School of Medicine, then Vice President for Medical Affairs, and then served as
President of the University. He became the Executive Director of the Association of American
Medical Colleges and during this tenure, from
1957 to 1964, the Association grew greatly in
stature and influence in medical education
throughout the world. He continues to serve as
the Executive Secretary of the National Intern
Matching Program and currently he is visiting
professor of medicine at the University of Colorado School of Medicine and consultant to several national medical and educational organizations. He has been the recipient of many honors,
one of the more recent ones being the Flexner
Award of the A.A.M.C. bestowed in November,
1965. He is an Honorary Fellow of the American

College of Hospital Administrators, and an honorary member of the American Hospital Association.

There is much that is implicit in this subject. First, it is implicit that
"education for health and medical service" means much more than the
education of physicians and that the word "service" includes much
more than the activity of physicians.

Next, it is implicit that as we consider "the long pull" we recognize
and plan for the inevitability of change. And in this planning, human
nature and educability being what they are, it must be remembered
that it takes time—much time—before changes in education can have
any appreciable effect upon the structure and function of any of the
elements of a society. Particularly in medicine, I believe this factor of
time is such that unless we can keep our system of education ahead of
the scientific and social pressures that are so rapidly changing our way
of life, any excellence or effectiveness that this system now has will be
but a point in time that will rapidly pass and leave us in the wake of
yesterday. In other words, we have no time to lose. The long pull in
medical education must get under way today.

As we look ahead to this long pull, I submit that all thinking and
planning should be in line with the best possible education and that
nothing should be considered or accepted that will compromise this
principle. This will permit a look at the future and at what the future
ought to be, without our being sidetracked by present confusions, ten-
sions, and problems.

NEW DEFINITIONS

To begin with, I suggest new definitions for the terms "medical care"
and "medical education." [1] It is important that the definition of medical
care encompass the field of total care—the evaluation and management
of health as well as of disease and the practice of both health management and disease management—utilizing supporting personnel, services, and facilities at the level of the practitioner and his patient. Medical education, then, must no longer be limited to the education of physicians. It must be considered as embracing education in all of the
disciplines, at all levels, in all of the professional and technical fields
that can contribute to the effectiveness of health and medical care.

The need for these new definitions has its roots in the increasing body
of knowledge and the new techniques that are becoming increasingly important to biology and human health and medicine. As new knowledge
and techniques have developed, and as the consequent demands and
the methods of delivering health and medical care have changed, the

field of medicine has necessarily been fragmented into learnable parts. The result is called specialization. This fragmentation of knowledge has been largely the result of research. But specialization stimulates more research which in turn produces more knowledge and more techniques, thus giving impetus to more specialization. Continued specialization, therefore, is inevitable. It follows, then, that if the new definitions of medical care and medical education are to be given meaning, specialization must be so manipulated that it can serve the purposes of both.

THE NEED FOR CONTINUING, COMPREHENSIVE PERSONAL AND FAMILY SERVICE

It is my thesis that our developing society needs a system of medical care based on the concept of continuing, comprehensive personal and family service, rendered by a well-balanced and well-coordinated core of professional, subprofessional, and technical personnel which, using facilities and equipment that are physically and functionally related, can permit delivery at a cost economically compatible with individual, family, community, and national resources.

I have used the word "system" purposely. The word implies organization and this implies institutionalization. Whether we like these words or not, I believe that the continued institutionalization of medical care and education—like specialization—is inevitable. Therefore, I believe that all of the nation's resources for health and medicine—personnel, facilities, and services—should be integrated to serve the purposes of continuing, comprehensive care.

Dr. Lester Evans amplified the concept of comprehensive care when he said:

> There is nothing new or complicated in the concept. Basically, comprehensive medical care is the kind of compassionate, personalized, birth-to-death attention—preventive, advisory, rehabilitative, as well as diagnostic and therapeutic—that the ideal family physician used to give (and sometimes still gives) within the limits of his knowledge and facilities.
>
> What is new and complicated is adapting the concept to the uses of urban society and specialized skills so that medical care does not become increasingly an episodic, impersonal, and even haphazard matter of a patient's shopping in bewilderment from specialist to specialist, none of whom know the emotional and environmental problems interacting with his organic complaint. The aim should be to combine the concentrated knowledge and skills of the specialists with the broad understanding, wisdom and continuing care of the generalist, to the end that the patient receives precisely as little or as much care as he requires. . . .[2]

Dr. Evans' statement implies that if continuing, comprehensive care is to be made available as a general pattern, two things must be different. First, there must be a new kind of general physician and second, the phrase "teamwork" must take on special meaning.[3]

The combination of the " . . . concentrated knowledge and skills of the specialists, with the broad understanding, wisdom, and continuing care of the generalist, to the end that the patient receives precisely as little or as much care as he requires . . ." will be the key to the effectiveness of comprehensive care. And the most important thing here will be the interest, knowledge, and judgment that will be required to decide between care that is precisely as little or precisely as much as the patient may need. The necessary judgments will not be resolved with an equation, a slide rule, or a computer. Judgments in health and medicine, even quick ones, are entirely dependent upon a high order of human cerebration. The ability to form adequate judgments must be common to all health professionals at a level that is consistent with the responsibility for which each has been trained.

Thus, the professional judgment of the first-contact physician, whether he be specialist or generalist, will be of tremendous importance to the initiation of the care of every single patient. Therefore, all physicians— in fact, all members of all of the health professions—should be oriented to the concept of comprehensive care. *But it is the general physician who must give substance to this care;* and if he is to have the broad understanding and wisdom required of the concept, he himself must be a specialist. I prefer to call this physician a "specialist in family medicine." His will be a special task involving responsibility that will require a special kind of training, particularly in psychiatry, pediatrics, internal medicine, preventive medicine, and rehabilitation. It will be these competences that will place him in a position to be effective in the evaluation and management of disease and also of health; to cooperate effectively with other specialists; to work with, even supervise, professional and technical personnel from fields ancillary to M.D. medicine and, consequently, to guide his patients through the ever-increasing maze of medical care. In other words, in spite of the inevitable increase in its institutionalization, a way must be found to offer medical care that centers around the patient and his family. The implication here is that *teamwork will dominate the future patterns of medical care;* and, if this is true, teamwork must also dominate the future of the clinical aspects of medical education.

Teamwork in these terms is difficult to define. By a team I do not mean a group of individuals organized for combat. Rather, I am speaking of a concept—a concept in which a physician can no longer function as an entrepreneur, or under conditions that are necessarily of his own creation or that are primarily adjusted to his own liking, or in which his relationships with other health and medical professionals depend entirely upon his own initiative. But I do mean a situation in which the physician is the acknowledged leader. And if this is to pertain, he must have some competence in personnel management. He must also have competence in the administrative aspects of medical care as well as in its science and art. The exercise of this leadership will involve teamwork at two levels: first, his relationship with other physicians of all specialties (including dentists), and second, his relationships with other professionals and subprofessionals who have been deliberately trained for lesser but nonetheless specific and important roles in medical care.

THE NEED FOR RESEARCH IN MEDICAL CARE

The only way I know to give meaning to this question of teamwork is to initiate more research in the field of medical care. There are many ways of approaching this kind of research. Some research, particularly the type that can establish bench marks against which changes can be measured, has been and still is being done. At least it has been demonstrated that methods for determining these bench marks are available or can be developed. Many of the deliberations of this conference (Medical Education in the Hospital, October, 1965), such considerations as the control of quality of medical care, the study of hospital utilization, the medical audit, and the transfusion, tissue, and patient care committees, have been closely related to opportunities for this kind of research. Also, these deliberations have reflected the close relationship between the evaluation of medical care on the one hand and its institutionalization upon the other. The kinds of evaluation considered at this conference cannot very well take place outside the hospital or outside a well-organized clinic or some other type of medical care organization.

But the kind of research that will be necessary for the evaluation of teamwork itself will be the establishment of experimental systems or models of medical care in which various concepts and combinations of teamwork can be evaluated against different combinations of community facilities and services, different patterns of organization, different methods of financing, and the different kinds of communities for which our medical establishment must be responsible. The role of hospitals—particularly the community hospitals—will be essential to this enterprise.

Before teamwork itself can be made subject to final evaluation, it will be necessary to establish the criteria that will describe effective teamwork and then to develop methods that will provide for these criteria measurements. Both the identification and measurement of criteria must be in terms of what happens at the level of the patient and the various individuals on the team who will be taking or sharing the responsibility for his care.

The research should lead to the answers of such questions as: What do the members of the team do or not do, or say or not say, that make the patient ill? Or stay ill? Or get well? Or stay well? Research that will permit the answers to such questions will not be easy, not only because the necessary criteria and the methods for their measurement have yet to be developed but also because the area in which they will be applied will involve the no-man's land between the variability, adaptability, and fallibility of human nature. These are the very reasons why this research is so important. It is in the environment of this no-man's land that patient care takes place. Therefore, research that will help define and measure the criteria that can describe this environment, and hence that can lead to its becoming more meaningful—to its deliberate use in the evaluation and management of both health and illness—will go far toward permitting us to measure the results of teamwork. This is teamwork which, in view of the inevitables I have just mentioned—specialization and institutionalization—must be harmonized with the structure and function of any system of medical care that is to answer human desires and human needs.

To attempt to keep research in medical care independent of education for medical care, would be unforgivable. In medicine, research and the care of patients will continue to be the most important teaching and learning tools that we have. Therefore, responsible educational experience that can combine both research and medical care should be the ultimate tool for the combination of teaching and learning. If the future patterns of health and medical care are going to call for a special kind of teamwork and if this in turn will call for a special kind of education, it is logical that the universities—particularly those with professional and technical schools in the health and medical sciences—should be looked upon as the principal resource for integrating teaching and learning into a common enterprise.

If the universities are to play this role in addition to their basic and clinical sciences in the various fields of health and medicine, it will be necessary for them to take their resources in the behavioral and social sciences—the sciences that will help solve the criteria problems of which I speak—and reach across their campuses into the surrounding communities, thus gaining access to the social laboratories in which students, faculty, the practicing health and medical professions, and the lay leadership representing the community's stake in medical care can all work together. Models of systems of medical care, and the research and education which they will house, must be operated in an environment where the vendors and the recipients of medical care are functioning under the conditions of everyday life. And if these efforts are to be attended with success, *the universities must provide opportunities for the continuing education of the health professionals* of these communities so that they can keep in step with progress, not only for the sake of progress itself but also to help them play their roles in assisting with the teaching and research activities of which they will be a part. It will also be important that the coordination of university and community effort involve the frequent use of the forum and the conference so that there is ample opportunity for the comprehension of research goals and the discussion and understanding of the meaning and application of research results.

In calling attention to the importance of community-centered research in medical care, I do not believe I am speaking idle words. As I have mentioned, work that is basic to research in medical care is slowly increasing, and a considerable literature has been the result. I believe that many of the intellectual and physical resources that are needed to accelerate this work now are at hand. Also, financing is beginning to appear. All that remains is the will. And the necessary will may now be forthcoming because social pressures, amply reflected in Medicare, and the national program for the conquest of heart disease, cancer and stroke, and the anti-poverty program, are demanding change. And if in medical care we are to have the kind of change we can call progress, our related research and education should be geared to the origination of change as well as its direction and control.

BIBLIOGRAPHY

1. Darley, W.: Implications of the Institute for the University, the Medical Profession, and the General Public, *J. Med. Educ.*, 40:387–393, Part II Jan.) 1965.

2. "Education for the Health Professions," State Committee on Medical Education. Albany, N.Y. 1963.

3. Darley, W.: Commencement Address, Medical Campus of the University of Illinois, June 11, 1965. Abstract: *SR*, 48:55–56 (Sept. 4) 1965.

35

Generic Problems in
Graduate Medical Education

By Walter S. Wiggins, M.D.

Walter S. Wiggins has been secretary of the
American Medical Association Council on Medical Education since 1959. He received the M.D.
degree from Jefferson Medical College and was
a member of the faculty of the State University
of New York College of Medicine at Syracuse
from 1949 until 1954 when he joined the AMA.
Dr. Wiggins in a Fellow of the American College
of Physicians, a Fellow of The American Association for the Advancement of Science, and a
diplomate of the American Board of Internal
Medicine.

The major purpose of this presentation is to define some of the fundamental problems which I believe to be generally pertinent to all internship and residency training. I should like to do this against a background of certain characteristics which appeal to me as necessary bench
marks of our profession. (ED. NOTE: *An earlier version of this material
was presented at the annual meeting of the National Board of Medical
Examiners in Philadelphia, Pennsylvania, in March, 1965.*)

MEDICINE IS A LEARNED PROFESSION

Physicians take just pride in being members of a *learned* profession.
With the prevalent practice of relating the term "profession" to almost
any type of human endeavor, there is danger that its necessary meaning
to medicine may be weakened or lost. If medicine is to remain a learned
profession, we are obliged to give thought and meaning to some of the
common duties membership in it imposes on us.

Latham has written: "Medicine, as it begins to touch upon higher

353

interests, even the interests of life and death, should feel itself in alliance with higher motives . . . it claims a sort of moral respect in the handling; it calls upon the conscience as well as the intellect. . . .[1] There is certain substance to *the profession* of medicine which calls upon the *conscience* of its members both collectively and individually to honor the common good of the public it serves. At the core of this substance and central to medicine's responsibility as a learned profession is the role of stewardship of a body of knowledge essential to the public welfare. Our value to society is measured ultimately by the extent to which we exercise our stewardship to the benefit of the society which has entrusted it to us.

To be worthy stewards of this essential knowledge, we are obliged to keep it a vigorous, living force in three significant ways. First, we must keep it alive by transmitting it to the generations of physicians who will follow us. Second, we must strive to advance the body of knowledge, that is, to enhance our stock of demonstrated truth. Finally, we are obliged to use available knowledge in a manner that will best benefit the health of our people. This is to say, then, we are responsible for teaching, research, and patient care.

By nature of endowed interest, ability, and opportunity, individual physicians direct their daily activities more toward one of these ends than to the others. However, no physician is free to divorce himself from a conscientious concern for any of these three roles of stewardship, for the privilege of wearing the professional mantle imposes on *each* of its wearers a responsibility for the performance of *all*.

The founding of the American Medical Association in 1847 and the evolution of its role in medical education reflect a response of the collective conscience of medicine worthy of the good stewardship which should characterize a learned profession. You are aware of the sorry nature of medical education in the United States before the present century. It was characterized initially by an unorganized apprenticeship system without intrusion of any meaningful educational standards. Later this was supplemented and eventually replaced by medical schools, in many of which the outstanding characteristic related to the exchange of money rather than knowledge between teacher and student.

This deplorable situation provided the common cause which excited and united the professional conscience of leaders of medicine and led directly to the formation of the American Medical Association. The preamble of the constitution of this new association declared its foremost purposes to be "for cultivating and advancing medical knowledge; [and] for elevating the standard of medical education. . . ."

There is logical reason to accept the establishment of the American Medical Association and the purposes ascribed to it as the beginning of the awakening of the profession's conscience. The statement of purposes acknowledges a recognition of the need to bring about improvement in the standards of medical education through a voluntary concerted action. The revolutionary change that finally resulted is a proud heritage from our forefathers. While taking pride in this heritage, it is of great importance to the present generation to be mindful of the obligation to keep alive our own collective conscience so that it acts responsively and responsibly in its stewardship role.

In today's turbulent scene, we are beset on every side by needs to adapt to a social environment that changes so rapidly that medicine's adjustments of yesterday are criticized today as evidence only of our determination to resist change. Certainly there is increasing reason for us to be more aggressively alert to the need for change so that we may help shape the change rather than succumb to it.

In the context of this background, I would propose to you certain generic problems in graduate medical education that require our studied attention. As you will note, these are focused primarily but not exclusively on the internship and residency years.

ADAPTATION TO SPECIALIZATION

With an ever-growing body of knowledge, medicine has become increasingly the province of physicians who know more and more about a smaller and smaller segment of the total body of knowledge. Specialism is an inevitable and basically sound process which has both resulted from and contributed to the advance of medical science and practice. It now poses significant problems to medicine because we have not taken into account all of the concepts important to the successful application of the process of specialism. We have given full sway to the concept of fragmenting medical knowledge into component parts without at the same time giving equal attention for the need to search among the parts for pieces of knowledge that can be synthesized and generalized.

In the structure of graduate medical education, the results of fragmenting without a concomitant concern for generalizing have recently become sufficiently evident to initiate beginning changes. For example, certain of the more highly specialized segments of surgery now require some training in general surgery prior to training in the limited subspecialty field. This alteration is far from complete and probably is more than offset by continued emphasis on early specialty training on a too limited general base.

As specialization progresses, there is need for greater and greater cooperative effort among specialists, yet there is little conscientious attention to this need in most graduate training programs.

With the vast majority of recent graduates seeking specialty training, the public is acutely aware that it is threatened with all specialists and no generalists. People are justifiably concerned that their vital need for a family physician, generalist, personal physician—call him what you will—may not be satisfied. Satisfactory adaptation to specialization falls far short of achievement in the present medical scene.

ABSENCE OF PRECISE OBJECTIVES

The specific goals of graduate medical education have never been defined adequately. For instance, the goals that differentiate the internship from the clinical clerkship on one hand and from the initial year of residency on the other are available only in vague terms. Such often heard expressions as "increased clinical competence," "graded patient responsibility," and "integration or correlation of fundamental concepts" undoubtedly serve as useful guides. However, they are not sufficiently precise to assure their meaningful application to the specific design of each of the several years of clinical instruction.

It is not possible to designate in what significant respects the first year of clinical clerkship differs from the second. Neither is it possible to learn of specific differences between the educaional objectives of the final clerkship year and the internship, even though between these years certain important events occur: the M.D. degree is awarded; the "student" becomes a "professional" who is legally eligible in many states to enter practice; and the locus of further learning often shifts to a nonuniversity environment.

There is not only a lack of specificity of goals within and among programs of graduate medical education, but also, and perhaps more importantly, an absence of clearly defined objectives for each of the yearly segments comprising the entire span of clinical instruction.

THE FUNDAMENTAL NATURE OF CLINICAL INSTRUCTION

Historically, preparation for medical practice in the United States was by apprenticeship, which represented vocational training in almost pure form. With advances in science and the university orientation of our medical schools, preparation for medicine has become increasingly science-based, but this transition is by no means complete. It is particularly within the area of clinical instruction that both science-based and empirical knowledge are essential to the achievement of clinical competence and skill.

From the earliest introduction to clinical medicine in the second medical school year, the acquisition of vocational skills in the examination of the patient is vital in the preparation of a physician. Thus, clinical instruction from its beginning involves a varied mixture of *scientific concepts, vocational training,* and *empirical knowledge.* Then, as the student advances, this mixture is further complicated by his involvement as a participant in patient care, requiring of him a need for artfulness in the application of his knowledge and skills to the problems of patients.

Perhaps this necessary complexity of approaches to the learning of medicine has inhibited a precise definition of goals. At the same time, this situation should compel a definition of objectives to the fullest extent possible to assure that the excuse of complexity does not mask poor pedagogy.

THE CONFUSION OF THE INTERN YEAR

Under present circumstances, the *rotating internship* most closely resembles the medical school clerkship years in design and content. The *straight internship* most closely resembles the first year of residency. The *rotating internship* and the *straight internship* resemble one another hardly at all.

If there is cause for the existence of these very disparate types of internship, the cause should be found in the disparate needs of our young graduates or in disparate means to achieve similar or deliberately differing goals for the first hospital year. I am doubtful that there can be demonstrated a cause for this degree of disparity except our own confusion.

THE APPRENTICESHIP SYSTEM IN GRADUATE MEDICAL EDUCATION

When house officer training programs were initiated early in this century, in essence the young physician apprenticed himself to learn through observation and supervised participation under an experienced clinician in his care of hospitalized patients. With the present, more organized approach, the young physician is apprenticed not to one but to a group of clinicians who constitute a hospital service in the particular field of the young man's career interest, thus affording him a broader and deeper experience. However, succeeding generations of specialists learn from their elders basically unchanging notions of the operating mores and the carefully guarded domain of their chosen field of medicine. By their nature and tradition, extramural bodies that influence training programs also tend to perpetuate the status quo. Nowhere is there built into the system of graduate medical education the distinctly different viewpoints that could be expected to challenge it.

It is in this regard particularly that graduate medical education in a university environment should be expected to upset tradition. However, like the community hospital, the design and conduct of a training program in the university hospital is vested wholly in one clinical department. Unlike the medical school curriculum, the content and format of graduate training programs are not subject to scrutiny and challenge by the diverse viewpoints of representatives from a community of scholarly disciplines. The residency program in surgery belongs only to surgery, and other departments may intrude at their peril. The same is true, of course, in all clinical fields, and graduate training inevitably must suffer the results of the nepotism that governs it.

SPONSORSHIP OF GRADUATE MEDICAL EDUCATION

The weight of opinion supports the belief that graduate medical education is generally better in university hospitals than in their community counterparts. Indeed, many have been tempted to the quick assumption that whatever the problems of graduate medical education, they would largely be resolved if all responsibility for it was assigned to university hospitals.

Among the significant weaknesses in such an assumption is that it would leave wholly unanswered a question as to whether the better conducted programs in university hospitals are in fact satisfactory or merely less unsatisfactory than programs in community hospitals. I happen to believe this is a pertinent question that presently requires an answer. There exists between these two types of hospitals more similarities than differences in the design and function of graduate programs. The differences that can be found appear to derive largely from the availability and concentrated efforts of full-time, clinical faculty of the university hospital as compared to the volunteer, practitioner-teacher of the community hospital.

Another factor that should be weighed in comparing the values of university hospital training with those of community hospitals is the intellectual ability of their respective resident staffs. It seems likely that university hospitals attract the more competent students. To the extent that this is true, university hospital programs have an inherent advantage over community hospitals.

There are not really fundamental differences between the two categories of hospitals in the basic nature, design, and conduct of training programs. With the primary educational mission and organization of the university hospitals and the primary service mission of the community hospitals in mind, it seems likely that the major differences that are not evident will be most crucial to a future improvement in graduate medical education.

Surely it is to be expected that university hospitals will feel a particular obligation to find better methods for graduate medical education through experimentation. Unfortunately, I am not aware that serious efforts of this kind either are in progress or planned. It would be more than negligent of us to recognize problems of the magnitude suggested, as well as other problems unmentioned here, and do nothing to secure resolution of them. After much study, discussion, and several false starts, the American Medical Association Council on Medical Education elected to approach the troublesome issues of graduate medical education in much the same fashion as the Council of an earlier day approached the inadequacies of undergraduate medical education. This, as you know, resulted in the famed Flexner study.

THE CITIZENS COMMISSION ON GRADUATE MEDICAL EDUCATION

Because of the greater complexity of the current situation in graduate medical education, it was concluded that it would be unrealistic to expect one man to point the way out of present difficulties. Accordingly, a Citizens Commission on Graduate Medical Education was created with a broad charge to study the training of young physicians and to recommend changes so that future physicians might be better prepared to serve the needs of society. The Commission is chaired by Dr. John S. Millis, President of Western Reserve University. Serving with Dr. Millis are 10 citizens whose accomplishments give them wide recognition as distinguished public servants. By deliberate choice, only a small minority are from the field of medicine; the others represent leadership in the worlds of higher education, business, science, and law. Thus medicine once again has turned to prominent citizens essentially outside its own ranks to assure a thorough and objective study for the advancement of medicine's service to the public.

The Citizens Commission became operative in October, 1963, and completed its task in late 1966. The Commission, of course, has full authority to conduct its study and report its findings and recommendations in whatever manner it believes will be most effective. The report is to be made to medicine, universities, hospitals, and the interested public. I am confident the Commission will provide us guidance and direction for an improved future in gratuate medical education. I also expect that achievement of the Commission's recommendations will not be without a degree of shouting and tumult.

CONCLUSION

May I remind you again that one of the most overwhelming characteristics of our time is the accelerated rate at which inevitable change takes place. This situation gives urgency to the need for identifying resolutions to our problems if we are to continue in the tradition of our forebears as worthy stewards of knowledge essential to the public good. At the same time we must be mindful that change is not synonymous with progress. It is our collective obligation to assure that the inevitable change is inevitably progress.

BIBLIOGRAPHY

1. Bean, W. B.: "Aphorisms from Latham," The Prairie Press, Iowa City, 1962.

36

The Posture of the Hospital Staff
As Influenced by Medical Education

By Robert L. Hawley, M.D.

Robert L. Hawley is pathologist at Mercy Hospital in Denver, where he served as chairman of the hospital's Education Committee for many years and where he is now chairman of the Patient Care Committee. Dr. Hawley received the M.D. degree from the University of Colorado, where he is now Assistant Clinical Professor of Pathology. He is a diplomate of the American Board of Pathology.

The Guide Issue of *Hospitals, JAHA,* August 1, 1965, gives the following data for New Mercy Hospital: Beds, 250; Admissions, 10,929; Census, 217; Bassinets, 17; Births, 964; Newborn census, 13; Total expenses, $3,470,000; Payroll, $2,253,000; Personnel, 553.

The most powerful force for the continuing education of the medical staff in the private hospital is the extern, the intern, and the resident. No planned program of lectures, conferences, or films can inspire continued learning by medical staff members equal to the stimulus set in motion by an intern or resident who is a potential source of searching and revealing questions. A graduate medical education program not only acts as a general educational stimulus but may also produce fundamental changes in staff organization and changes in staff policy and procedure. Medical staff standards are constantly raised to satisfy the needs for good training programs. The following case describes the evolution of a medical education program and demonstrates some of the changes that occurred in a medical staff secondary to the upward driving force of medical education.

The hospital in this illustration has been approved for internships and some residencies for many years; but the educational program was generally weak and poorly organized, and the recruitment of house staff was scanty. The staff of the hospital was made up of physicians who were generally quite passive about their responsibility to the house officers. At the same time the staff organization itself was amorphous. The executive board presided over a disinterested staff which seldom questioned any action taken by the board. Chiefs of the major services were elected in a limp popularity contest. Both the teaching program and the medical staff were in the doldrums. In a period of 10 years a series of significant changes were effected.

Initially, the internship and residency programs received only minimal supervision. A part-time director of medical education was then employed, and he visited the hospital a few hours a week. This arrangement was quite unsatisfactory, and he was replaced by a *director of medical education* who spent full time in the hospital. It readily became apparent to the new director that some definitive and even drastic steps needed to be taken. He recognized the need for delegation of teaching responsibility and for supervision on the major clinical services.

The more concerned members of the medical staff were then organized into an *education committee* which became a sounding board for pertinent issues and a focus of concern for the quality of the teaching program. Initially the committee made all major decisions for the medical education program.

The next step was to establish a *teaching staff organization*. At first this included essentially all physicians on the active staff. There followed a period of evaluation of the performance of each physician with regard to his interest in the house staff, the amount of time given to teaching, and his teaching effectiveness. Those who did not meet the criteria were not reappointed to the teaching staff although they continued to be active members of the medical staff. This created a considerable reaction in the staff, and as a result a greater premium was placed on being a member of the teaching staff. Year by year, the teaching staff appointments became better defined with higher standards, and they became ever more sought after by the members of the medical staff.

The next move was to *diversify the responsibility of the medical education program*. A medical education committee was then organized on each major service. To these formal committees was delegated the responsibility of the supervision of the interns and residents on their own service. A medical education committee for each major service placed more responsibility in the hands of appropriate staff members.

After some time, it became apparent that the medical education committee needed more effective teeth to properly supervise and control the level of education on their service. In the next organizational change, the committees were converted to *service committees,* one on each major service. These committees were given extensive prerogatives in addition to supervision of intern and resident training, including the review of credentials of new staff physicians, the review of surgical privileges of staff surgeons, decisions concerning house staff versus nursing service problems, the quality of patient care, and the evaluation of the performances of members of the teaching staff.

These organizational changes led to detectable improvement in the general staff posture, more effective control over medical education, and concomitantly improvement in the staff organization. Democratization evolved with many more physicians being incorporated into the active staff program.

The next step toward building a still better medical education program was the *recruitment of able and qualified physicians for the teaching staff*, especially to fill specific needs. This was pursued vigorously and was aimed particularly at young men fresh from residency programs. In interviewing applicants, the credentials committee and the appropriate service committee discussed with them medical staff responsibilities as well as teaching responsibilities. It is felt that this encouraged certain physicians to become active members of the staff.

To facilitate the use of the hospital by new physicians and by those physicians who were aggressive and effective teachers, *the admissions policy* was redefined with admission privileges being higher for those physicians on the teaching staff and highest for those who were new on the teaching staff. The medical staff constitution and bylaws were revised, incorporating provisions to strengthen the staff organization and to buttress the medical education program. All these changes in different areas of hospital policy and staff organization have increased interest and effectiveness of medical education and medical staff function.

These changes, stimulated largely by the needs of a medical education program, have raised the medical staff of this hospital from a nearly recumbent position to a much more productive one. The drive of medical education continues to affect the medical staff, and further goals lie ahead.

For an effective, growing, alert medical staff, it is vitally important to integrate medical education of our juniors into the staff philosophy and into the total program.

From the Latin, "doctor" means "teacher." By being a teacher, the physician improves himself. By dedication to medical education, the medical staff organization similarly improves.

37

The Director of Medical Education

By William S. Vaun, M.D., and John C. Leonard, M.D.

William S. Vaun is the director of medical education at Monmouth Medical Center in Long Branch, New Jersey. He was formerly assistant director of medicine at St. Luke's Hospital in Cleveland, where he was also chairman of the House Staff Committee and performed many of the duties of a DME. He received the M.D. degree from the University of Pennsylvania. He is a diplomate of the American Board of Internal Medicine and an associate of the American College of Physicians. He is a member of the Executive Committee of the Association of Hospital Directors of Medical Education and also clinical assistant professor of medicine at the New Jersey College of Medicine and Dentistry.

The Guide Issue of *Hospitals*, *JAHA*, August 1, 1965, lists the following data for Monmouth Medical Center: Beds, 450; Admissions, 15,676; Census, 403; Bassinets, 40; Births, 1,825; Newborn census, 22; Total expenses, $5,643,000; Payroll, $2,872,000; Personnel, 731. The population of Long Branch is 28,000.

John C. Leonard was the director of medical education at Hartford Hospital from 1947 until his death April 26, 1966. His position was the first of its kind in the United States. He held many important posts during his very active career, including associate director of education programs for rural hospitals of the Commonwealth Foundation, associate director of the Bingham Foundation, and associate director of the Joseph H. Pratt Diagnostic Hospital in Boston. He received the M.D. degree from Yale University and

served there as clinical professor of medicine. Dr.
Leonard was a member of the Advisory Committee on Internships of the AMA Council on Medical
Education, a member and chairman of the AMA
Residency Review Committee in Internal Medicine, and chairman of the AMA Committee on
Postgraduate Medicine. He was vice-president
and regent of the American College of Physicians
and had been Governor of the College for Connecticut.

The Guide Issue of *Hospitals, JAHA,* August
1, 1965, gives the following data on Hartford
Hospital: Beds, 800; Admissions, 30,584; Census, 723; Bassinets, 150; Births, 5,411; Newborn census, 82; Total expenses, $15,207,000;
Payroll, $10,626,000; Personnel, 2,082. There
are three other short-term general hospitals in
Hartford with 144 beds, 189 beds, and 654 beds.
The population of Hartford in the 1960 census
was 162,178.

For several years, in the hope of attracting interns and residents,
community hospitals have been modifying their medical education programs in the direction of more formalized academic activity. The increasing interest of responsible medical organizations as well as lay
groups in the continuing education of the practicing physician has augmented the trend. Efforts in graduate and postgraduate education have
made increasingly apparent the need for a director of medical education
(DME) in hospitals that wish to continue to participate in these activities.

EVOLUTION OF THE DME CONCEPT

In recognition of the increasing complexity of educational programs
for interns and residents and the relatively small number of experienced
educators in community hospitals, the Commission on Graduate Medical Education predicted the need as early as 1940 and recommended
the creation of the position of director of education.[1] Within a decade,
several DME's appeared on the hospital scene. With the growing shortage of interns and residents, however, the educational intent of the DME
was sublimated by the exigencies of recruiting house staff. The success
of some of the early DME-directed programs stimulated other well-
intentioned institutions to create such positions, hoping to alleviate their
house staff shortages. As might be anticipated, the results have been

success and failure, dependent not so much on the qualifications of the DME as on those of the institution, its medical staff, and their willingness to support the serious and heavy responsibility of educational programs. Given adequate financial resources, a satisfactory physical facility, sufficient depth in patient material, a devoted teaching faculty augmented with salaried personnel where needed, and a research arm, the DME has the ingredients to blend a successful educational program. What he makes of them depends on his capabilities as a clinician, administrator, and educator. Without them, regardless of the DME's qualifications, the programs are doomed to failure.

Sound graduate programs in community hospitals, organized and directed by capable DME's, continue to attract able students despite mounting pressures to divert them to university programs. It is not so much a university or non-university hospital scene that makes the difference; it is rather the recognition of responsibilities to young physicians in training and the availability of educators capable of implementing programs.

The DME continues to evolve from the original concept of an interested physician through the recruiting-sergeant phase to the position of a sophisticated educator and administrator on the hospital scene. Natural selection ultimately eliminates defective programs, DME-directed or not, university or non-university; and the capable DME will survive, modified somewhat by local collateral factors, to pursue the goal of physician education.

Not all hospitals can or should aspire to the development of graduate and postgraduate educational programs complete with full-time DME's. Where the prerequisites and motivation are present, they should be developed to maximum potential. Where they are not present or cannot reasonably be anticipated, the educational spectrum must be restricted accordingly but not abandoned. A part-time or voluntary DME may be just as important to his particular hospital in organizing continuing education programs as is the full-time DME in commanding a full spectrum of educational activities. Each hospital should realistically evaluate its own potential and design a DME position appropriate to its needs.

FUNCTIONS OF THE DME

The functions of the DME described here encompass activities in a large hospital—400 beds or more; but it is our sincere belief that some modification of this position has a place in every hospital. In the past, the functions of the DME have been considered in the broad categories of educational and administrative activities, together with interface and collateral responsibilities.[2] Recent and dynamic changes in the hospital scene and in the spectrum of medical education, superimposed on a

period of great socio-economic ferment, have markedly altered the profile of the DME within each category, and perhaps have created a few
more categories.

Educational Functions

Stimulated by the discrepancy between house staff positions available
and those filled, and perhaps by an increased understanding of the
learning process together with the need to train a different type physician, the graduate educational experience in successful hospitals has
changed. It has evolved from the concept of hands for service functions—
histories, physical examinations, operating room and emergency room
assistance—to a curriculum of integrated patient responsibilities, conferences, rounds, and laboratory and research exposures with defined
objectives that complement the undergraduate years and prepare for
specialty practice. To move from the concept of a distributor of hands
to that of a DME who is expected to administer the educational needs of
graduate students is hardly enough to serve the purpose. The DME must
be an educator, coordinating the curriculum not only at the graduate
level, but also at the increasingly important postgraduate level.

As mentioned initially, the complexity of the programs in a large hospital dictates that the DME be a full-time position. But even in the
smaller hospital that is involved only with *continuing education of the
staff*, voluntary appointees cannot usually commit the needed time without some compensation. Again reflecting the complexity of the programs,
the DME needs special training and experience in educational methods.
Unfortunately, there are very few opportunities available for such instruction, but they are beginning to appear.

Apart from his contribution to the programs in his own field of clinical
competence, the DME has no greater teaching role than other clinicians
except for the *communication of knowledge regarding teaching techniques and materials*. Unfortunately, it is often assumed that a professional degree carries with it an ability to teach. Would that this were
so! With better evaluation techniques, knowledge of the learning process
and educational methods must be a major concern of the educator.

Some physicians predict the doom of the DME with the advent of
full-time clinical chiefs. This is hardly a logical conclusion when the
evolution of full-time chiefs is carefully analyzed. It was the DME who
first recognized the need for full-time chiefs. Appreciating his limitations
in the clinical fields and recognizing the urgent need for more assistance
in developing specialty training, the DME has promoted this progressive
idea to his staff and his trustees. The spectrum of activities of the DME
and the full-time chiefs may indeed overlap initially, but when the full-

time chief modifies the DME's departmental functions, and it is ridiculous to consider that he would not, the DME is able to devote more time to coordinating overall hospital activities in harmony with administrative and staff needs and less time to worrying about individual clinical specialties and their inherent problems.

We concur with Dr. John Freymann that a new breed of physician is due on the hospital scene.[3] *The director of clinical services,* described by him, characterizes many current DME's and perhaps represents the evolutionary direction that many more will follow.

Most of the discussions in this area involve problems in semantics. The large hospital we have depicted will continue to need the DME. We further predict that full-time chiefs will enhance the need for the DME; and every chief added to the staff, if his qualifications are what they should be, will be another needed educator in the hospital. It would appear mandatory that activities of full-time chiefs be coordinated through the DME to avoid the service insularity which is all too often present.

Whether a director of clinical services will be needed apart from the DME depends largely on the degree of interface and collateral activities he is required to undertake; on whether the hospital administrator is a physician or whether there is a medical director; on whether other employed physicians share responsibilities in patient care; and also on the complexity of educational needs.

Medical School Relations

Despite the schism between the academic and the practicing medical worlds, the "town-gown syndrome," there are signs that the rift is healing. There are a few medical schools and community hospitals which, having recognized the needs of all phases of medical education, have joined their efforts to the advantage of all concerned, not the least of whom is the patient. To suggest that all graduate education will ultimately be conducted in university hospitals is not a mathematically sound conclusion when one considers faculty shortages, commitments to research, the increasingly large number of graduate students, the growing number of medical school graduates, and the great number of foreign medical graduates in the United States for graduate training. On the other hand, to suggest that the community hospital can sustain adequate graduate and postgraduate programs without the assistance and cooperation of medical school faculty is equally unrealistic.

To continue to *bridge the gap between the medical school and the community teaching hospital,* the DME must be a member of the medical school faculty. He must be aware of undergraduate curricula to be able to effectively program the needs at the graduate and postgraduate levels. He must encourage his hospital teaching staff to participate in medical school activities and maintain close medical school ties.

A good DME-directed community hospital program offers much to a medical school and vice versa. It is hoped that the Coggeshall Report[4] will stimulate and augment a combined effort on the part of medical schools and teaching hospitals, be they university or private. Affiliations established with an educational objective must be encouraged. Affiliations entered into for recruiting advantages have no lasting benefit to either party and should be discouraged. The participation of community teaching hospitals in medical education, commensurate with their educational resources rather than their service needs and in concert with university medical centers, will play an increasingly important role in the future. The need of the DME in this role is apparent.

Recruitment of House Staff

An excellent teaching program is the finest recruitment device available; and when the DME and the attending staff work together to develop sound programs, neither need be procurement officers. Apart from this, the DME is involved with recruitment by preparing brochures and informational materials, processing applications and correspondence, and scheduling interviews. Brochures must be accurate, truthful, and realistic. In all these activities, the DME needs the full cooperation of his chiefs and the teaching staff. Many recruitment methods have been described, but each hospital must use those best suited to its needs. No recruitment device will continue to sell an educationally unsound program.

Most hospitals fail to maintain adequate *alumni relations*. This is tragic, for it is one of the most legitimate and effective of all recruitment media. Satisfied house staff, like college graduates, will fondly remember their alma mater. The DME should be alert to this resource.

Administrative Functions

Within this category is the "house mother" capacity of the DME. In addition to the administrative aspects of the training programs and guidance in the collateral needs of house staff (housing, uniforms, board, health care, recreation, etc.), the DME has a great responsibility in *counselling* young house officers. A DME not conversant with current trends in medical practice, residency, licensure, military obligations, and specialty board requirements cannot objectively counsel young physicians.

As the graduate educational programs become reoriented with a shift of house staff away from important service needs in patient care, the

DME has an important role in helping the attending staff and the administration to solve the resulting problems. Although it is included under administrative functions, this duty might better be categorized as educational because it represents a reorientation of attitudes of administrators and medical staff in the incorporation of paramedical personnel into the health care team. These interface activities of the DME in patient care may be modified by the presence of full-time chiefs, physician-administrators, medical directors, outpatient chiefs, directors of clinical services, and others.

Evaluation

Evaluation—of programs, of participating house officers, and of teaching faculty—is an important function of the DME. Unfortunately, in the current house officer market, satisfactory completion of programs and awarding of certificates is too often taken for granted. This attitude also seems to penetrate the undergraduate years. Although admittedly it is a difficult chore, the DME nevertheless must persistently and objectively evaluate his students, faculty, and program. New techniques for evaluation are appearing; more objective ones are needed.

Requirements for the Future

Last but not least, the DME must project educational requirements for the future. Progress and success as an educational institution does not simply happen. It must be planned, with the definition of objectives, an inventory of assets, a recognition of needs, and delineation of methods.

CONCLUSION

The need for the DME is apparent. The advent of full-time chiefs augments the need of the DME rather than detracts from it, although these people will without doubt modify his functions. The insularity bred by capable and efficient chiefs must be tempered for the common effort. The DME and the full-time chiefs coexist somewhat akin to the relationship of the Secretary of Defense and his Navy admirals. The admirals have a specific and crucially important duty, but they may sometimes lose sight of the overall objective.

Apart from full-time chiefs, the changing spectrum of professional personnel being incorporated into the hospital scene will definitely have a modifying influence on the functions of the DME. This can hardly be denied when we consider the evolutionary pattern already experienced. Though he may be called by a different name in the future, the DME

372 GRADUATE MEDICAL EDUCATION AND THE HOSPITAL

will not become extinct. On the contrary, as he is relieved of many responsibilities such as managing specific clinical services and outpatient departments and directing research programs, he will become what he was intended to be, a professional educator in the hospital.

BIBLIOGRAPHY

1. "Graduate Medical Education," Report of the Commission on Graduate Medical Education, The University of Chicago Press, Chicago, 1940.

2. Guide Committee of the Association of Hospital Directors of Medical Education, The Director of Medical Education in the Teaching Hospital; A Revised Guide to Function and Status, *JAMA* 192:1055–1060 (June 21) 1965.

3. Freymann, J. G.: Whither the Director of Medical Education? *New England J. Med.*, 273:1253–1257 (December 2) 1965.

4. Coggeshall, L. T.: Planning for Medical Progress Through Education, A Report Submitted to the Executive Council of the Association of American Medical Colleges, April, 1965.

38

The Physician's Responsibility
for Nursing Education

By L. Joseph Butterfield, M.D.

L. Joseph Butterfield is director of the department of neonatology and coordinator of postgraduate education at Children's Hospital in Denver. He received the M.D. degree from the University of Colorado and serves there as assistant clinical professor of pediatrics. He has been active in nursing education not only in his own hospital but also in the University of Colorado School of Nursing and in continuing education for nurses throughout the Rocky Mountain region.

The Guide Issue of *Hospitals, JAHA,* August 1, 1965, gives the following data for Children's Hospital: Beds, 222; Admissions, 13,600; Census, 169; Bassinets, 0; Births, 0; Newborn census, 0; Total expenses, $3,643,000; Payroll, $2,410,000; Personnel, 607.

The importance of the nurse in the care of sick newborn infants is a widely acceptable fact among experienced physicians. This theme was candidly supported by a prominent educator who once remarked that if a premature infant had his choice between the team of a smart doctor and a dumb nurse or the reverse combination, he would live a lot longer if his team included the smart nurse.

In the Newborn Center of Children's Hospital, the physician is encouraged to take an active part in nursing education. This is not only proper for the sake of optimum patient care but essential for nursing morale, and it promotes the eagerness with which each new problem is faced. To provide a practical example of the several ways in which the physician participates in nursing education, an outline of the activities of the Newborn Center is presented.

The Newborn Center is an intensive care facility for babies with medical and surgical problems relevant to the newborn period. The Center is a recent extension of the premature infant center concept which has spread throughout the country in the past 43 years. Although premature infants are admitted to the Center, they constitute only 20 per cent of the admissions. The remainder of the babies referred to the Center are full-term infants with a variety of challenging problems. These babies come from throughout the state of Colorado and the surrounding states. The most common problems leading to admission are metabolic and immunologic disorders, birth defects, respiratory distress syndromes, and atypical gestations. These cases, 50 per month, provide the case material for the teaching experience in the Newborn Center.

Nursing rounds are made daily by pediatricians from private practice and by full-time staff members of Children's Hospital. The charge nurse takes an active part in these rounds and is encouraged to participate by emphasizing nursing problems. The dialogue between the physicians and the nurses on these rounds becomes both an integral part of patient care and a teaching experience for both. Other staff nurses and student nurses in training who are working in the Newborn Center are likewise encouraged to participate in these teaching rounds.

Grand Rounds are held weekly. Cases from the various departments of the hospital are discussed for their educational value. These sessions are well attended by the nursing staff.

Child Health Day is a 4-hour postgraduate session that is held once each month. Nurses from throughout the community and the state attend this meeting. The greatest advantage of the dual attendance at these sessions of both physicians and nurses is that new concepts in patient care are extended to both professions at the same time.

A Perinatal Conference is held each Tuesday by the director of the Newborn Center and other members of the full-time staff or by a visiting obstetrician. Cases with perinatal problems are discussed to provide an educational experience for residents and nurses as well as an acquaintance with the Newborn Center facilities for obstetricians and pediatricians from the metropolitan area.

A conference on maternal and child health is held on the first Friday of the month and is considered "Grand Rounds for nurses." Both physicians and nurses speak at these conferences on a wide range of subjects which include medical as well as surgical concepts of maternal and child care. Notices of these meetings are distributed to hospitals throughout the state of Colorado, and it is gratifying to see nurses from as far away as 200 miles attend these conferences. These, as much as anything else, have demonstrated the interest of the nursing profession in exercises in which the physician takes an active role. During these conferences, the nurses have been queried about their desires and interests in postgraduate education. One of the most common requests has been for more nursing education on a basic medical level and for the allotment of definite times for such education in their work schedule. A few of the areas in which specific interest was expressed included (1) new procedures and laboratory tests; (2) information about instruction in prenatal and postpartum care; (3) basic science topics; and (4) ways of improving communication with the physicians. The design of the conference has been altered from time to time in recognition of these requests.

A new traineeship in newborn care is being planned. This 5-day course of advanced training in the care of newborn infants will be offered by arrangement to a small number of staff nurses who are currently at the head nurse level of responsibility. This course will consist of newborn care experience, crib-side conferences, and discussions specifically oriented to the needs of the nurse trainee. We feel that there is a need to update the knowledge of the head nurse from the general and community hospitals where she is given a remarkable degree of responsibility in the total care of newborn infants. Facing the increasing demands for better trained nurses in the newborn area, it is hoped that such a training experience will provide a better appreciation of the available laboratory techniques and therapeutic procedures which are available today. Further, it is reasonable to expect that the experienced head nurse who has been given additional training in the recognition of neonatal diseases will be able to accept increasing responsibility for actual newborn care with a greater degree of confidence than is possible today.

Throughout the above learning opportunities the basic responsibility of the physician is to present the medical, surgical, and humanistic facets of patient care so that the nurse's approach is on a more solid footing. (ED. NOTE: *Dr. Butterfield's paper is oriented toward the milieu of the newborn service of a children's hospital. However, many parts of his discussion can be readily applied to similar situations in general hospitals.*)

Part VI

*Continuing Education of
the Staff Physician*

39

Continuing Education in the Non-teaching Hospital

I. IN A MINNESOTA HOSPITAL

By Jo E. Anderson, M.D.

Jo E. Anderson is a general practitioner in a small group practicing in Le Sueur, Minnesota. This agricultural community of 3,310 (1960) is located 60 miles southwest of Minneapolis. The Minnesota Valley Memorial Hospital, the only hospital in the community, is relatively new, having been established in 1960. It has 39 beds, and in 1964 there were 870 admissions, 135 births, an average daily census of 17, and 34 personnel (Guide Issue, *Hospitals, JAHA*, August 1, 1965.) The *American Medical Directory*, 23rd edition, 1965, lists three general practitioners in the town, one of whom has a secondary specialty of pediatrics, and a general surgeon. Dr. Anderson received the M.D. degree from the University of Kansas School of Medicine in 1954; following a rotating internship, he served a two-year general practice residency at the University of Colorado School of Medicine.

(ED. NOTE: *This chapter consists of three sections written by three physicians with different viewpoints. The first two sections by Dr. Anderson and Dr. Sadler reflect their experiences in small, rural hospitals. Educational programs in these hospitals are largely confined to the continuing education of the attending staff and inservice education for nurses and other paramedical personnel. There is perhaps an occasional extern*

*on a medical school preceptorship or a general practice resident rotating
for a brief period from a university hospital. In the third section Dr.
Rosenow approaches the problem from a different viewpoint. In his discussion he considers the non-teaching hospital to be a non-university
hospital or a hospital not affiliated with a medical school, but one in
which interns and residents may be trained.*)

In 1960 the citizens of Le Sueur, Minnesota, decided that they must
have a community hospital. (ED. NOTE: *In Dr. Anderson's section of
Chap. 30, "Special Problems of Small Hospitals," additional information
is given on the Minnesota Valley Hospital and the community.*) The
project was encouraged by the four physicians practicing in the community. Until that time all patients requiring hospital care were taken
to St. Peter or Mankato (10 and 20 miles away) or into the Minneapolis-
St. Paul area, some 60 miles distant.

A NEW RURAL HOSPITAL

In spite of statistics which indicated that an adequate number of
hospital beds were already available for the area and without Federal
funds to help in the construction, the people of Le Sueur decided to go
ahead. They obligated themselves to a bond issue and constructed a
modern 39-bed hospital. A representative hospital board was chosen,
and they quickly realized that for a new hospital to be a success a good
administrator was essential. The one who was selected viewed the hospital as the start toward the development of a rural health center, the
general acute hospital serving as the nucleus.

The next step was to get the physicians in the community to adopt
similar views and to stimulate in them a desire for a better than ordinary
hospital. One of the four physicians then retired, and another left for
specialty training. Two new physicians were attracted to Le Sueur by the
excellence of the hospital and its plans for the future.

THE RURAL HEALTH CENTER

The problem of adequate medical and hospital care in a rural area
was the concern of the health planners in Le Sueur. They believed
that the health needs of the community could best be satisfied by a cen-
trally located rural health center coordinated with a large regional medical center.

The United States Public Health Service granted funds to "demonstrate
those accomplishments that lead to improving the quality and increasing the availability of hospital and medical care through the development of a health center with the general acute hospital serving as the
nucleus and affiliated with a large metropolitan teaching hospital." It

was envisioned that the health center might include, in addition to the hospital, clinical office space for physicians, outpatient consultants' offices, a convalescent and nursing care unit, a home for the aged, and clinical facilities for dentists, mental health teams, public health workers, and other social agencies concerned with the health of the community.

Affiliation with a Metropolitan Teaching Hospital. The next step, then, was an affiliation with Mount Sinai Hospital of Minneapolis. (ED. NOTE: *Mount Sinai Hospital is affiliated with the University of Minnesota School of Medicine. According to the Guide Issue of Hospitals, JAHA, August 1, 1965, Mount Sinai has 305 beds, 9,662 discharges, and 712 births. The hospital is approved for 14 rotating internship positions and 18 residency positions in medicine, surgery, and pathology, as indicated by the Directory of Approved Internships and Residencies, published by the American Medical Association in 1965.*) Although the full potential of the affiliation was not then apparent and has not yet been completely realized, it has proved to be a significant aid in the development of the Minnesota Valley Memorial Hospital at Le Sueur.

Of particular significance to the staff physicians was the feeling that the affiliation could make the practice of medicine in a small community more attractive and even exciting. Some of the things which make small town practice difficult and unattractive are the lack of good hospital facilities, the lack of ready consultation, and the lack of opportunity for continuation of study at the postgraduate level to meet the challenge of keeping abreast of expanding medical knowledge. The affiliation with Mount Sinai Hospital in Minneapolis offers qualified consultants in the various specialties who are willing and even eager to come to Le Sueur for consultation and participation in the continuing educational program.

POSTGRADUATE EDUCATION

Seminars. During the three years that the affiliation has been in operation, 12 postgraduate seminars have been held at our rural hospital, in the areas of general surgery, general medicine, cardiology, pediatrics, obstetrics and gynecology, psychiatry, physical medicine, urology, and dermatology. The sessions have been conducted by 16 specialists from the Mount Sinai Hospital staff. The general format has included a presentation of one or more cases for the visiting consultant to examine and to use as the basis for teaching. Some of the cases are diagnostic problems, others are representative cases that demonstrate specific aspects of a disease process. Following an informal staff dinner, the visiting consultant presents a formal paper.

Teaching Consultations. A significant secondary gain from these seminars has been the development of a close working relationship between the Le Sueur staff physicians and the Mount Sinai consultants. After becoming acquainted with the staff physician of the hospital and seeing the type of work he does and the facilities at his disposal, the consultants have found that many problems can be handled by telephone consultation. If the situation can be handled locally, this is done; but if the consultant feels further care is needed beyond the scope of the small hospital, he quickly arranges for this at Mount Sinai Hospital.

In a progress report of the project, Dr. Reuben Berman, an internist who is chairman of the Mount Sinai Hospital Project Clinical Directors, cited an individual patient problem which demonstrated the working of the affiliation. He wrote as follows:

> Mrs. E. W. suffered a cerebral hemorrhage which was thought possibly to be amenable to surgery. This occurred at the time of the flood. Le Sueur was beleaguered by the Minnesota River. The patient was seen at the Le Sueur Hospital by me, utilizing an airplane and landing at an officially closed Le Sueur airport. She was then evacuated to Mount Sinai Hospital by Navy helicopter and Navy ambulance. She was seen by neurologic and neurosurgical consultants within an hour after she left Le Sueur. Unfortunately, the eventual surgery was not helpful. However, the entire case points out the arrangements that can be made between affiliated institutions, mobilizing a large force of professional and other help, in a very short time.

Staff Meetings. In addition to the formal teaching seminars, the Mount Sinai staff frequently participates in the scientific portions of the regular Minnesota Valley Memorial Hospital medical staff meetings. Twice a year the pathologist reviews the pathological specimens and slides of the interesting cases from the Le Sueur Hospital. Other special programs have been presented in radiology, obstetrics, pediatrics, cardiology, and resuscitation techniques. The hospital has hosted the county medical society meeting on one occasion and the district chapter of the American Academy of General Practice on three occasions.

As evidence of a sustained interest in postgraduate education, every member of the Minnesota Valley Memorial Hospital staff has attended at least two postgraduate scientific meetings during the past three years in addition to those held at the hospital. These have included postgraduate courses at the University of Michigan, the University of Minnesota, and the University of Colorado, and the annual review seminars at the Mayo Clinic as well as scientific meetings of state and national medical societies.

Other Educational Benefits. There are other aspects of the affiliation which may be considered a part of the continuing education of the staff physicians. Regular *weekly cardiac and tumor clinics* are held at the affiliate hospital throughout the year. Referral of patients to the cardiac clinic is readily accomplished by a telephone call to the appointment desk of the Mount Sinai outpatient department. The patients are presented to the specialists attending the clinic, specific recommendations are formulated and discussed with the patient, and a written report is submitted to the referring physician. At the tumor clinic, pathologists from several Minneapolis hospitals meet to review sections from puzzling cases. The consensus of this conference is then reported to the referring physician.

The outpatient service for indigent care and the free bed service at Mount Sinai have been very helpful. Patients referred to the free bed service participate in the teaching program of Mount Sinai Hospital—the affiliation thus benefits both hospitals.

The availability of a good *medical library* and librarian has helped the Le Sueur hospital in maintaining its own library and in extending library facilities through interlibrary loans.

One of the Le Sueur staff physicians, after the affiliation had been in effect for one year, took a leave of absence from his practice and participated in a *medical residency at Mount Sinai Hospital.* He subsequently returned to Le Sueur and limited his practice to internal medicine. The fact that an affiliation existed with Mount Sinai Hospital undoubtedly contributed to his choice of residency. Robert Smith says, in his Master of Science degree thesis, "An Urban-rural Hospital Affiliation and Its Effects on the Medical Care of Patients in a Rural Hospital," "Furthermore, his desire for more training was more than likely increased by the stimulation of the early 1963 clinical conferences held at Le Sueur." Each year Mount Sinai Hospital provides a *residency training program for a graduate student in hospital administration* from the University of Minnesota. Through affiliation, the Minnesota Valley Memorial Hospital has been able to participate in the hospital administration resident training. Mr. Smith spent two weeks at the Le Sueur Hospital as a part of his rotation, and he became sufficiently interested in the program to write his thesis on this project. The rotation to the Le Sueur hospital has become a regular part of the administrative residency program of Mount Sinai Hospital.

SUMMARY

The building of the Minnesota Valley Memorial Hospital in Le Sueur, Minnesota, in 1960 was the initial step in establishing a rural health center in the community to provide health care services approaching those available in metropolitan areas in an up-to-date manner. It was the desire of the health planners for Le Sueur to make the hospital the nucleus of a rural health center and also to provide a stimulating medical atmosphere for the physicians of the area. A demonstration project was developed with a United States Public Health Service grant to demonstrate the value of an affiliation with a large metropolitan teach-hospital. An affiliation with Mount Sinai Hospital in Minneapolis has been developed to provide quickly available consultants in all the specialties and to provide leadership in postgraduate education. These and many other aspects of the affiliation have aided in attracting and retaining qualified physicians for the community. Out of the affiliation has emerged a sense of responsibility and a willingness on the part of Mount Sinai Hospital to advance rural health care.

II. IN A COLORADO HOSPITAL

By Jackson L. Sadler, M.D.

Dr. Jackson L. Sadler is in general practice with a specialty interest in pediatrics in Fort Collins, Colorado. He received the M.D. degree from the University of Colorado, where he is a faculty associate. He was a resident at Children's Hospital in Denver. He is a member of the Executive Committee of the Poudre Valley Memorial Hospital in Fort Collins, and he was formerly chief of staff. For many years, he was chairman of the Education Committee which supervised the training of a general practice resident who rotated to their hospital from the University of Colorado and which also arranged the educational program presented at the hospital each month by two members of the Medical School faculty.

The Guide Issue of *Hospitals, JAHA,* August 1, 1965, gives the following data on the Poudre Valley Memorial Hospital: Beds, 128; Admissions, 5,414; Census, 78; Bassinets, 12; Births, 924. The population of Fort Collins in the 1960 census was 25,027.

For the past 18 years, the University of Colorado School of Medicine has sponsored a monthly visit of two consultants to the Poudre Valley Memorial Hospital in Fort Collins, Colorado. These consultants represent the various specialties of medicine and surgery and are selected from the full-time faculty of the University and the volunteer clinical faculty, which is comprised largely of specialists practicing in Denver.

This program of continuing medical education was begun in 1948 when the University of Colorado School of Medicine, in conjunction with the Colorado Medical Society, selected this community hospital as one of several to participate in the Medical School's General Practice Residency program. A resident is assigned to the Poudre Valley Memorial Hospital for 3 to 4 months during either the first or second year of his training, and he is the only house staff physician in the hospital.

Consultant teams arrive at the hospital about 11:00 A.M., and on arrival they make teaching rounds with the resident physician. Then they have lunch with interested members of the hospital staff in the hospital dining room.

A portion of the time of each consulting team is spent in discussing cases and problems with the resident. The consultants also confer with any member of the attending staff regarding hospital patients or outpatients who are brought to the hospital for this purpose. Cases of special interest are presented to the entire staff and to the consultants, who conduct bedside teaching seminars. Each consultant also presents a lecture, followed by a question and discussion period.

An important part of the program is the social hour held in the late afternoon at the home of one of the staff members, followed by a dinner in a private room of a restaurant. At first, these social activities were unscheduled and spontaneous. But increased attendance now requires prior scheduling and supervision by a committee of the hospital staff. It is an excellent opportunity for the staff and the visiting consultants to develop rapport.

The consultants are selected by the Office of Postgraduate Medical Education of the University School of Medicine in conjunction with the requests of the Medical Education Committee of the Poudre Valley Memorial Hospital. An attempt is made to pair consultants representing different disciplines of medical practice in which there may be related clinical problems. During the 18 year period, approximately 180 programs have been presented by about 150 different consultants. Some consultants return annually; many others have made two or more visits.

When the program was begun in 1948, there were 22 members on the active staff, 16 of whom were in general practice. The specialties were represented by one radiologist, one clinical pathologist, one orthopedic surgeon, and two ophthalmologists. Six of the general practitioners professed a specialty interest and had received some specialty training. The average attendance at the postgraduate sessions was maintained at 70 per cent through the first 10 years of the program. The population of Fort Collins has grown from 15,000 to 30,000 over the 18 years, and there are now 52 members on the attending staff, 26 of whom are engaged in specialty practice. Recent attendance at the monthly postgraduate sessions has fallen to about 30 per cent.

The decline in the percentage of staff attendance and participation in the postgraduate program results from many factors. It can be explained only partially by the increase in the number and percentage of specialists on the attending staff. It has been noted that several of the younger and better trained specialists attend nearly every session; but on the other hand, there are several of the younger general practitioners who rarely attend.

Some believe that one of the contributing factors to decreased attendance is the increased use of consultants from the full-time faculty. Since these physicians are not in private practice and many are new to the community, they are not as well-known to our staff, and this results in some loss of interest and loss of rapport.

Perhaps one of the strongest influences accounting for the decline in interest is the irregular assignment of general practice residents to our hospital in recent years. This has been caused by a decrease in the total number of residents in the program. Also, some residents select assignments in other community hospitals more conveniently located to Denver, which would make commuting possible and avoid the problems of moving a family. When general practice residents were regularly assigned to our hospital, there was deeper involvement of staff members in the education program.

Along with the decreased attendance, there has been a recent decline in the number of cases presented to the consultants for discussion. This detracts from the broad interest in the program. We are hoping to improve this part of our monthly sessions by asking each of the clinical committees of the staff to select suitable cases for presentation to the consultants.

It is my personal belief that this program has greatly improved the quality of medical practice in our hospital. Many patients have benefitted directly, and many more indirectly, from the improvement in our skills and in our staff organization.

As our hospital and staff increase in size and as the staff becomes more specialized, new problems will develop. It is our hope that these can be solved and that an active postgraduate program will continue. Some type of affiliation with the Medical School will continue to benefit our hospital and, I believe, the University.

III. IN THE NON-AFFILIATED HOSPITAL

By Edward C. Rosenow, Jr., M.D.

Dr. Rosenow is the executive director of the American College of Physicians. He received the M.D. degree from Harvard Medical School and was a fellow in internal medicine at the Mayo

Graduate School of Medicine. He is a diplomate of the American Board of Internal Medicine. He was in private practice in Pasadena, California, for 17 years and was clinical professor of medicine at the University of Southern California School of Medicine. Presently, he is an adjunct clinical professor of medicine at the University of Pennsylvania. He has held many important offices, being past president of the Los Angeles County Medical Association, the Los Angeles Society of Internal Medicine, and the Los Angeles County Heart Association. He was chairman of the Committee on Postgraduate Activities of the California Medical Association and editor of *Audio-Digest*.

(ED. NOTE: *As mentioned at the beginning of this chapter, Dr. Rosenow approaches the problems of education in the non-teaching hospital from a different viewpoint. He considers the non-teaching hospital to be a non-affiliated hospital, but one in which interns and residents may be trained. This is in contrast to the viewpoints of the other two contributors to this chapter who consider the non-teaching hospital to be one without interns or residents, the educational program thus being confined to the continuing education of the attending staff and to the inservice education of nurses and other paramedical personnel, and perhaps to an occasional medical school preceptee.*)

There are several types of so-called non-teaching hospitals. They are not affiliated with a medical school, but sometimes they are hospitals where medical school faculty members hospitalize their private patients. Government hospitals and special hospitals of various kinds constitute another group. The largest group includes the free-standing community hospitals, whose main purpose is to provide service of high quality on as comprehensive a basis as possible.

These hospitals face a number of current problems. Many are not able to attract interns or residents. It is difficult to get staff members to take part in programs; and although foreign interns may be accepted at these hospitals, too often they are not given an educational experience. Doctors are so busy that they are unable or unwilling to set aside time for continuing education. Too few of these hospitals have done any effective work in medical audit or in utilization review.

A few suggestions are in order. Realistically, most of these hospitals should forget about intern training programs. Unless they have staff and resources to justify approved residency programs also, they are really only deluding themselves. Many of these hospitals can attract only foreign house staff. Nothing does more harm to the reputation of medical education in the United States than the exploitation of the foreign intern. The only education he may get is the realization that there is a great shortage of doctors for emergency work. Too often, unfortunately, he does not get the kind of training he needs for this activity.

These hospitals should concentrate on the education of their own staff; however a primary problem is to convince the members of the staff that they need continuing education.

Much more attention must be given to evaluating the performance of staff members. This can be done through an active medical audit, and through the record and tissue committees. Through programs like those of the Commission on Professional and Hospital Activities, the committees can determine how their staff compares with the staffs of similar hospitals. The board of directors, by whatever name, must be included in evaluation planning so that they will know what is going on.

Physicians have often been reluctant to let the lay members of the board know much about professional aspects of the hospital. This may result in duplication of facilities in neighboring hospitals with inordinate expenditure of community resources. For example, more than 700 hospitals in this country are fully equipped to perform open heart surgery, yet the average frequency of use of these facilities is only once in two weeks. Medical center hospitals commonly perform heart surgery daily; therefore some hospitals must perform heart surgery about once in six or seven weeks. This is hardly an economical or efficient use of medical talent and costly facilities, and difficult surgery performed infrequently is apt to be performed incompetently.

The hospital board and staff must achieve a friendly, understanding relationship if anything is to be accomplished. Recently, at a meeting of the Joint Commission on Accreditation of Hospitals, we were all distressed to have the chairman of the board of a hospital which was seeking approval appear as the champion of his community's cause. He stated that the medical staff was so indifferent to the problems of the hospital that he was unable to get the chief of staff to join him in a common plea.

There is an increasing trend for hospitals of adequate size to employ a director of medical education. He should be a seasoned, scholarly man with experience in clinical practice and a real interest in teaching. The title this man bears is not as important as the type of man. The whole teaching program should center about day-to-day interchanges between the various specialties and the full-time staff, including the pathologist, the radiologist and the director of medical education. Some type of incentive must be applied. If this can be done without punitive measures, well and good. If not, the staff should have the courage to make even the recalcitrant individuals cooperate.

Finally, the community hospital is an excellent place for the physician to educate ancillary personnel and the public itself.

40

Experiences with Two-way Radio Conferences

By Henry S. M. Uhl, M.D.

Henry S. M. Uhl is associate professor of post-graduate medicine at the Albany Medical College and assistant director of the Albany Regional Hospital Program. He was formerly the director of medical education at the Worcester City Hospital and then at the Springfield Hospital, both in Massachusetts. He is a past president of the Association of Hospital Directors of Medical Education. He received the M.D. degree from Harvard Medical School and is a diplomate of the American Board of Internal Medicine and a Fellow of the American College of Physicians.

In the past 10 years the department of postgraduate medicine of the Albany Medical College has perfected the use of educational FM radio in continuing medical education. The Albany Medical College maintains and operates an educational FM radio station, WAMC, licensed by the Federal Communications Commission. In recent years several other medical centers have developed similar radio conference networks. These include the University of North Carolina, Ohio State University, the Pennsylvania Hospital in Philadelphia, the University of California in San Francisco, and the University of Utah. Additional networks are in the process of organization.

TECHNICAL REQUIREMENTS

The technical arrangements of an operating two-way FM radio educational network are basically simple. There is a central broadcasting studio at the medical center with its associated transmitting facilities. In each participating community hospital there is a standard FM receiver and a remote transmitter. A special antenna is required which will not only receive a signal from the transmitter but also transmit in line of sight back to the transmitting and receiving equipment of the radio station. In each community hospital the remote transmitter is equipped with a standard broadcasting microphone which is operated by the local moderator. Not only will all participating hospitals hear the broadcast of the program from the medical center studio, but all hospitals as well as the studio will hear the questions or comments transmitted by individual hospitals. What is achieved, in effect, is a simulated classroom in which faculty and students alike hear and see everything that transpires in the educational program. Each hospital in the program is provided with a complete set of visuals, 2 x 2 slides, mimeographed information, or other types of reproductions. Each remote transmitter is provided with an alert signal button which, when pressed by the hospital moderator, flashes a light in the medical center studio, indicating that the hospital wishes to ask a question or make a comment.

The broadcast programs of WAMC encompass an area of approximately 22,000 square miles. In addition to the medical college transmitting facilities, WAMC is linked to WGBH in Boston, WFCR in Amherst, Massachusetts, and WRVR in New York City. These cooperating educational stations make it possible for the programs to extend from the metropolitan region of New York City and northern New Jersey to distant hospitals in the state of Maine. At the present time there are more than 60 hospitals in the educational network of the Albany Medical College. These hospitals are located in eastern New York State and Long Island, northern New Jersey, Connecticut, Massachusetts, Vermont, New Hampshire, and Maine. Since a maximum of 12 hospitals can participate in any one conference, it is necessary for the department to produce six radio conferences each week during the academic year from the first of October until the first of April.

FACULTY

It is clearly beyond the scope of a single medical school faculty to present 48 different conferences each year on a schedule of six conferences per week. Fortunately, the department has developed an effective working relationship with 22 other medical schools in the production of the programs. Electronically and technically it is simple and relatively inexpensive to link the studio at the Albany Medical Center with any other medical college through the use of class D telephone lines. This provides a satisfactory audio quality for the broadcast. In this way, the faculty can remain "at home," for example, in Columbus, Ohio, at the Ohio State University School of Medicine. In fact this procedure underwent its ultimate test in October of 1965 when a two-way FM radio conference was held with a faculty participating at the University of Sidney in Australia.

COSTS

What is the projected cost of the basic equipment for a medical center and 20 hospitals? The information is provided in Table 40-1 for esti-

TABLE 40-1. Cost of FM Equipment for a Medical Center and 20 Hospitals

	Minimum	Maximum
Master transmitter	$ 5,000	$12,000
Antennae, towers, studio equipment, etc.	8,000	14,000
Remote pick-up transmitters ($700 each)	14,000	14,000
Other costs, including technical assistance	5,000	10,000
	$32,000	$50,000

mated minimum and maximum cost. The total annual figure may vary from $32,000 to $50,000. In addition to these items the medical center will have to provide an engineering staff to maintain the equipment, both at the transmitter site and in the individual hospitals. This department installs a remote transmitter and receiver in the community hospitals, installs the antenna, checks out the transmission and reception, and periodically visits each hospital to check out all aspects of its operation. Each hospital in the conference network pays an annual fee of approximately $800 to the Albany Medical College. This fee includes 24 radio programs, the installation of the receiver and transmitter, the installation of the antenna, and the maintenance of the equipment on an annual basis. This is indeed an educational bargain!

AUDIENCE

Some overall statistics concerning physician attendance at these conferences are given in Table 40-2. The sharp increase in physician attendance between 1955 and 1965 does not indicate a dramatic rise in the

TABLE 40-2. Physician Attendance per Week

	1955–1960	1960–1965	1964–1965
First half of season	203	524	721
Second half of season	201	501	587
Total (24 weeks)	202	512	653
Total physician attendance	4,748	12,295	15,690
Others (nurses, technicians, etc.)	439	1,160	1,688

NOTE: The first two columns represent annual averages.

average attendance by physicians at each hospital but rather reflects the increased number of hospitals participating in the network. The average physician attendance at individual hospitals has not changed significantly and varies a great deal from one hospital to another. In recent years an average of slightly over one hospital per year has withdrawn from the network. Many hospitals have continued to participate over a period of 5 or more years.

The type of practice among physicians who attend these conferences is shown in the Table 40-3. It is clear that the widest appeal is to physi-

TABLE 40-3. Type of Practice Represented at Conferences

	1955–1960	1960–1965	1964–1965
General practice	29.2%	25.1%	29.2%
Internal medicine	15.5%	15.3%	14.9%
Surgery	9.2%	9.3%	9.2%
Other specialties	20.2%	27.1%	20.1%
House staff	25.9%	23.2%	26.6%

NOTE: Table 40-3 indicates the percentage of physicians in the various categories who attended the Albany Two-way Radio Conferences. The first two columns represent annual averages.

cians who are basically involved in the practice of general medicine, whether as internists or family physicians. This is related in part to the fact that there are many more such physicians in the practice of medicine in community hospitals and also to the fact that the programs produced deal primarily with topics in general medicine, especially in the adult.

SUBJECT OF CONFERENCES

The categories of subjects presented on two-way radio conferences over the past 10 years is summarized in Table 40-4. Medical topics predominate, although surgical topics are not neglected by any means.

EVALUATION OF CONFERENCES

The department has for years distributed evaluation cards to each hospital for the use of physicians in attendance. These cards are collected by the local moderator and returned to the department. Through the years the rating of individual conferences has been predominantly in the range of good to excellent. The return of these cards has also made it possible to have an accurate counting of physicians and other

TABLE 40-4. Categories of Two-way Radio Conferences, 1955–1965

Category	Number
General medicine	42
Cardiovascular disease	39
Metabolic disease	11
Endocrinology	16
Gastrointestinal diseases	7
Pulmonary disease	10
Renal disease	15
Antibiotics and infection	8
Neurology	5
Psychiatry	10
Pediatrics	13
General surgery	11
Special surgery	11
OB-GYN	13
EENT	6
C.P.C.	20
D & T conference	14
Unclassified	12
Physical medicine & rehabilitation	6
Total	259
Total number of conferences	883
Total physician attendance for all conferences (1955–1965)	93,211

individuals attending the programs. Table 40-5 summarizes the results of over 88,000 conference ratings by physicians.

TABLE 40-5. Results of 88,000 Conference Ratings by Physicians

	1955–1960	1960–1965	1964–1965
Excellent	49.4%	40.1%	35.2%
Good	46.6%	50.8%	55.3%
Fair	3.8%	8.1%	8.3%
Poor	0.2%	1.0%	1.2%

CONFERENCE HOUR

Each conference is held at 12 o'clock noon Monday through Friday, except for one broadcast at 10:00 A.M. Tuesday to the metropolitan New York City area. Two different programs are broadcast weekly; each program is repeated three times. There are two networks, designated network I and network II. Programs are broadcast to the hospitals in network I on Tuesday, Wednesday, and Friday at 12:00 noon and to network II on Monday and Thursday at 12:00 noon and at 10:00 A.M. on Tuesday. It is not uncommon for an individual hospital to serve a buffet luncheon on trays in the room where the conference is held.

SUMMARY

Two-way FM radio conferences are a proven method for the continuing education of practicing physicians and house officers in community hospitals. The technique provides a great saving in time for both faculty and audience. It is one imaginative approach to solving some of the pressing problems of postgraduate medicine, by bringing a high-quality program each week to the busy physician in his own hospital.

41

The Medical Audit Is Postgraduate Education

By C. Wesley Eisele, M.D.

C. Wesley Eisele is associate professor of medicine and Associate Dean for Postgraduate Medical Education at the University of Colorado School of Medicine. He received the M.S. and M.D. degrees from Northwestern University and served on the faculty of the University of Chicago before coming to the University of Colorado School of Medicine in 1951. He is a diplomate of the American Board of Internal Medicine and a Fellow of the American College of Physicians. In 1961, he received a Certificate of Meritorious Service from the American Academy of General Practice, and in 1966 he was awarded an Honorary Fellowship by the American College of Hospital Administrators.

Dr. Eisele has long been active in postgraduate education. He was a member of the AMA Residency Review Committee for Internal Medicine and served as chairman of the Continuing Education Committee of the Association of American Medical Colleges. He was a founding member of the Board of Trustees of the Commission on Professional and Hospital Activities, and he is past president of the Commission. He has also acted as a consultant in medical audit activities and evaluation problems in many hospitals. Through his efforts and enthusiasm, three postgraduate courses have been given by the University of Colorado on the Hospital Medical Staff and Medical Education in the Hospital. This volume is the product of those postgraduate courses.

Physicians are often criticized for their failure to keep up with scientific advances and for the gap between the research laboratory and the bedside. But there have been great gains in the number, variety, and quality of short postgraduate courses offered throughout the country as well as gains in the number of registrants at these courses. In the year 1965–66, there were 1,641 postgraduate courses in the annual list of the American Medical Association Council on Medical Education. They were offered by 252 primary sponsors, with 863 (53 per cent) of the courses sponsored by medical schools and 351 (21 per cent) sponsored by hospitals. The number of courses has increased almost 50 per cent in the past 5 years, and the number of registrants has increased more than threefold.[1]

Impressive as these gains are, critics have rightfully found many faults with our current offerings in postgraduate courses. Often they are archaic, inappropriate, and ineffective. Rarely is the registrant given an opportunity to participate actively. The lecture method, which has been largely abandoned in undergraduate medical education, remains the backbone of postgraduate programs. It has been clearly shown that retention of material from lectures is generally poor. Subject matter and presentation may not be pertinent to the practicing physician's needs or interests and may be tangential to his experience. The curriculum is usually fragmentary and not planned systematically.

In a survey conducted by the American Medical Association,[2] eight major deterrents to the continuing education of the practicing physician were found:

There is no one to take care of his patients while he is away.
The courses are held at unsuitable times.
The cost in money and the time away from practice are prohibitive.
There is a multiplicity of other meetings.
The subject matter is not suited to the physician's needs.
There is a lack of courses in the physician's area.
There is previous unsatisfactory experience with poor courses.
There is lack of information about courses.

There are two paramount questions which we must ask ourselves: Are our postgraduate programs reaching the physician who most needs help? Are we providing educational opportunities which will alter the physician's way of practice and elevate his standards? These questions are perennial topics for discussion whenever medical educators consider postgraduate education.

We are impressed with the physicians whom we see at our postgraduate courses year after year, earnestly and conscientiously listening to lectures and panels; but we doubt that they are the ones who need continuing education the most. Certainly there are many practicing physicians who have never been seriously involved in any form of continuing education—no postgraduate courses, irregular attendance at hospital staff meetings, unopened medical journals, and attendance at medical society meetings only for their social functions. They may see an occasional pharmaceutical detail man on whom they rely for virtually all their continuing education. I know of no reliable data on how many such physicians there are in our communities; one can only guess.

The other question is even more thorny. Are our traditional efforts in postgraduate medical education achieving their goal with those who do participate? Do they actually effect changes in the physician's pattern of practice and elevate his standards? Are the physician's basic attitudes improved? Efforts to evaluate the effectiveness of postgraduate courses have not been very fruitful; and again, one can only guess.

ACCEPTANCE OF THE MEDICAL AUDIT CONCEPT

The phenomenal growth of the recognition and acceptance of the concept of the medical audit is one of the more significant developments on the continuing education scene. In essence, the medical audit is the only situation in the practice of medicine which provides an element of compulsion for continued learning—a compulsion which is palatable and may be imperceptible. The medical audit is a way of life in many hospitals, and many more are coming to realize that the unacceptable alternative is compulsory periodic examinations by state licensure boards.

Most physicians practice in a hospital setting. The psychiatrist is perhaps the only specialist who may conduct his practice successfully without a hospital affiliation. Hospital practice, therefore, is the only medium available for establishing and assessing professional standards in medicine. A systematic analysis of the competence of the medical staff is highly superior to the surveillance that is possible by a medical society or a state licensure board. The necessity of documenting the care of the patient for his own benefit sets the entire process in motion.

Although hospital practice constitutes only a part of a physician's total practice, it is difficult to believe that the quality and standards of care rendered in the hospital do not carry over into his outside practice. The physician does not become a different kind of doctor when he goes from the hospital to his office.

But these are negative aspects of the medical audit, and they are greatly overshadowed by the positive attributes—the opportunity to provide an ever better standard of patient care; the opportunity for physicians to learn by their errors and shortcomings so that they may do better in the future; and the opportunity for physicians to continue to grow in knowledge, judgment, and skill. It profits one but little to repeat the same experience 20 times if that experience is inferior when measured against realistic progressive standards.

For 20 years, some of us have advanced the concept that the prime function of the medical audit is education and not control, discipline, or regulation. Acceptance of this concept grew slowly in the early years, but more recently, at an accelerated rate. Many physicians continue to cling fearfully to the misconception that the medical audit is "to regiment the practice of medicine," "to beat down the general practitioner," or "to give the boys who are 'in' an excuse to cut my privileges." Unhappily, on rare occasions such motives may indeed have been associated with the abuse of the medical audit, particularly in the early years. But I know of no instance in which such tactics have had notable success, certainly not for long.

We have now come to a crossroads. Utilization review—quality control of some sort—has become mandatory through Medicare. In effect, the government has placed the public's stamp of approval on quality control. Utilization review has also become a requirement of the Joint Commission on Accreditation of Hospitals. The medical staff must now make a choice: Will it follow the educational, comprehensive medical audit route, or will it take the path which may appear to be easier—the control approach?

The concepts underlying the medical audit are in the finest tradition of medicine and go back to the very beginning of the profession. Medicine is a true, learned profession. The physician is unselfishly dedicated to the welfare of his fellow men. Now that the term "professional" is applied loosely to almost anyone who is paid for whatever he does, it is important that the attributes of a learned profession be clearly defined. High on the list is the willingness to engage in self-evaluation, self-criticism, and self-discipline.

No other learned profession has the opportunity for self-evaluation that is so easily available to the medical profession, for no other profession has its documentation in order and in a central location. Dentistry, law, architecture, the clergy—none have anything approaching the hospital patient's clinical record as a tool for professional self-appraisal and self-discipline.

One must decry the failure of the medical schools to introduce this philosophy to the student and to largely ignore the facts of the important functions of the hospital medical staff. Nor are these things communicated very well in the internship and residency years because the house staff function is separated from the attending staff function.

In spite of the criticisms and shortcomings, medicine is far ahead of almost every other profession in its efforts in continuing education. But more effective approaches and new methods must be constantly sought.

THE EDUCATIONAL VALUES OF THE MEDICAL AUDIT

The educational aspects of a well-conducted medical audit answer many of the major criticisms of traditional continuing education surprisingly well, and the uses of this new tool should be thoroughly explored by medical educators who until now have failed to appreciate its significance and usefulness. The medical audit satisfies the special educational needs of the practicing physician in seven ways.

1. *The educational benefits of a medical audit are universally available.* The medical staff of any hospital that wants it, regardless of size or remoteness from a medical center or a metropolitan area, may have the unique benefits of a medical audit program. The only limiting factor is the motivation of the medical staff. Among the more than 800 hospitals across the country that participate in the Professional Activity Study and the Medical Audit Program of the Commission on Professional and Hospital Activities, several dozen have only 20 to 40 beds, many are in isolated communities, and some have fewer than 1,000 annual admissions. There are hundreds of hospitals of less than 100 beds that participate. I have observed one rural hospital with less than 100 beds that has had an active medical audit committee since 1950, and all members of the staff work on the committee in rotation.

2. *The medical audit utilizes the highly esteemed self-education principle.* This is becoming the ultimate goal of all formal education. More and more, the better liberal arts colleges are introducing tutorial and thesis courses similar to many graduate level courses. The student is stimulated to seek knowledge on his own initiative. As William Saltonstall has said so poignantly, "In the last analysis, our job as teachers is to make ourselves dispensable. We cannot give the student an education, but we can help him find out how to get one—assuming that he wants it."

3. *All members of the staff are involved.* Those who serve on the medical audit committees reap the greatest educational benefits. It is therefore wise for all members of the staff to serve on the committees in rotation. The review of medical audit results with the staff is an additional learning experience. The reluctant physician may shun postgraduate courses and may avoid scientific meetings in his own hospital and county medical society, but he will be hard put to escape the impact of the medical audit, especially as it involves his own patients.

4. *The medical audit utilizes the physician's own patients and his own experience.* It starts where the student is—another cardinal principle of education. Learning proceeds best and retention is greater when the student's own experience is the base line.

5. *The medical audit engenders motivation for formal as well as informal continuing education.* There is nothing more effective in making one hustle to the library than being faced with one's own errors and deficiencies. The motivation is especially great when one sees his record compared objectively with those of his fellow staff members, and especially when anonymous interhospital comparisons show that his own mediocre work caused his whole hospital to suffer by comparison.

Once the physician begins to revisit the library and the learning process is again set in motion, it is an easy step for him to seek more formal instruction.

6. *The findings of the medical audit committee define areas of greatest need for the formal continuing education programs of the staff.* Deficiencies in performance in specific disease areas may become obvious when the practice of the entire staff in a given area is reviewed. The process becomes especially sharp when there are interhospital comparisons, such as those provided by the PAS-MAP programs. An area in which the practice of the staff differs from that in other hospitals is a clear signal for investigation and frequently for specific educational efforts.

7. *The medical audit, more than most other educational processes, achieves the ultimate goal of continuing education—the improvement in the quality of patient care.* It has been the common experience of hospitals of all types and all sizes that when a well-motivated and a well-conducted medical audit program is introduced the standards of care are elevated and conformity to the standards are improved. These desirable effects are less noticeable if the motivation is control rather than education.

SUMMARY

The benefits of an educationally oriented medical audit are often subtle and, in many respects, unique. The gentle compulsion for continuing education is palatable and often imperceptible. A medical audit is available to any hospital that wants it, regardless of size or location; it utilizes the self-education principle to a high degree; all members of the staff are involved; it uses the physician's own patients and his own experience as a base line; it engenders motivation for formal as well as informal continuing education; it helps define the areas of practice in the hospital in greatest need of educational programs; and it influences the physician's patterns of practice and elevates his standards—the ultimate goal of all continuing education.

BIBLIOGRAPHY

1. Continuing Education Courses for Physicians, *JAMA*, 193:447–536 (Aug. 9) 1965.

2. Vollan, D. D.: Postgraduate Medical Education in the United States, Report of the Survey of Postgraduate Medical Education carried out by the Council on Medical Education and Hospitals, American Medical Association, 1952–1955.

Part VII

Internships and Residencies

42

Mechanisms for the Approval of Internships and Residencies

By John C. Nunemaker, M.D.

John C. Nunemaker is the associate secretary of the Council on Medical Education and Hospitals of the American Medical Association. Prior to taking this post in 1958, he served as director of the Education Service in the department of medicine and surgery of the Veterans Administration from 1952 to 1958. He received the M.D. degree from Harvard Medical School, and he is a diplomate of the American Board of Internal Medicine. He is also a lecturer in medicine at Northwestern University Medical School.

HISTORICAL INTRODUCTION

Although our present concern with graduate medical education as a formal matter dates from about the beginning of the present century, it is important to note that a house staff was employed with the first hospital in the United States, the Pennsylvania Hospital, since its founding in 1751. The year 1889 is an important bench mark in the history of graduate medical education in this country, for that date marks the opening of the Johns Hopkins Hospital and the employment of a graduate resident staff. With the graduation of the first class at Hopkins in 1897, interns were selected and appointed to a rotating service in the hospital.

It is convenient to divide the modern history of graduate medical education since 1900 into four eras, the first three of which are each roughly 20 years in length.

The Internship Era

The first 20 years may be identified as the Internship Era, since it was during that period that lists of approved programs and standards were first published. Within the first few years of the 20th century, there was a reorganization of the American Medical Association itself. By 1904 the previous committee on medical education had been abolished, and the Council on Medical Education was established with a full-time staff. The first Education Number of the *J.A.M.A.* was published in 1901, and by 1913 the Council had initiated its first study of facilities for advanced training in medicine. In 1914, it published the first list of hospitals approved for internships, but this was not a very selective list inasmuch as it included programs in specialty hospitals as well as in general hospitals, varying in lengths from 6 to more than 30 months. A second survey of facilities for graduate education in 1919 revealed that they were entirely inadequate, and accordingly the first standards were established and published as the *Essentials of an Approved Internship.*

By the time the first list was published in 1914, approximately 70 per cent of medical school graduates were taking internship training. In 1915 there were 96 medical schools with approximately 15,000 students. There were approximately 600 hospitals offering about 3,000 internship positions to some 3,500 annual graduates.

The Residency Era

The Residency Era, involving the 20 years between World Wars I and II, saw further developments in the area of graduate education for the specialties; and because of increasing attention to hospital facilities for this purpose, the name of the Council was changed in 1920 to the Council on Medical Education and Hospitals. In that same year the Council organized 15 committees in 11 clinical and 4 basic science areas for the purpose of recommending "what preparation was deemed essential to secure expertness in each of the specialties." It is of considerable interest that the following year the recommendations of these committees were reported at the annual Congress on Medical Education, specifying that in a few specialties there should be two additional years of graduate study beyond the internship, but that for most specialties, three years of additional graduate study was recommended. The Council minutes give us no indication of the basis upon which this three-year recommendation was made more than 40 years ago, and it is somewhat surprising that this general pattern and duration of training has persisted.

That *hospital service requirements* played some role in matters relating to intern and resident training has been clear since the first editorial on the shortage of interns was published in 1921. In 1923 the Congress on Medical Education included a paper on "The Role of Non-medical Clinical Assistants in Hospitals without Interns." Here again we see early recognition of the fact that the intern delivered valuable services and that it was desirable that hospitals develop additional categories of persons to assist the physician in clinical care of patients.

As was true in the earlier era for internships, the first list of approved residencies was published before the publication of standards. The list was published in 1927, and the *Essentials of Approved Residencies* was published in 1928, even though they had been adopted by the House of Delegates five years earlier. With the availability of statistics on the number of residencies available, we were thus able to calculate that in the 13-year period between the establishment of lists of internships and the establishment of the list of residencies a pattern of graduate education had developed relating interns to residents by a ratio of 3:1, establishing a pyramidal pattern.

By 1930, a resolution had been presented to the House of Delegates calling for the creation of a national accrediting body to recognize specialists. During the next three to fours years of intense activity, the Advisory Board for Medical Specialties was established in 1933 and 1934, and it included the four existing boards. At that time, the *Essentials for Approval of Examining Boards in the Specialties* was prepared jointly by the Council and the Advisory Board and approved by the American Medical Association House of Delegates. By the end of this era in 1940, 10 additional boards had been formed, thus bringing to fruition the recommendations of the 15 committees which the Council had appointed 20 years earlier.

Another significant activity at the end of this era was the creation in 1937 by the Advisory Board of a Commission on Graduate Education and the publication of its report in book form in 1940 under the title *Graduate Medical Education*. Much of the basic philosophy contained in that publication is fully current after more than 25 years, and that book was probably the first true guide to supplement the relatively meager material published in the *Essentials*.

Throughout the entire first 20 years and most of the second 20 years, the approval of internships and residencies was entirely in the hands of the Council and carried out by its staff.

The Hospital Era

The period during and after World War II may be identified as the Hospital Era because there was a marked growth of hospitals in connection with government-assisted building programs, a rapid increase in prepaid hospital and medical care insurance with an accompanying increase in hospital utilization, and a rapid rise in hospital service needs.

By 1941 the increase in residencies was sufficient to produce a ratio between internships and residencies of 1.5:1. By 1946 there were more residencies than internships, and for the next several years the increase in available residency positions was explosive. This increase was condoned by the Council because of the thousands of veteran physicians who wished to resume their interrupted residency programs and for whom such positions had to be created hastily. Accordingly, for several years residency programs were approved on a paper basis and without survey.

Even the Council was unprepared for the continued subsequent growth of residencies; and in 1947 a statement was published suggesting that when the acute demand by veteran physicians had subsided, the total residency positions should be reduced to a lower level in order to maintain high educational standards. The Council did state, however, that certain of these newly developed training facilities should be continued so that they would be available to physicians from foreign countries who might be expected to come here because of our world leadership in medicine. The Exchange-Visitor Program was implemented in 1949 when, for the first time, the Council files began to report a surplus of available residency positions.

By 1950, there had been a definite decrease in the number of American graduates seeking residency training, but by 1953 the increased numbers of foreign graduates coming to this country had restored the total number of residents on duty to a figure which was in excess of the number of American residents in training in 1948. Thereafter, the columns continued to lengthen each year, and no one knows where it will end.

Because of the increasing concern of authorities in this country not only over the standards for approval of training programs but also over the qualifications of the trainees, a list of foreign medical schools was published in 1950. This was an advisory list, prepared jointly by the Executive Council of the Association of American Medical Colleges and the Council on Medical Education of the American Medical Association. At no time was this considered to be a list of approved foreign schools.

By 1951 the National Intern Matching Program had been inaugurated to allow recent graduates to choose internships free of some of the pressure generated earlier by hospitals' desires for assistance with their service problems.

By 1957 the Educational Council for Foreign Medical Graduates had been established; and by 1960 the advisory list of foreign medical schools was withdrawn. At this time, the continued increase in residencies of nearly 600 per cent compared to 1941 had far outstripped the increase in internships of only 50 per cent. As a result, the pyramid became inverted, and the ratio of internships to residencies became 1:3.

The Era of Crisis in Medical Manpower

With the end of the Hospital Era about 1960, we moved into the Era of Crisis in Medical Manpower. Many of our efforts today to maintain and elevate the standards of medical education conflict with the desires of the medical profession and society for additional medical manpower.

THE DEVELOPMENT OF REVIEW COMMITTEES

In 1928, a field staff was first employed for the specific purpose of surveying educational programs in hospitals. Until that time, those surveys of internships and residencies which had been performed were largely done by the small full-time staff of the Council.

In 1939, toward the end of the Residency Era, the Secretary of the Council met with the Regents of the American College of Physicians and later with the Board of Trustees of the AMA to discuss better collaboration in the evaluation and approval of residency programs.

Because of the established interests of the various national groups, the Council approached this matter delicately and went through the formality of a supplementary report to the House of Delegates as follows:

> The Council has found it desirable to confer with the examining boards in several of the specialties, and some of the specialty societies, such as the American College of Physicians and the American Psychiatric Association, concerning problems of graduate medical education, relating to the training of specialists, and requests permission of the House of Delegates to explore the possibility of cooperative relationships with other organizations.

This was approved by the House of Delegates, and it is reported here only to indicate that some of the well-established working relationships which we all understand and take for granted did not come about easily and without considerable negotiation on the part of many dedicated men representing various national groups.

The cooperative plan for the joint study and appraisal of programs in the specialties developed in 1939 was first endorsed by the boards of anesthesiology, pediatrics, pathology, and radiology; and by June of 1940, 10 boards had endorsed it. The plan would provide that:

1. After conference with the respective specialty board, a suitable application blank be prepared in triplicate so that one copy would be available to the Council, one to the specialty board, and one for the hospital files.

2. An inspection be carried out by the Council staff to confirm and amplify the information submitted by application.
3. An inspection report be prepared emphasizing objective data that could subsequently be utilized in the evaluation of the education program.
4. Copies of the application and inspection report be forwarded to the secretary of the board for further evaluation.
5. Subsequently the application be submitted to the Council with the recommendation of the board.

Shortly, all boards except ophthalmology were cooperating in this type of evaluation. The American Board of Ophthalmology supplied information but felt it was not in itself an evaluating or approving agency.

It is important to mention at this point that *the American College of Surgeons inaugurated a survey of selected hospitals* in 1937, and in 1939 it published its own list of approved hospitals, confining its attention to those with three-year programs in surgery and placing particular emphasis on instruction in the basic sciences. The College also published its fundamental requirements for training in surgery. It was not until 1948 that the American College of Surgeons and an AMA Joint Committee agreed to a collaborative effort. This was known as the Joint Committee on Hospital Problems, and it provided a single standard and a single list of approved programs published by both the Council and the American College of Surgeons.

While the above activities were being pursued by essentially all the boards in collaboration with the Council, further developments were being made in the field of internal medicine. In 1940 a tripartite body known as the Conference Committee on Graduate Training in Internal Medicine was organized, representing the American College of Physicians, the American Board of Internal Medicine, and the Council on Medical Education. This committee met to review programs, and it was the first departure from the pattern of evaluations and recommendations being made by the board or a committee of the board alone. World War II caused a suspension of the Conference Committee's activities, and the Council and the Board continued to evaluate programs as did all other Boards until the committee was reactivated in 1949.

As mentioned, it was not until 1948 that the American College of Surgeons and the Council on Medical Education and Hospitals agreed that desirable economies of effort, time, and money could be accomplished by the organization of a single acceptable procedure. Between 1948 and 1950, representatives of the American College of Surgeons, the American Medical Association, and the American Board of Surgery developed a tripartite committee known as the Conference

Committee on Graduate Training in Surgery, which functioned similarly to that in medicine.

My predecessor, the late Dr. Edward Leveroos, joined the Council staff after the War and was directly concerned with Council relationships with the Boards and the Conference Committees in the evaluation of residency programs. As a result of the experience in the fields of medicine and surgery, he was able to recommend to the Council in 1952 the establishment of *residency review committees in other fields*. The proposal was for the Council to establish administrative procedures in its office and to provide a secretary for each committee. The chairman of the committee was to be selected from the specialty board represent-atives, and the representatives of the Council and the Board need not necessarily be members of either organization but should be specialists in the field involved. The Council minutes do not indicate the extreme delicacy with which some of these negotiations were carried on; but many difficulties were encountered during this period by certain of the specialty groups which had long had vested interests which they were reluctant to share until they were assured that the newly proposed procedure represented a true improvement. By 1953 five boards had indicated an active interest in the new proposal, and the Conference Committee on Graduate Training in Internal Medicine officially changed its name to the *Residency Review Committee in Internal Medicine*, in keeping with the belief that this name more adequately described its activities. The title "Residency Review Committee" has been used in all other specialty areas except in surgery where that tripartite committee prefers to retain the original Conference Committee title.

By 1954 it was possible to establish an Internship Review Committee, and by 1958 the 18th Residency Review Committee was established in obstetrics and gynecology. Only the American Board of Pathology and the Board of Thoracic Surgery prefer to continue the Joint collaborative activities along the 1939 pattern outside the Residency Review Com-mittee structure.

ORGANIZATION AND ADMINISTRATION OF REVIEW COMMITTEES

In 1952 one secretary from the Council staff served all committees; it has now become necessary to provide three physicians for this function in addition to three administrative assistants who act as recorders for the meetings and manage the host of administrative details relating to them. While the committeemen representing the Council usually are not Council members, representatives of the specialty board on most committees are board members.

It is the established policy of the Council that no review committee shall consist of more than three sponsoring organizations and that no committee shall have more than 12 voting members. The cooperating organizations have agreed to these standards. The two basic sponsors of any committee are the Council and the Board.

Committee Membership. While the majority of committees are bipartite, six of the committees are tripartite. There are two to four voting members from each organization, so the total committee membership varies from six to twelve. The responsible staff officials of the sponsoring organizations also usually attend the meetings in an ex officio non-voting capacity. The committee size may fluctuate, and one six-man committee has recently been increased to eight because of the increased scope of the review activities. Actually some of the non-voting ex officio secretaries of the specialty boards also assist in the review procedures even though they have no vote in policy matters.

In the case of the Residency Review Committee for General Practice, since there is no board, the American Academy of General Practice provides three representatives and the Council provides three representatives. In this case the representatives are members of the Council although they are not necessarily general practitioners.

The Internship Review Committee was established with somewhat different sponsorship than the Residency Review Committees, and it was determined that no individual specialty groups should be represented. Accordingly, representation on the Internship Review Committee is from the Council on Medical Education, the American Hospital Association, the Association of American Medical Colleges, and the Federation of State Medical Boards. There is also a representative from the field of general practice. The Academy of General Practice is not specifically included because other specialty groups would likely feel that they were also entitled to membership. A representative from the field of general practice is therefore picked by the Council with the approval of the Academy of General Practice, which pays his expenses to the meetings.

Most committees meet twice a year, but some meet three times a year. The meetings are of one- to two-days' duration, depending upon the number of cases to be reviewed.

Tenure of Committeemen. In the case of the Council representatives, the committeeman is appointed for a three-year term and is eligible for one reappointment. There is some variation in the case of members from the boards or specialty societies; some adhere to the three-year appointment scheme, but others cannot since, according to their own rules, their representatives serve by virtue of their particular appointment on the board. For instance, some boards have a rule that the president and certain other officials are automatically members of the residency review committee. When they relinquish their office on the board, even though they remain as members of the board, they automatically go off the review committee. Nevertheless, there is an orderly turnover of members on all the committees.

Authority of Review Committees. Because of the nature of the sponsoring bodies for the Internship Review Committee, the nature of the internship itself, and the extreme concern shown by the House of Delegates for internship matters, the Council has chosen to retain for itself the responsibility for final approval of programs recommended by the Internship Review Committee. In other words, the Internship Review Committee does not have final authority to approve or disapprove and to recommend listing in the *Directory* but only makes recommendations to the Council.

In the case of the Residency Review Committees, with few exceptions the sponsoring groups have delegated full authority to their representatives on the Committee for final action. In one or two instances, a committee of the specialty board meets on the same day or the day following the meeting of the review committee to review the actions of its representatives. In no case, however, may the specialty board reverse the actions of the review committee although conceivably they could ask the review committee to reconsider action in a specific case.

There are certain activities which the committees can take in their own names and others on which they can only make recommendations to sponsoring bodies. They have final authority for all actions relating to approval, disapproval, or probation of specific programs, and they make final recommendations on the manner in which programs are listed in the *Directory*. They have full authority to develop their own forms for evaluating programs, and they are fully responsible for establishing the procedures by which their committee operates.

The areas in which they *cannot take final action but must first make recommendations to the parent bodies* relate to the production of guide books as supplements to the *Essentials,* proposals for revisions of standards which would be incorporated in the *Essentials,* and the nomination of members of the committees. About a third of the committees have produced guide books, and several are now in the process of making revisions. Any revised standards for incorporation in the *Essentials* must be approved not only by the Council but also by the AMA House of Delegates. In securing panels of names for consideration for appointments to the committees, the Council uses a variety of sources, including nominations from the Council itself, from the residency review committees, from the boards, and from the national specialty societies in the area concerned. The Council attempts to maintain a balance on the committees by considering the geographic source of the members as well as the stature of the member from the professional and educational standpoint, whether or not he is a department head in a medical school.

THE REVIEW PROCEDURE

The initial application for an approved internship or residency may be a letter, a phone call, or a personal visit to the Council office. The Council provides application forms and, in the case of residencies, uses what we call a two-page "short form" to supply basic statistical information. This is returned to the Council office with a narrative description of the proposed operation of the programs and information relating to the staff, library, and other facilities. After a preliminary review in the Council office and if it appears that the program meets the basic requirements stated in the *Essentials,* the application is accepted and the hospital is notified that a survey by a field representative is being scheduled.

Survey by Field Representative. Schedules of the field representatives are usually established several months in advance, and a hospital should not expect a survey before three to six months. Occasionally, a program may be surveyed earlier if a field representative has scheduled a visit to the hospital for the purposes of surveying an existing program. Sometimes requests are received to change the dates for a scheduled survey because the administrator or some other hospital official will be absent. Usually dates cannot be changed, and we feel that no program should be so dependent upon the presence of any one man that it could not be appropriately reviewed. In other words, besides the director, there should be assistant directors and others sufficiently conversant with the program so that it could be reviewed effectively even in the absence of a chief. A change in the dates may affect many other hospitals, thus disturbing plans made by a variety of other individuals.

Regional Evaluation. In recent years, some of the review committees have arranged for particular programs to be surveyed by experienced specialists as well as the Council field representatives. These are called regional evaluations since they involve specialists in the same general geographic region. In the case of the surgery committee, any new application or any request for extension of approval from three to four years must automatically be surveyed by a specialist after it has been surveyed by the Council field representative. This, of course, may mean several more months delay before the matter can come before the committee.

The "Long Form." Each hospital is notified approximately one month before the actual date of the survey, and at that time it is given a "long form" to be completed and held for the surveyor's visit. This varies from as few as 4 pages to as many as 10, depending upon the specialty. Several review committees are now developing more comprehensive forms based on many years of operating experience, but ordinarily the forms do not entail a total revision of the manner in which the hospital keeps statistics.

Most of the committees feel that the statistics they need may not necessarily relate to the standard overall hospital statistics kept by the medical record librarian; and, in fact, many of the data are best collected in the clinical department by the program director. Several committees demand absolute adherence to the long form and will not accept additional material. The long forms enable the surveyors to spend more time evaluating the program and verifying the data on the form and less time in writing voluminous reports of their own.

The Council representatives are basically reporters, but at the time of the survey they may also act as *consultants*. They can be very helpful in interpreting policies of the Council and the review committees as well as the standards as published in the *Essentials*, but they are not expected to visit hospitals for the primary purpose of assisting the hospital staff to organize acceptable programs. If a hospital staff is not fully qualified to organize an acceptable program on the basis of its own knowledge and experience, it is felt that no amount of consultation with field representatives will be effective.

The material on the long forms and the field representative's report are given a preliminary review in the Council offices and then mailed to committee members for review. Deficiencies in the application may lead to a request for additional information from the hospital.

The evaluation procedure at the time of the review committee meeting is initiated by a detailed discussion of the program by one or more members of the committee who have reviewed the program in depth. For some of the committees, the Council staff has made statistical extracts of the programs up for review.

Committee action on each program may be one of the following: (1) provisional approval (in the case of a new program); (2) full approval; (3) confidential probation if there are deficiencies which do not merit continuation of full approval; (4) withdrawal of approval for a program that has been unable to remedy the deficiencies; or (5) deferral of action for additional information. No public announcement is ever made of the confidential probational status of any program, and it remains listed in the Directory as approved. Such a program is allowed 12 to 18 months for correction of the deficiencies before a final decision is made. Programs which have been inactive for two successive years are considered individually for withdrawal from the list of approved programs.

The *Annual Report of the Council*, which is published in the *Directory of Approved Internships and Residencies* and also in the Education Number of the *J.A.M.A.*, includes a table which shows the activities of the various Residency Review Committees for the previous year. For the period July 1, 1964, to June 30, 1965, 37 committee meetings were held, and 2,470 programs were reviewed. There were 127 programs added to the approved list, and by pure coincidence an identical number of programs had approval withdrawn. There were 72 new programs on which approval was withheld because requirements were not met for even provisional approval; there were 226 placed or continued on confidential probation; there were 1,258 granted continued full approval.

SOURCES OF CONFUSION AND CONCERN

At the conclusion of the review committee meeting, the minutes are completed, and the Council staff begins to prepare *notification letters* to the individual program director and the hospital administrator. Difficulties sometimes arise because of delays in notifying hospitals of committee action. It is our policy to attempt to make notification letters as helpful as possible. Many committees make suggestions even though they give full approval to a program. Often they ask for progress reports for consideration at the next meeting, and they frequently recommend an early resurvey. Routinely, every fully approved program is resurveyed every three years, but we find more and more frequent surveys being made because of committee concern over some aspect of a particular program.

When programs are placed on *confidential probation,* there is often a rather severe emotional reaction on the part of the program director and the hospital administrator. If a program director feels the action of the committee was inappropriate, he may appeal for reconsideration; and he is given an opportunity to submit additional material in support of his appeal. The committee considers such appeals at their next regularly scheduled meeting but rarely takes action between meetings. An exception is the rare case in which the Council staff discovers that a committee took action in the absence of all available data because of a breakdown in the communications chain or because of an accidental misinterpretation of some of the submitted material. When the Council discovers such an error, it is usually possible to secure ad hoc committee action by a subcommittee of the review committee, thus preserving the previous status of the program until the next regular meeting of the full committee.

In the case of programs from which approval has been withdrawn, the letters of notification carry specific statements permitting trainees in the program to finish the current year without prejudice and with full credit toward board certification. Residents are advised to communicate immediately with the board to ascertain their status, but the Council's policy is directed at protecting the trainee where he clearly was not responsible for the defects in the program and obviously could not have known in advance of the action of the review committee.

The review committees do not permit personal appearances of program directors, for an eloquent personal plea is no substitute for a factual site visit where a competent surveyor can observe the program in operation and interview all concerned including the residents.

A point of some confusion on the part of hospital personnel relates to the fact that *committees in the varying specialties may take somewhat different points of view* on individual programs. In one instance, a hospital received letters from three different committee secretaries with the information that each committee had taken a different type of action from full approval to probation to withdrawal of approval. In the opinion of the hospital staff the three programs had equal merit. Considerable correspondence and personal consultation was required before the hospital staff understood that these three separate actions were taken by three totally different committees and were based on quite unrelated factors involving each individual specialty.

CONCERNS OF THE COUNCIL

The Council has shown continuing concern for *improving methods of evaluation,* and this has been echoed by all of the review committees. With the advent of sophisticated data processing methods, a greater degree of uniformity may be developed in some of the committee procedures. Record keeping and computer programming would be considerably simpler, but at the hospital level, activities of the medical record librarian and the department heads would also be greatly facilitated. When computer facilities are fully developed, the scheduling of surveys, the preparation of material for committee meetings, and the preparation of the *Directory of Approved Internships and Residencies* will be greatly facilitated.

In the past year, we have been fortunate in adding more personnel to the staff of the Section on Graduate Education. Each of the review committees can now be served more effectively, and hospitals can receive notification of committee actions considerably sooner than in the past. There is still the problem of approximately 20 different committees setting meeting dates quite independently of each other so that it is rarely possible to arrange an even flow of work a year in advance.

We are gratified that most directors of medical education are quite cognizant of these problems, but we feel a vast amount of education and orientation is yet to be done not only with program directors but particularly with representatives of county and state medical societies to whom the complexities of our evaluation procedures are largely unknown.

The Council endeavors to hold meetings with representatives of state medical societies in various regions of the country at least four times yearly. At each of these meetings, the Council members and staff describe the general area of the Council's total responsibilities and then in-

vite discussion. Almost without fail, the subjects of greatest concern revolve about the approval of internships and residencies. Actually, a high
proportion of the time of the Council staff and of each of the review
committees is devoted to two major problems in community hospital programs—the dependence of many community hospitals on foreign-trained
physicians and the conflict between the standards for education and the
hospital's service requirements. It is believed that the message is finally
coming home to hospital staffs, their administrators, and governing bodies
that a fully satisfactory program which will attract well-qualified trainees
year after year cannot be maintained without a degree of support which
many are unwilling or unable to give. The true worth of a program is not
measured by its successful evaluation by one of the review committees
nor by its listing in the *Directory of Approved Internships and Residencies;* rather, it is measured by successful recruitment year after year,
based largely on the word-of-mouth advertising of satisfied customers.

43

What Makes a Good Internship?

By Jesse D. Rising, M.D.

Jesse D. Rising is chairman of the department of postgraduate medical education, professor of medicine, and professor of pharmacology at the University of Kansas School of Medicine. He received the A.B. and M.D. degrees from the University of Kansas. He has long been active in the field of postgraduate medical education, having served on the Advisory Committee on Internships and Hospital Services of the AMA, the Commission on Education of the American Academy of General Practice, the AMA Residency Review Committee for General Practice, and the Committee on Continuation Education of the Association of American Medical Colleges. He is chairman of the AMA Commission on Medical Practice and a member of the Internship Review Committee. He is also chairman of the Preceptorship Committee at the University of Kansas School of Medicine. He was engaged in the private practice of general medicine in Kansas City, Missouri from 1939 until 1953.

It is probably fair and accurate to state at the very beginning that no one really knows in any objective sense how to answer the question posed by the above title, but the subject is important and warrants thought, study, and discussion.

EVALUATION OF INTERNSHIPS

Evaluation of an educational experience presupposes that clear criteria are available against which to measure the experience. Such clear criteria have not been developed for the internship.

It is reasonable to say that the best internship is one that turns out the best doctors as measured by the quality of their practice and patient care, but everyone is aware of the difficulties in evaluating the quality of physicians' work. The well-known study by Osler Peterson attempted to correlate the quality of practice with the kind of training that physicians had received both in medical school and afterwards, and the only significant finding was that the more training a man had had in internal medicine the better he practiced medicine.[1] This study has been the subject of much debate; but until better information is available, we must keep in mind its one outstanding finding. The study of family physicians conducted by the Health Insurance Plan of New York, under the direction of Morehead, had as its significant finding the fact that the quality of care given by physicians who had two or more years of training was superior to that of those who had less.[2] The importance of this will be discussed later. Finally, Kenneth Clute in his Canadian study found that the quality of care was better among physicians who had had at least part of their training in a teaching hospital and that the length of training in non-teaching hospitals was not correlated with increasing quality of patient care as he measured it.[3]

To avoid some of the value judgments inherent in the more or less subjective studies mentioned above, Edith Leavit and her group undertook to use *standardized, objective examinations* to evaluate the effectiveness of internships.[4] The National Board Examination Part III has been well standardized and is commonly accepted as a fairly valid measure of a young physician's clinical competence, and this examination was used to evaluate "graduates" of various types of internships. In order that the findings not be biased by the quality of physicians entering the internship, the National Board Examination Part II was used as a measure of input, and the final results were corrected for this factor. Concerning the caliber of intern obtained they found that (1) affiliated hospitals got better interns than non-affiliated ones; (2) hospitals filling over 75 per cent of available positions got better interns than those that did not; (3) hospitals offering straight internships got better interns than those offering only rotating internships; and (4) the amount of the stipend did not correlate with the quality of the input. Of more importance in relation to our current question is the matter of the quality of the product of the internship. In this regard they found that (1) the quality of the "input" was a determinant of the competence of the physician at the end of the internship, but not to the degree expected; (2) affiliated hospitals that filled less than 75 per cent of their positions graduated poorer quality interns than those that filled well (but this was not true of non-affiliated hospitals); (3) interns of non-affiliated hospitals offering a lower stipend tested better than those from non-affiliated hospitals paying high stipends (but this was not true of affiliated hospitals); and (4) no other identifiable characteristic showed significant relation to competence of the graduating intern.

The findings of these studies are of great interest and deserve close study. One must remember, however, that the criteria used are open to some question, and, even if they were not, the studies deal with statistical means, variations, and correlations. I am sure that each of us knows, even if it is only a clinical impression, that there are some straight internships in affiliated hospitals that are utterly miserable and there are some rotating internships in non-affiliated hospitals that pay high stipends that are superb. Furthermore, no study can take into account the individual requirements of all the trainees. For this reason it may be worthwhile to give some consideration to what the internship looks like from inside the American Medical Association Internship Review Committee —or at least what it looks like to one person on the committee.

THE AMA INTERNSHIP REVIEW COMMITTEE

In the first place the members of the *hospital's staff should have high qualifications in medicine and its specialties.* They should also have interest in the internship program of the hospital. This should be true even of staff members who are not directly concerned with the teaching of interns. And those who instruct interns should have a demonstrated ability to teach.

In recent years many hospitals seem to have concluded that to attract interns they must have a director of medical education (DME). It has become obvious to most of us that a DME is not a cure-all, but it is most helpful to have a good, full-time DME who knows medicine and medical education (i.e., one who is a professional medical educator). Furthermore, he must not only have prestige among the staff but must also be given the necessary authority to conduct a first-rate educational program. Such a man can do a great deal toward improving all the educational activities of the hospital.

The educational program should of course conform to the *Essentials of an Approved Internship* published by the Council on Medical Education of the American Medical Association. But this is not enough. It should show evidence of imagination and planning that capitalizes on the strengths of the hospital and its staff that caters to the individual needs of the interns. *It should show no evidence of purely service objectives,* such as excess scrubbing in surgery (i.e., scrubbing on more patients than an intern can work-up, follow, and study), doing histories and physical examinations on patients who are not subsequently followed by the interns, and arranging schedules to get coverage of the "work services" such as the emergency room, the operating room, and the birth room. The service load of the intern should be commensurate with the *educa-*

tional objectives of the internship, and the intern should have reasonable responsibility for patient care, including private patients. There should be adequate opportunity for interns to follow discharged hospital patients on an ambulatory service. There should be an abundance of well-organized and well-attended clinical conferences, journal club meetings, grand rounds, and clinicopathological conferences. Finally, there should be both special medical and cultural programs for foreign graduates on the house staff as well as ample opportunity for interplay between American interns and the foreign graduates.

It goes without saying that the hospital facilities should be adequate in both the clinical and the laboratory areas and that there should be a first-class medical library that is easily available to all members of the house staff. The clinical records should be above reproach both to document good patient care and to serve as a basis for evaluation and for clinical research.

There are, in addition, some characteristics of the "total" internship that are of supreme importance in judging whether it is really a good one. It should have good consumer appeal (Campbell's Law), that is it should fill through the National Intern Matching Program without an excessive stipend. There should also be an adequate house staff complement (including residents if residencies are offered) to allow for interaction among physicians-in-training.

Since virtually no one considers a one-year internship an adequate preparation for practice, *the internship should form a smooth transition between the medical school and residency training.* In other words, it should be a logical first year of training for the type of practice in which the young physician intends to engage; it should not stand alone as a "strange interlude" or a "brief encounter." It does not seem proper today for the internship to be designed as a terminal experience. Indeed, there is increasing appreciation of the fact that all formal training in medicine both undergraduate and graduate should form the basis for the lifelong study of medicine.

BIBLIOGRAPHY

1. Peterson, O., et al.: An Analytical Study of North Carolina General Practice, 1953–1954, *J. Med. Educ.*, 31:1–165 (Part 2) 1956.

2. Morehead, M. A.: Quality of Medical Care Provided by Family Physicians As Related to Their Education, Training and Methods of Practice, quoted by Peterson in *New England J. Med.*, 269:1174–1182 (Nov. 28) 1963.

3. Clute, K. F.: "The General Practitioner; A Study of Medical Education and Practice in Ontario and Nova Scotia," University of Toronto Press, Toronto, Canada, 1963.

4. Leavit, E. J., et al.: The Internship: An Evaluation of Input and Output, *JAMA,* 189:299–305 (July 27) 1964.

44

The Future of the Internship

By James A. Campbell, M.D.

James A. Campbell is attending physician, president, and formerly chairman of the department of medicine at Presbyterian-St. Luke's Hospital in Chicago. He is professor of medicine at the University of Illinois School of Medicine and formerly was dean of Albany Medical College. He received the M.D. degree from Harvard Medical School and served residencies at Boston City Hospital. He is a diplomate of the American Board of Internal Medicine.

Dr. Campbell has contributed substantially to medical education and medical practice in the United States, and he holds many posts in national organizations, particularly posts relevant to the internship. He is a member of the AMA Internship Review Committee and is Vice-Chairman of the Board of Directors of the National Intern Matching Program. He serves on the AMA Review Committee on Internships and the AMA Task Force on Internships. He was a member of the National Board of Medical Examiners Part III Committee and a Member of the Planning Committee for the Association of American Medical Colleges Institute on Clinical Teaching. He has recently been appointed Planning Director for Education in the Health Fields for the State of Illinois Board of Higher Education.

The Guide Issue of Hospitals, JAHA, August 1, 1965, gives the following data on Presbyterian-St. Luke's Hospital: Beds, 856; Admissions, 23,810; Census, 722; Bassinets, 77; Births, 3,051; Newborn census, 46; Total expenses, $20,413,000; Payroll, $12,909,000; Personnel, 2,866.

The future of the internship will be fashioned in great measure by the same factors which have shaped its past. Although many elements in varied assortments have served to modify the nature of the internship, several basic formative factors have been most persistent. Among these, four are certainly well recognized.

First, there is the need felt by newly graduated physicians for increased postdoctoral training before entering practice.

Second, there are the requirements of licensing groups, certifying boards, and various professional associations for postdoctoral training usually well beyond the internship year as evidence of meeting their particular demands for competence.

Third, there is the feeling by more and more hospitals, those composites of laymen and health professionals, including physicians, that an atmosphere conducive to medical education, particularly demonstrated by an approved internship, improves patient care and, hence, is to be sought and striven for.

Fourth, there is the knowledge that any medical educational process, particularly at the postdoctoral level and most notable in the acquisition of skills, is dependent in great measure upon an increasing participation by the trainees in caring for patients. Indeed, this direct service to patients has been traditionally equated with the "tuition fee" for house officers, and their stipends have been likened to "fellowships."

The interactions about these four forces have produced some fascinating, albeit traumatic, incidents in the evolution of the internship. Balance between the first two forces, the perception of the need for more education and training by the students and their certifying groups to be achieved through some degree of service, and the second two forces, the expectation that service to patients, doctors, and hospitals can best be met through some degree of education, has not been particularly well achieved; and the advocates of each force tend to grow increasingly vocal and opinionated as they near their particular polar position. In terms of commerce, the sought after market balance in the internship seems to be determined on the one hand by absolutely "giving the lady what she wants," and on the other by resolutely "charging what the traffic will bear."

To predict the future of the market it seems well to examine a few past and recent trends. It is of particular interest to review some early reactions to the need for postdoctoral training clearly stated by the newly graduated physicians themselves. It was discovered in 1913 that, despite the broad legal acceptance of the M.D. as prima facie evidence of training as a physician, 70 per cent of the graduates of United States schools were seeking more hospital training here or in Europe. In 1914 the first list of "Approved Internships" was published. Although there continued to be an increasing demand by students for the post M.D. internship as a preparation for practice, it was not until 1926 that there actually were as many approved internships as there were candidates to fill them. The need for internship training was given further encouragement by state licensing agencies, and by 1915 seventeen states had followed Pennsylvania's lead in requiring an internship, usually rotating, as an essential for medical licensure.

The relative numbers of internships and candidates remained sufficiently close through the 1930's to sustain the rise of specialty boards and the founding of residency programs as the ascendant postdoctoral educational goal of the students; and thus a semblance of balance was kept in the market. By the late 1940's, however, other forces seemed to have taken over. Internship positions exceeded applicants by roughly two to one. By 1953 intern recruiting tactics resembled a cross between rushing for a college fraternity and shanghaiing sailors along the Barbary Coast, and the National Intern Matching Program was brought into being. Although this has made intern recruitment more orderly, the disparate ratio of positions to candidates has served to make hospitals and their internship programs more and more responsive to the needs and wishes of the potential candidates. Included in these has been the increasing stipends, which are rapidly approaching the levels of a living wage.

What are some of the major trends which apparently reflect a responsiveness to this "buyers' market"? The type or content of the internship is changing. Initially almost all internship programs offered were of the "rotating type." That is, a rotation through each one of four clinical service areas—medicine, surgery, obstetrics, and pediatrics—was required. It was apparently felt that the applied knowledge gathered in this twelve-month rotating internship adequately prepared the new M.D. to handle virtually any type of practice, and licenses to practice as "Physician and Surgeon" were appropriately issued.

It is interesting that in 1960 75 per cent of the internship programs were still of the rotating type, but by 1966 this number had decreased to 50 per cent. In 1960 "mixed" internships (usually experience on two or three clinical services, frequently with a "major" or emphasis on one) made up 3 per cent of the programs. These had increased to 14 per cent by 1966. In 1960 only 22 per cent of all programs were "straight" internships (a program offered by a single service in medicine, surgery, pediatrics, obstetrics, or pathology and, therefore, under a single director, although often including some experience in another clinical area). By 1966 the number of these straight programs had risen to 35 per cent of the total internships offered.

A further indicator of the continuation to this trend of changing types of internships is the degree to which these programs are filled. In 1966 78 per cent of the rotating internships were filled, 82 per cent of the mixed internships were filled, and 84 per cent of the straight internships were filled.

A second major trend worth noting is that all intern candidates, particularly those graduates of United States schools, are seeking internships in medical school affiliated hospitals more and more. For example, in 1953 a little over half of the U.S. graduates interned in major or minor affiliated hospitals. By 1966, however, 62 per cent interned in affiliated and only 27 per cent in non-affiliated hospitals.

As is readily apparent, these two important trends tend to reinforce one another. In 1966, although non-affiliated hospitals offered 61 per cent of *all* approved internships, they offered 71 per cent of the rotating internships. Affiliated hospitals offered only 39 per cent of all internships, but they offered 68 per cent of the straight internships. Moreover, 88 per cent of the straight internships in all categories in affiliated hospitals were filled. Of additional interest and, of course, of great importance is the fact that 84 per cent of all foreign-trained physicians were in non-affiliated hospital internships; indeed, 40 per cent of all non-affiliated hospital internship positions are occupied by foreign graduates.

To underscore this further, in 1965 only six programs in major medical school affiliated hospitals failed to match a single student, whereas there were 196 programs offering over 2,000 positions in non-affiliated hospitals which failed to match a single candidate.

These trends emphasize the current "buyers'" position, which is distinctly favorable for the United States graduate. In addition to knowing what he wants with respect to type and affiliation of his internship, the present newly graduated M.D. also plans to take certainly one, and usually two or three additional years of postdoctoral training as a resident or fellow. Currently, at least 90 per cent of all interns are planning or are actually committed to further training. This appetite for continued education, reinforced by many outside agencies, has added a further factor which, in essence, has reduced the internship from its original single year of total clinical experience to but an initial step in the sequence of preparing for practice.

The terms "internship" and "rotating internship" are firmly established in the language of graduate medical education as well as in the language of a majority of state medical licensure acts (although in 1962 Pennsylvania and Illinois modified their rigid rotating internship requirements to more flexible requisites for licensure). A task force of the Council on Medical Education of the American Medical Association recently recommended that the terms "internship" and "rotating internship" at least be kept in our medical glossaries but that the definition of the rotating internship be modified. In June 1966 the House of Delegates concurred. Fundamentally, the Council

. . . determined that the simplest and most effective solution is to re-define the rotating internship to include the program flexibility now permitted for the mixed internship, and to eliminate the mixed internship as a separate entity. This will permit hospital staffs to continue to offer whatever type of rotating internships may be required by the laws or regulations of particular states. It will also permit hospitals to vary their programs from year to year in accord with the varying desires of their interns.

A rotating internship is defined as one which provides supervised practice in internal medicine and at least one of the following: surgery, pediatrics, obstetrics and gynecology, psychiatry, pathology, radiology or anesthesiology. Interns ordinarily should not be assigned to more than one of the above services at a time. Even though a formal full-time assignment might be offered in the fields of laboratory diagnosis or radiologic interpretation, these disciplines also should be included through integration with the interns' activities on other services.

In rotating internships of 12 months' duration, the time allotted to internal medicine may in no case be less than four months. No assignment may be of less than two months' duration, and in such cases, the two months' assignment must be consecutive. Block assignments of two months each in internal medicine are acceptable, but assignments of four or more months consecutively are preferable. If an intern desires experience in a specialty not included in his rotation schedule, such training may be offered through appropriate outpatient assignments or by participation in consultations on his own and other patients conducted by members of the department concerned. Too frequent a rotation of assignments, and hence too short a time on a service, is inconsistent with the conduct of a good internship.

The greater flexibility permitted in these revised standards for a rotating internship permits hospitals to capitalize on their strengths and eliminate weak services from a required rotation. A rotating internship may consist of as few as two services or as many as five.

It should be clear that in recognizing the trend to limit the internship to a twelve-month period, the Council does not consider this period sufficiently long to prepare the young physician for practice. Physicians who take only a twelve-month internship should supplement this educational experience with at least one additional year spent in a residency preparing for a specialty or general practice.[1]

This represents, in my opinion, the major indicator for the future of the internship year. It should also be noted that at no point in this historic decision did the Council get enmeshed in the old semantic trap of arguing whether or not a straight internship is not in reality a first-year residency. It does not, however, come to grips with the problems of affiliated versus non-affiliated hospital programs.

So much for trends in actions which have been primarily responsive to buyers' demands. There has been and still is pressure, however, for "charging what the traffic will bear."

There are "prestige" internships which are not considered to be top flight experiences by the very persons who are enrolled in their programs, and yet which are filled each year. The candidates who seek these spots continue to do so because they believe, rightly or wrongly, that a particular internship is an essential prerequisite to a subsequent residency under the same department head's direction.

In Richard Saunders' still classic study of the "University Hospital Internship in 1960" [2] he noted that only 65 per cent of all straight surgical interns felt that their internship had been a clinical experience significant beyond medical school clerkships. (This contrasted to 76 per cent in rotating internships and over 90 per cent in both straight medicine and pediatric internships who felt their programs were so.) Despite this, 81 per cent of the same straight surgical interns indicated it was clearly the attractiveness of the residency program which "recruited" them to the internship. These abuses are by no means limited either to surgeons nor to university hospitals. As the new graduates more and more frequently pick internships with residencies in mind, so the service chiefs pick interns with residents in mind. Indeed, some of the tactics earlier applied to internship recruitment are now being used at the residency level. It is hoped that the attempts by the directors of the psychiatry residencies to institute a Residency Matching Program presages progress for additional specialties as well.

The offering of a stipend which is too high or too low, each in its own fashion pressure on the new graduate, is another force applied in the internship market place. The threat of withholding staff appointments or the promise of a particular research job are similar devices for persuading candidates of the value of particular internships.

But, by and large, it remains a buyers' internship market for all except the graduates of foreign, that is non-United States or non-Canadian, medical schools.

In the following tabulation there have been put together some data from 1965–66 [3] associated with some of the major, as well as less well accepted, variables that might be used to derive profiles of the internship either "most likely to succeed" or "most likely to fail" as an indicator for future programs. (The overall "average" is 79 per cent filled.)

For some further basic data for readers who may wish to extend the profile, a partial set of factors listed by Saunders[2] as of stated major importance are herewith included.

From these data one might infer that to create the profile of the "internship most likely to succeed" it would be best to offer a straight medical internship, which is already well recommended by its former interns, in a larger than 500-bed university-affiliated federal hospital, located in

TABLE 44-1. Internships in 1965–66

Type	Per cent filled
Straight	84
Mixed	82
Rotating	78
Family or general practice program	51
Service, if straight internship	
Medicine	93
Surgery	84
Pediatrics	71
Pathology	58
Obstetrics & gynecology	42
Support	
Federal	88
Government (non-federal)	80
Non-profit corporation	78
Church	74

	Medical school	
Size of hospital (beds)	affiliated	Non-affiliated
500 or over	87	80
300 to 499	80	73
200 to 299	76	77
200 or less	47	77

Location	
Pacific	87
New England	85
Mid Atlantic	84
South Atlantic	78
East North Central	78
Mountain	74
West South Central	72
East South Central	71
West North Central	69

California, Washington, Oregon, or Hawaii. Such a hypothetical internship could be expected to have 87 per cent of its positions filled and to have 85 per cent of the interns be graduates of United States or Canadian medical schools. A close second would be a surgical internship in a similar hospital, but it would depend a great deal for its success on the reputation of the surgical residency.

From similar extrapolations the profile for internship failure seems most likely if a straight ob-gyn internship is offered in a non-medical-school affiliated, small, church-supported hospital located in the Dakotas. It could expect about 36 per cent of the positions to be filled with interns, 85 per cent of whom are graduates of foreign schools. A rotating intern-

TABLE 44-2. Major Factors Influencing Internship Selection

Factor	Type of internship and per cent
	Rotating
Recommendation of former interns	67%
Section of country	65%
Number of ward patients	65%
	Straight surgery
Attractiveness of residency	81%
Recommendation of faculty	55%
Recommendation of former interns	52%
	Straight medicine
Recommendation of former interns	72%
Recommendation of faculty	63%
Opportunity to work with senior staff	62%

ship in a similar hospital has a slightly better chance, but only if there has been a significant increase in ward patients or perhaps a change of geographic location.

It is apparent that manipulation of the data used to develop the above hypothetical profiles reflects an internship's success or failure only in quantitative terms. In reality, of course, numerical success is no absolute guarantee of superiority either of the programs or of the interns who fill them. Per contra, numerical failure does not necessarily deny potential excellence of an internship program. It must be recognized, however, that in a buyers' market the odds for any kind of success remain distinctly in favor of those programs certified not just by the standards of appraisal of the AMA, but those which have, in addition, gained that extra seal of approval achieved only by being filled by young physicians who have chosen the internship and who have been gratified by the training and experience provided.

In view of the cumulative forces producing changing patterns in graduate medical education and since success can neither be totally assured nor can failure be entirely thwarted by any rigid formulae, with some trepidation, but nonetheless with rather full expectation of their eventuality, the following speculations on the future of the internship are ventured:

1. The recognition of the internship as a separate, free-standing year will disappear.

2. The internship will continue as a convenient legal and traditional term to describe the first of several years of programmed graduate education in preparation for practice of any of the several specialties including

that of family practice, and an internship will be active and function only if it is part of such programs.

3. Straight or specialty internships will become appropriately recognized as an integral part of most graduate specialty training programs. Just as the American Board of Pathology now gives full credit toward board certification for an internship in pathology, other specialties will begin to include specific internship programs as recognized specialty board training. Indeed, pediatrics has recently made such a move. Through such recognition of and thence responsibility for such programs these internships may well have their content more sharply defined, their clinical bases broadened beyond their present services, and a more optimal total training program developed.

4. The recently redefined rotating internship with its broad base in internal medicine and multiple electives may well mutate into the first year of a family practice specialty program and hence be under the guidance of this "board." This presupposes the establishment of such a "family practice board" either as a separate entity or a creature of another board's creation, and this is a speculation willingly included.

5. Affiliation with medical schools and/or larger non-medical-school hospitals with more extensive facilities and senior faculty-level personnel will become an increasing requisite for success in graduate medical education; and, as a corollary, medical schools will take an increasing responsibility for community hospital educational efforts. As solo internship years tend to disappear unless they are related to a broader program of at least two more years of postdoctoral training in a related hospital or school, integrated programs for graduate medical education may be developed on a state or regional basis with intern and resident rotations through various centers and a counter flow of faculty through member hospital units as common patterns.

6. Hospitals in which internships alone can be offered will have even less expectation of success in the future than at present. Smaller hospitals will have greater difficulty than ever in internship competition, and *consolidation* as well as affiliation will become increasingly popular, following patterns of such programs for graduate medical education as those in Jacksonville and Pensacola, Florida, and Cedar Rapids, Iowa.

7. Costs for these programs will increase through increasing needs for full-time directors of laboratories, service chiefs, and research personnel. A broader support base must be found than is currently available in many hospitals which are trying to compete for trainees in internship and residency programs.

8. A Foreign Intern Matching Program will be developed which will greatly assist in making peer contact possible between graduates of both United States and foreign schools in internships throughout this country, with a resultant improvement in both medical education and interna-

tional understanding. "Matching plans" will probably also be forthcoming for many residency programs as well.

9. Finally, on an attempted lighter note, unless an "astrodome" of such gargantuan proportions can be built so that an entire city with controlled sunshine or powdered snow covering ivy can be offered by a hospital as a fringe benefit along with a superb educational opportunity, it is doubtful that anyone can compete with ease against California, Colorado, or New England in the internship market of the future.

BIBLIOGRAPHY

1. Revision of the Essentials of an Approved Internship, AMA Council on Medical Education Special Announcement, June, 1966.

2. Saunders, R. H., Jr.: University Hospital Internship in 1960, *J. M. Educ.*, 36:561–676, 1961.

3. Nunemaker, J. C., Thompson, W. V., Mixter, George, Jr., and Tracy, R.: Graduate Medical Education in the United States, *JAMA*, 194:15 (Nov.) 1965.

45

What Makes a Good Residency in Medicine?

By John C. Leonard, M.D.

John C. Leonard was the director of medical education at Hartford Hospital from 1947 until his death April 26, 1966. His position was the first of its kind in the United States. He held many important posts during his very active career, including associate director of education programs for rural hospitals of the Commonwealth Foundation, associate director of the Bingham Foundation, and associate director of the Joseph H. Pratt Diagnostic Hospital in Boston. He received the M.D. degree from Yale University and served there as clinical professor of medicine. Dr. Leonard was a member of the Advisory Committee on Internships of the AMA Council on Medical Education, a member and chairman of the AMA Residency Review Committee in Internal Medicine, and chairman of the AMA Committee on Postgraduate Medicine. He was vice-president and regent of the American College of Physicians and had been Governor of the College for Connecticut.

The Guide Issue of *Hospitals, JAHA,* August 1, 1965, gives the following data on Hartford Hospital: Beds, 800; Admission, 30,584; Census, 723; Bassinets, 150; Births, 5,411; Newborn census, 82; Total expenses, $15,207,000; Payroll, $10,626,000; Personnel 2,082. There are three other short-term general hospitals in Hartford with 144 beds, 189 beds, and 654 beds. The population of Hartford in the 1960 census was 162,178.

THE RESIDENCY REVIEW COMMITTEE IN INTERNAL MEDICINE

The Residency Review Committee in Internal Medicine is made up of four representatives each of:

1. The American Board of Internal Medicine
2. The American College of Physicians
3. The Council on Medical Education of the American Medical Association

It was organized with the objectives of (1) constantly improving existing residencies and (2) encouraging the establishment of new residencies if basic essential criteria are met. This committee has constantly recognized the need for changing criteria and guide lines as the field of internal medicine broadens its horizons.

Under the aegis of its three sponsoring organizations, the Residency Review Committee in Internal Medicine reviews and approves qualified residency programs in internal medicine according to their educational and training value. It also provides the basis for the listing of such programs in the *Directory of Approved Internships and Residencies*, published annually by the American Medical Association.

There is no official connection between the Residency Review Committee in Internal Medicine and the Joint Commission on Accreditation of Hospitals (JCAH). Before applying for approval of their residency training programs, however, hospitals should first meet the requirements of the JCAH.

The Residency Review Committee in Internal Medicine utilizes the administrative facilities of the Council on Medical Education, which provides the secretariat and the field staff for the detailed, time-consuming, and highly valuable work of gathering the data necessary for the evaluation of residencies. The committee meets regularly three times each year and reviews the data on residencies in internal medicine collected from the hospitals under consideration. The committee also enlists the services of ad hoc committees and individual distinguished consultants in internal medicine for additional consideration of special and urgent problems.

Programs for approval are limited to the standard three-year training program. One- and two-year programs were discontinued for approval on July 1, 1965. No group of rigid criteria are used, but the following essentials are basic to any good training program:

1. Adequate numbers of patients for whom the resident is responsible
2. Increasing responsibility for the resident from year to year
3. A competent and highly motivated attending staff

Programs limited to ambulatory clinics cannot be considered for approval. If two years of the program are devoted to the broad field of internal medicine, one year of the three-year program may be devoted to a medical specialty of the resident's choice.

BASIC SCIENCES

Basic sciences may be provided separately, or they may be incorporated in the clinical training of the resident. However, if the latter method is used, the attending staff must carefully guide and supervise this important part of the resident's learning opportunity. Purely didactic lectures in which the resident does not participate usually have little value and should not occupy an excessive portion of any training program.

In general, basic science instruction can be better afforded in an integrated manner at the patient's bedside. This obviously means that the teachers must be involved constantly in their own continuing medical education.

PATHOLOGY AND ROENTGENOLOGY

The clinical laboratory, the x-ray department, and other diagnostic services constitute an important part of a residency program. The quality of these and the adequacy with which they are correlated with clinical medicine are considered carefully in the evaluation of a residency.

It is helpful to have the attending physician, at the end of ward rounds, take his residents to the x-ray department to view the films of the patients just seen. Similarly, they should visit the clinical pathology department to see bone marrow and other microscopic and laboratory examinations dealing with the patients just seen on the wards.

RESEARCH

Under suitable circumstances, a portion of the residency may well be allocated to a research problem. Such research should be *inspired rather than required*. Where investigative facilities and competent guidance are available, this part of the program may be very valuable. Ability in research varies widely from person to person; therefore, to force research upon one who has no talent for it may only waste time that would be better spent at the patient's bedside. However, an active productive research program conducted by competent investigators provides a healthy climate for an educational experience whether or not the individual resident participates directly.

MEDICAL LIBRARY

The medical library should be readily accessible to the resident staff, both day and night. A locked library has no value! The textbooks should be kept up to date, and there should be an adequate number of domestic and foreign journals devoted to internal medicine, its subspecialties, and the basic sciences.

When a comprehensive library is not available in the hospital, an active reference lending system should be provided through larger medical libraries.

OUTPATIENT DEPARTMENT

Many of the patients seen in the hospital outpatient department are comparable to those seen later in private practice. It is essential therefore to include in the program closely supervised training in an active outpatient department. This assignment should be one of increasing responsibility under the conscientious guidance of a qualified attending staff. Well-balanced training in internal medicine cannot be achieved with ambulatory patients alone, but it is also true that experience limited to acute and chronic disease in hospitalized patients is equally incomplete.

Medical records in the outpatient department should be as complete and as carefully supervised as medical records for the inpatient service.

NEUROLOGY AND PSYCHIATRY

Much of the medical resident's later experience in practice will contain a large number of neurologic and psychiatric patients. It is important that adequate, supervised experience in these fields is included in the training program.

Internal medicine in its broadest sense includes knowledge of all the organ systems included in the medical subspecialties. The residency training program should include training in many of these special disciplines such as cardiovascular disease, pulmonary disease, gastroenterology, endocrinology, hematology, and allergy.

RESPONSIBILITY: ATTENDING AND RESIDENT STAFFS

The Residency Review Committee recognizes that no resident training program can possibly succeed unless the attending staff has ability, motivation, enthusiasm, and a sense of responsibility for teaching. The medical staff should make the above listed attributes prerequisite to active staff membership.

A keen sense of responsibility for patient care on the part of the resident staff is essential. No amount of scheduled rounds and conferences or devoted teaching by the attending staff can produce well-trained graduates if the residents insist upon excessive "time off" or minimal contact with patients. The Residency Review Committee in Internal Medicine recommends that residents who are on active inpatient care service ideally should be on duty a minimum of alternate nights and weekends or the equivalent and that "time off" should begin only when proper patient care and welfare are assured. A good training program will automatically provide the best in patient care.

A residency is a full-time training position, and there must be no outside jobs attempted concurrently. This is emphasized because many residents have complained of excessive work under the above system; and when the requirements were lessened by some hospitals, many residents resorted to "moonlighting." The result was that the residents involved returned to their program too fatigued to learn or to take adequate care of their assigned patients. Today's resident salaries have improved so rapidly that "moonlighting" should not be permitted.

The importance of taking and recording a good medical history and performing a careful and complete physical examination cannot be overemphasized. Experience indicates that these fundamentals are woefully neglected in favor of important but nevertheless supplementary information supplied by a multiplicity of clinical laboratory procedures. A reliable index of the quality of a medical residency is found in the quality of the hospital records, which should include frequent progress notes by both staff and residents as well as a concise discharge summary.

The medical residency should constitute a progressive educational experience and should never be permitted to deteriorate into a purely service activity.

"It is not essential, or even desirable, that all hospital residencies should adopt exactly the same program or that they should offer a rigidly uniform sequence of experience. It is essential, however, that all hospitals participating in graduate training should be able to meet the fundamental essential requirements for our approved program and, either alone, or in collaboration, should attain comparable results in the quality of training and amount of experience obtained." [1]

Finally, if we of the attending staff in internal medicine wish to apply the acid test of the real quality of a program, we should ask ourselves, "Is this the type of program in which I would wish my nephew or my son to seek his training?"

BIBLIOGRAPHY

1. "Essentials of Approved Residencies," Council on Medical Education, American Medical Association, Chicago, 1960.

46

What Makes a Good Residency in Surgery?

By George H. Yeager, M.D.

George H. Yeager is in the private practice of general surgery in Baltimore. He received the M.D. degree from the University of Maryland where he is professor of clinical surgery and director of professional services at University Hospital. He is a diplomate of the American Board of Surgery, and he is the representative of the AMA Council on Medical Education to the Conference Committee on Graduate Training in Surgery. He is the editor of *The American Surgeon* and of the *Maryland State Medical Journal*.

Two types of surgical residency training programs are recognized by the Conference Committee for Graduate Training in Surgery. Satisfactory completion of either type qualifies an applicant to be considered for examination by the American Board of Surgery.

In view of the increasing influence of this certifying board, it can be assumed that the young surgeon seeking surgical training ultimately hopes to achieve certification. Some hospitals demand certification before they consider an applicant for hospital privileges. The government has added specific incentives for board certification when it considers physicians for commissions in the military service and the Public Health Service, and salary levels in Veteran Administration hospitals are geared to certification.

In view of this emphasis, guide lines established by the Conference Committee and the American Board of Surgery must be given respectful attention. In weighing the merits of a specific program, some of the guide lines can be identified and evaluated specifically. This phase of the program represents the tangible element. Intangible factors, however, frequently comprise a more important phase. Unfortunately these factors occasionally do not lend themselves to simple analysis and evaluation.

PROGRESSIVE RESPONSIBILITY

The basic principle of a good residency is graded, progressive responsibility under supervision, terminating with at least a year as chief resident with responsibility for the management and operation of clinic patients. Confidence, judgment, and technical skill cannot be acquired without a system of graded, progressive responsibility.

The Conference Committee has adopted the following definition of the term "responsible surgeon" as it relates to surgical residents in training:

> The resident can be considered to be the "responsible surgeon" only when the patient has been placed in his care so that he has made or confirmed the diagnosis, selected the appropriate operative procedure, been responsible for preoperative care, acted as the surgeon, cared for the patient postoperatively, and seen the patient at a follow-up visit, so as to know the end result. All this must be under the supervision of the responsible member of the senior staff.

SUPERVISION

Supervision may need further definition. Obviously, the senior staff member must be satisfied that the resident properly accomplishes each step in the care of the patient before he proceeds to the next. When a particular operative procedure would likely present complications, the senior staff member, in the interest of the patient, may choose to perform the operation himself or to act as first assistant. Supervision during the operation often need be no more than observation. Generally, the well-prepared senior resident may be allowed to proceed with most operations on "service cases" without immediate observation by the senior staff member, provided the latter is readily available for prompt consultation if the resident asks for it.

Training must include education in the total surgical care of the patient and not merely in performing surgical procedures. This includes accurate diagnosis, preoperative preparation, the operation, postoperative care, and rehabilitation. The exercise of independent judgment for making decisions and independent action based on such decisions is essential in the latter stages of training.

SIZE OF SURGICAL SERVICE

It is agreed that a hospital should have 300 to 500 surgical admissions annually to support a surgical residency. The number of service or ward beds assigned to the resident is more important than the total bed capacity. Patients admitted to these beds may come from any source.

The important feature is that these "service beds" are set aside for the senior resident and the resident controls admission to these beds. Diversification and magnitude of the material available and follow-up results are more important factors than excessive numbers. By these criteria, a program of 7 to 10 assigned beds, is frequently excellent, whereas a program of twice the number of beds is occasionally unsatisfactory.

The record of patients in which the resident was the "responsible surgeon" is one measure of the graduated, progressive experience afforded the resident.

SURGICAL STAFF

The surgical staff should be composed of surgeons who are highly qualified in both surgical skill and judgment. The members of the staff should have a real interest in teaching and must be willing to give the time and effort required by the educational program if it is to be effective. The supervising staff should be enthusiastic and able and willing to impart their knowledge to others. The remaining staff, even though they may not have supervising responsibility, should also reflect enthusiasm for the program.

OTHER ESSENTIALS

Conferences should be frequent and participation by the entire staff should be anticipated.

Clinical material should be of sufficient scope and diversity to enable residents to observe the principal manifestations of major disease entities.

An opportunity should be presented for adequate *follow-up of patients.*

A *library* should be available with current journals.

Stimulation should be afforded to *original investigation.*

An active *outpatient clinic* is essential. This should be considered complementary to the inpatient service. It also may serve as a follow-up clinic in which the results of surgical care may be evaluated by the resident staff.

Emergency room service should be separated from the outpatient clinic; this insures better occupancy of the "service beds" and better experience for the resident.

Opportunity should be afforded for study of the *surgical pathology* of all tissue removed.

The percentage of *autopsies* should be maintained at a high level.

SUMMARY

It is difficult to evaluate the essential requirements for a good and rewarding residency in surgery. Certainly no one factor can be used as a gauge. The tangible components, such as the number of operations performed and the duration of the training period, lend themselves to the yardstick of evaluation. The intangible factors are more significant and are more difficult to evaluate. These include (1) the professional competence and the integrity of the senior staff and their ability and willingness to teach; (2) the responsibility given the resident; (3) the attitude of inquiry pervading the service; and (4) the opportunities afforded the resident for study, investigation, and teaching.

BIBLIOGRAPHY

1. "Guide Book for Residency Programs in General Surgery," Conference Committee on Graduate Training in Surgery, Chicago, 1961.

2. Firor, W. M.: Residency Training in Surgery; Birth, Decay and Recovery, *Rev. Surg.*, 22:153–157 (May–June) 1965.

3. Pearse, H. E.: Can Certification be Separated from Graduate Education in Surgery, *Surg. Gynec. Obstet.*, 106:97–99 (Jan.) 1958.

4. Pearse, H. E.: The Effect of Specialization on Graduate Education in Surgery, *J.A.M.A.*, 170:301–309 (May 16) 1959.

5. Rives, J. D.: The Impact of the American Board of Surgery upon Surgical Education in the United States, *Ann. Surg.*, 149:609–616 (May) 1959.

47

What Makes a Good Residency in Pediatrics?

By R. James McKay, Jr., M.D.

R. James McKay, Jr., is professor and chairman of the department of pediatrics at the University of Vermont, and in 1960 he was a Fulbright Lecturer at the University of Groningen in the Netherlands. He received the M.D. degree from Harvard Medical School, and he was a resident in pediatrics at Babies Hospital in New York and at Children's Hospital in Boston. At the time this article was written, he was vice chairman of the AMA Residency Review Committee for Pediatrics, president of the New England Pediatric Society, chairman of the Medical Education Committee of the American Academy of Pediatrics, and a member of the editorial board of *Pediatrics*. He is currently on the Executive Board of the American Academy of Pediatrics.

In view of the carefully prepared pamphlets, *Essentials of Approved Residencies* and *Guide for Residency Programs in Pediatrics,* both published by the American Medical Association, the fact that this paper has been requested implies a need for further clarification of the contents of these two booklets. This need arises because certain hospitals, particularly community hospitals not under direct or indirect control by a medical school, frequently find it difficult to obtain or maintain approval for a residency program in pediatrics, even though their staffs and administrations may feel that the requirements laid down or implied by the *Essentials* and the *Guide* have been reasonably, if not fully, met. Obviously, in such cases there must be a discrepancy in interpretation of the material contained in the pamphlets between the hospital and the reviewing agency, the Residency Review Committee for Pediatrics. What does the Residency Review Committee look for in evaluating an application for initiation or continuation of a residency in pediatrics?

The Residency Review Committee for Pediatrics, as does any approving agency, has many critics; and they are about equally divided between those who feel that the Committee is too strict and those who feel that it is too lenient in its decisions. Many who disagree with the decisions are ignorant and accordingly suspicious of the composition and functioning of the committee. Therefore, it is worthwhile to review its history, composition, and function.

THE RESIDENCY REVIEW COMMITTEE FOR PEDIATRICS

Originally the Council on Medical Education and Hospitals of the American Medical Association was immediately responsible for approval of all residency programs, with advice from the respective specialty boards. After World War II the great expansion in the number of residency programs made it necessary for the Council to establish residency review committees, of which the Residency Review Committee for Pediatrics is one. On it are two representatives each of the American Academy of Pediatrics, the American Board of Pediatrics, and the Council on Medical Education of the American Medical Association. Care is taken to maintain a balance between practicing pediatricians and academic pediatricians.

Each member of the committee is appointed for a three-year term with the possibility of reappointment for a second term. The two members from the American Medical Association Council on Medical Education are pediatricians appointed by the Council rather than members of the Council itself. The six representatives are the voting members of the Committee, and there are two ex officio members, the secretary of the American Board of Pediatrics and the committee secretary from the AMA staff.

The *purpose* of the Residency Review Committee is to approve new pediatric residency programs and to review old ones periodically to make sure that they are qualified to provide adequate training to prepare men and women as specialists in the practice of pediatrics. Basically, the committee's function is to see that residency programs meet, within reason, the standards set forth in the *Guide for Residency Programs in Pediatrics* and in *Essentials of Approved Residencies*. Since the purpose of the American Board of Pediatrics is to certify men and women as specialists in the practice of pediatrics, rather than as pediatric consultants, it should be emphasized that the Review Committee approves residency training programs with this aim in mind.

Committee Operation

The committee meets semi-annually to review those programs, both new and old, which have been surveyed by the AMA field staff. Approximately 70 programs are reviewed each time. Before the meeting, each member of the committee receives a sheaf of data and inspection reports on each program to be reviewed. Each member is responsible for a special examination of the data on several of the programs assigned to him for detailed review and recommendation. At the meeting he recommends approval, probation, or disapproval and backs his recommendation with specific information, some of which he may have gathered personally. The entire committee then decides on the action to be taken. If the committee is not satisfied that it can make a reasonable decision on the basis of the data and inspection report available, it may request the American Board of Pediatrics to send a pediatrician to the hospital for a more searching inspection.

New programs, if they are not disapproved immediately, are invariably given provisional approval. Usually after two years, to allow the program to get under way, reinspection is made to see how the new program is functioning. At that time it may be continued on provisional approval, be fully approved or disapproved. Similarly, when a previously approved program seems shaky or inadequate, it is put on confidential probation and reinspected in one or two years to see if the deficiencies have been remedied. Absence of residents in a program for two years renders it inactive, and this may be considered in itself adequate reason for withdrawal of approval. Actually, approval is rarely withdrawn purely on the basis of inactivity of a program. There are usually other reasons for the committee to be dissatisfied with the program, even though these reasons may at times be difficult to define.

The committee is interested in helping programs, both by criticisms and by imposing probation. Probation may help the program director, the hospital administration, or the medical staff to effect needed reforms which, in many instances, have been recognized by some but blocked by others.

KEY AREAS OF REVIEW

The Survey Questionnaire. It is a widely held misconception that the questionnaire which must be completed before each AMA inspection is an accurate guide to what the Residency Review Committee is looking for as criteria for approval. Actually, the questionnaire is designed only to record, insofar as possible, the documentable aspects of the general and special requirements outlined in the *Essentials of Approved Residencies*. Although the documentation is reviewed in its entirety, as is the report of the inspector, the committee focuses its attention on certain points which it feels are more important than others in judging the quality and variety of precept, example, and clinical experience to which the resident is exposed.

The Pediatric Attending Staff. The most important single component of a good residency program is *daily rounds conducted by a well-qualified, stimulating teacher* who has the authority to make effective suggestions, who is immediately available to the residents for consultation, and who is backed up by a staff of able consultants in subspecialty areas as well as by first-rate pediatrically oriented laboratory and radiologic facilities and personnel. Put more succinctly, the Residency Review Committee is interested primarily in the *quality* and *availability* of the pediatric attending staff and in the quality of its teaching performance. These difficult-to-measure factors are usually satisfactory in hospitals with a well-qualified, geographically full-time chief of service who has real and ultimate authority over the entire conduct of the service. They are usually unsatisfactory in hospitals where the position of chief of service is rotated among a voluntary or part-time staff of practicing pediatricians who have their chief base of operations outside of the hospital, particularly if the staff is heavily loaded with pediatricians and general practitioners who are not board certified. The presence of such geographically full-time staff members as a pediatric surgeon, a pediatric pathologist, a pediatric psychiatrist, a pediatric neurologist, a pediatric radiologist, a pediatric allergist, and a pediatric cardiologist usually signifies adequate quality. Absence of staff members with special interests *and* qualifications in *any* of these fields may warn the Review Committee of inadequate teaching and consultation in subspecialty areas. The same warning is given by a list of well-known consultants who have full-time primary obligations in other institutions so that it seems unlikely that they are in fact "staff members in pediatrics under whom the work of the resident is performed." The current residents will certainly be asked by the inspector whether or not they ever have contacts with these consultants.

Director of the Pediatric Residency. The person in active charge of the residency program should be a well-qualified, interested pediatrician who functions preferably on a geographically full-time basis. He is most effective when he is either the chief of service or is the direct delegate of the chief of service so that he carries virtually the same authority as does the chief in matters concerning the operation of the residency program.

The Current Residents. The Review Committee also examines the list of current and recent residents and fellows with interest. Usually, but not necessarily, if all positions are filled by graduates of American medical schools and the surveyor's report indicates high morale and satisfaction among the resident staff, the quality of the program is satisfactory. On the other hand, the committee is well aware that outstanding institutions may deliberately draw a significant number of outstanding foreign residents, and that high pay and broad perquisites may make a resident reasonably well satisfied with a mediocre or even below standard program.

Laboratory and X-ray Facilities. The presence of certain x-ray and laboratory facilities is important in a good residency. First, all such facilities should be available on a 24-hour basis 365 days a year for major emergencies. Determinations of serum electrolytes, serum bilirubin, and blood sugar, blood typing and cross matching, blood counts, urinalyses, and bacteriologic determinations should be available on a 24-hour basis as a routine. Micro methods for electrolytes, pH, and bilirubin and glucose determinations are highly desirable, if not indeed mandatory. A reliable method for testing sweat sodium or chloride content must be available in the hospital laboratories, and certain other tests, such as those for 17-ketosteroids, protein-bound iodine, and screening for aminoaciduria should be available on a basis practical for diagnostic use. An image intensifier and facilities for cineangiography and voiding cystourethrography by the cine method are highly desirable and indicate the completeness and sophistication of the diagnostic facilities available to the resident. Cardiac catheterization and cardiac surgery should be available, but referral to first-rate facilities is better than dependence on second-rate or seldom used facilities available locally.

Outpatient Clinics. Skilled supervision in outpatient work is important for a good pediatric residency. The Review Committee is less interested in the number of specialty clinics which may be staffed by persons unskilled in the field in question than it is in the qualifications of the staff members or consultants to whom the resident can turn for immediate advice or teaching in the management of patients in special categories.

Library. The 24-hour availability of a basic pediatric library, which includes the latest editions of the major pediatric and pediatric specialty texts plus bound volumes of at least the three major American pediatric journals for the past 5 or 10 years, encourages the resident to read and adds significantly to the effectiveness of his training.

Didactic Teaching. Contrary to impressions which might be gained from filling out the descriptive form required by the Council on Medical Education and Hospitals and from the questions asked by the AMA field inspectors, the Review Committee does not consider didactic teaching sessions of any kind to be an essential component of a good pediatric residency. In fact, it definitely considers them deleterious to a program which has too many of them, especially if they are not conducted by highly qualified individuals with *pediatric* orientation. Frequently scheduled didactic sessions, with the general hospital pathologist for instance, are generally considered by the committee to suggest a weak, unsophisticated program with inadequate pediatric staffing, leadership, and participation.

Patient Material. From the standpoint of patient material, the *Essen-*

tials of Approved Residencies points out that there should be a minimum of approximately 400 general medical pediatric admissions annually to provide sufficient variety and volume for a residency program. The character of patients admitted to a hospital is also pertinent. For instance, hospitals which refer all or most cases of infectious disease elsewhere have inadequate patient material unless the deficit is made up by an affiliation with an approved infectious disease unit. Specialty institutions (heart hospitals, tuberculosis hospitals, institutions for the mentally retarded, cancer hospitals, orthopedic hospitals, etc.) do not usually offer a sufficient variety of case material to support a pediatric residency program, although what they have to offer might be valuable as a rotation for a few months in affiliation with a good general program.

Children's hospitals need *an affiliation with an obstetrics unit* to provide training in newborn care. Community hospitals near medical centers or children's hospitals may have *an inadequate load of seriously ill patients* because the latter are mostly referred to the medical or pediatric centers. A small number of deaths on a particular pediatric service may be an indication of too few seriously ill patients. Conversely, too large a number may indicate poor standards of patient care.

The *autopsy percentage* is a reasonably accurate reflection of the interest taken by the staff in maintaining the quality of care. It is an even more accurate indicator of the interest of the staff in learning. The committee looks with favor upon autopsy rates on the pediatric service of 80 per cent or more.

The availability of patients for teaching is subject to frequent misinterpretation by hospitals with large private patient loads. From the standpoint of resident training, *a patient is available for teaching only if the resident has the opportunity to take at least some real responsibility.* The right to discuss private cases, the right to examine the hearts, lungs, eyes, or abdomens of private patients, or even the right to do the history and physical examination for the attending physician or to check the patient when it is inconvenient for the attending physician to do so—these are not enough. The resident must have the opportunity to arrive independently at his own diagnostic impression, to write his orders based on such an impression, and to carry out any procedures he is qualified to do. In case of procedures he is not qualified to do, he should be given the opportunity to become qualified by doing them under supervision.

The Residency Review Committee examines with interest the *balance of clinical material*—the relative numbers of medical, surgical, and tonsillectomy and adenoidectomy patients. A very high proportion of T&A patients may not only represent too high a service load for the pediatric resident staff but also tends to reflect a poor level of pediatric practice in the hospital. A high proportion of T&A cases combined with deaths of T&A patients, and a significantly higher proportion of private to total T&A admissions (as compared to the ratio of private to total general pediatric surgical admissions) are almost synonymous with a low standard of pediatric practice. An exception may be the rare instance in which all T&A's in a large community are done in one hospital.

Related Specialties. Finally, a good residency should include supervised experience in pediatric psychiatry, growth and development, orthopedics, mental retardation, allergy, and adolescent medicine. Growth and development tends to be the weakest part of many pediatric residency programs, and it also tends to be a section of the examinations of the American Board of Pediatrics which is often failed.

SUMMARY

The size and variety of case load, the variety and number of specialty clinics and consultants, the variety and number of conferences, the teaching of basic sciences, the laboratory and x-ray facilities, research programs, and library facilities are all important to the arch which forms a good residency program in pediatrics. But the keystone is high *quality of the teaching and pediatric practice* to which the resident is exposed. If this keystone is present, the other stones in the arch are rarely far out of place. Correspondingly, if other stones in the arch seem to be missing or far out of place, there is often something wrong with the keystone. Therefore, the Residency Review Committee for Pediatrics examines the presence and position of the visible stones of the arch as a guide to what really concerns it, the condition of the invisible keystone of quality.

48

What Makes a Good Residency in Obstetrics and Gynecology?

I.

By Clyde L. Randall, M.D.

Clyde L. Randall is professor and chairman of the department of obstetrics and gynecology at the State University of New York at Buffalo. He received the M.D. degree from the University of Kansas and served residencies in pathology and surgery in Kansas City before a residency in gynecology at the University of Buffalo. He is past president of the staff of Buffalo General Hospital. He was a member of the AMA Residency Review Committee for Obstetrics and Gynecology for six years and has been a director of the American Board of Obstetrics and Gynecology since 1960, serving as secretary-treasurer of the Board since 1964.

It is difficult for me to believe that a good residency in obstetrics and gynecology could be developed or maintained without three essentials: first, a favorable hospital environment in which the physical plant, the numbers of patients, and the personnel—the medical staff aside from the department of obstetrics and gynecology as well as the administration and governing board—all support the development of a good program in obstetrics and gynecology; second, a competent chief of service and departmental staff who are willing and able to train, discipline, teach, and inspire residents; and third, residents who possess the essential characteristics—honesty, industry, motivation, and dedication.

These three essentials cannot be listed in the order of their relative importance because hospital environment, departmental staff, and good residents are so interdependent that I believe all three are necessary if we are to develop a good residency. Too often the chief and his staff accept credit for a result which is impossible without good residents, for good residents, of themselves, bring out the best side of hospital personnel just as they bring out the best in their departmental staff and their chief.

Balance between Educational and Training Aspects

Current emphasis by the Residency Review Committee and the American Board of Obstetrics and Gynecology on the educational rather than the training aspects of the residency experience suggests the importance of efforts to assure a teaching-learning atmosphere throughout the departmental program. Perhaps the most difficult, but a most desirable achievement, is to strike a balance between an emphasis of patient care and the study of the patient's disease. Failure to achieve a proper emphasis of both is likely either where the departmental program goes all out in the development of research effort or where there is virtually no research by staff members and residents are almost entirely occupied by the care of patients. A resident may become preoccupied with patient care at the expense of learning how to keep aware of the scientific progress related to obstetrics and gynecology, especially where there is responsibility for the care of a heavy service load as well as in institutions where the residents are largely occupied in the care of private patients. It is not easy to maintain a desirable balance, but an attempt to do so is perhaps the chief's most important responsibility.

It is important for *the chief and the staff of obstetrics and gynecology to participate in the responsibilities assumed by committees of the staff,* be they charged with credentials, records, discipline, public relations, or long-range planning. Only by such participation can the obstetrics and gynecology department, when attempting to gain support for an expansion of departmental program or facilities, convincingly insist that "what is good for obstetrics and gynecology is good for the hospital."

A good residency in a good general hospital is likely to be superior to a residency in the relatively isolated environment of a so-called "woman's hospital," an environment that does not necessarily provide the best experience in obstetrics and gynecology.

Mechanisms of Residency Approval

Dr. Nunemaker clearly outlined the provisions and mechanisms currently responsible for the evaluation and approval of a residency program. (See Chap. 42.) I have experienced the anxieties of a chief whose program is being inspected. Since 1958 I have also observed the evaluation of residencies in obstetrics and gynecology by the Residency Review Committee. When a residency is disapproved, the Residency Review Committee is fully aware that the hospital administrator as well as the obstetricians and gynecologists often seem to regard the committee as a group of highly opinionated academicians with limited clinical interests because of limited clinical experience. Their "arbitrary" decisions seem to suggest an inability to recognize the virtues of the program surveyed—virtues which might well have compensated for the apparent weaknesses in the residency. I am personally convinced, however, that the evaluation and review of residencies is conducted in a manner not only fair to the program, but also less critical to it than the importance of such approval should demand.

At least three years of residency has been required by the American Board of Obstetrics and Gynecology since its organization in 1930. During the 1930s and 1940s, a large proportion of the candidates applying for certification had only a year or two of residency. The majority of these were seeking credit for several years of preceptorship experience with a Board-certified obstetrician-gynecologist as a substitute for the required years of residency. Although time in an approved preceptorship under specified conditions was, for many years, accepted as a substitute for one or two of the required years of residency, the acceptability of time in a preceptorship was gradually eliminated as the number of approved residencies increased. Finally in 1958, the annual *Bulletins* of the Board announced that after July 1, 1962, neither time in practice, in a preceptorship, in military service, or in an unapproved residency would be acceptable as a substitute for any portion of the required *three* years of residency in a program approved at the time the candidate was in the residency.

It is only since 1963 that the programs approved for three or more years of obstetric and gynecologic residency have provided the only opportunity for physicians to fulfill the requirements of the Board and gain admission to the examinations leading to certification as an obstetrician-gynecologist. It has been suggested that a brief review of the actual procedure by which approval of a residency in obstetrics and gynecology may be gained would be of interest. I shall try to keep repetition at a minimum.

Procedure of the Residency Review Committee for Obstetrics and Gynecology. The first step is usually a letter from the hospital administrator to the secretary of the Council on Medical Education or to the secretary of the Residency Review Committee for Obstetrics and Gynecology indicating that the hospital has organized, or reorganized, a residency program which they believe fulfills the requirements as detailed in the *Essentials*.

The secretary then sends to the hospital copies of the forms by which formal application for approval of the residency may be made. The chief purpose of these forms is to inform the director and the service chief of the information that should be made available to the field representative of the Council at the time the residency is surveyed. Usually the letter accompanying the forms indicates the date when the field representative's inspection will be made.

When the representative of the Council inspects the residency, the inspector fills out a worksheet which supplements the information provided in the forms already filled out by the hospital and the department.

After the inspector completes his visit, he writes a report of his findings and recommendations. The secretary of the Residency Review Committee then sends a copy of all data, reports, and correspondence to one member of the Review Committee who examines all the information received and records his own considered evaluation of the program.

When the Residency Review Committee meets, the member of the committee who has reviewed a given program presents to the entire committee his report and recommendation—this report may or may not be in agreement with that of the field representative who inspected the program.

The member of the committee who reviews a residency must not reside within the same geographic area or have any interest in or connection with the program. After he makes his recommendation to the committee, however, he must defend his conclusion in the face of whatever additional information and knowledge of the situation any other member of the committee may express. This is done before the vote of the entire committee is recorded.

Types of Action Taken by the Residency Review Committee. The action taken is either to (1) approve, (2) give provisional approval (for new programs), (3) place on confidential probation, or (4) disapprove. Not infrequently the vote of the committee does not support the recommendation of the member of the committee who reviewed the program. The field representative of the Council may not be an obstetrician-gynecologist; whenever the Residency Review Committee is in doubt regarding the merits of a program, an obstetrician-gynecologist who is experienced in the conduct of a residency program is asked to revisit the hospital and prepare an independent and supplementary report. Such a supplementary or "regional" evaluation is done by an obstetrician-gynecologist not acquainted with the community or the staff of the hospital in question. The Review Committee does not disapprove a program without considering a "regional evaluation" by an obstetrician-gynecologist in addition to the report of the field representative of the Council.

When the program is approved for the first time or when approval is questioned, the hospital and the chief of the residency are advised that the program has been given *provisional approval*. At the same time, the director of the program and the administrator of the hospital are advised that the residency will be re-evaluated in two years.

Approval of a residency program may not be withdrawn until after the program is inspected and placed on *probationary status*. At the time the residency program is placed on probation, the director is advised that re-evaluation and a final decision will be made in approximately one year.

Relationship between the Residency Review Committee and the American Board of Obstetrics and Gynecology. All matters pertaining to the content of a residency program are the responsibility of the Residency Review Committee, whereas the Board is concerned only with the qualifications of the individual physician and the conduct of the examinations by which the physician may become certified. Decisions of the Board do, however, affect the requirements of an approved program. At the present time, the Board requires a minimum of 18 months of residency in clinical obstetrics plus 18 months of residency in clinical gynecology, including the usual period in that program as senior or chief resident. Should the Board change the minimal requirements, it is expected that the evaluation criteria of the Review Committee would be changed to conform to the altered requirements of the Board.

The establishment of tenure on the Residency Review Committee seems to assure that individual opinions will not dominate or become long lasting. With a constantly changing committee of 12—on which each member usually serves a six-year term—there is a good chance that committee decisions will be unbiased and will be a continuing influence for the betterment of residency programs.

The objective of the committee is to encourage all of us to develop the best residency we can with the opportunities we have available to us. The characteristics of an approvable residency are clearly indicated in the pamphlet entitled *Essentials of Approved Residencies* issued by the Council on Medical Education of the American Medical Association. Additional information is given in the yearly *Bulletin* published by the American Board of Obstetrics and Gynecology. The characteristics of an approved program which make it a "good residency" have been discussed in the booklet entitled *Guide for Residency Programs in Obstetrics and Gynecology*, formulated by the Residency Review Committee and also published by the Council on Medical Education of the AMA.

In view of the available help there seems little justification for the statement that a hospital or service chief "can't find out what the Residency Review Committee wants." The administrator or service chief who desires to develop an approvable residency can, for the asking, obtain adequate information in regard to the requirements to be fulfilled.

What Does the Residency Review Committee Look For?

The Review Committee tends to look for certain *critical areas*—recognized as such because of the frequency with which weaker programs seem to rise or fall on the basis of their relative success in fulfilling the committee's concept of the minimum that is acceptable in these critical areas. Unfortunately for the administrator and service chief whose program is being surveyed, however, these critical areas are not emphasized in italics in the *Essentials,* the *Guide,* or the *Bulletins* of the Board.

What are some of the currently critical areas? In my opinion, questions that not infrequently determine the acceptability of a program include:

1. What are the qualifications of the chief of the department? How much of the chief's time is spent in this hospital? Particularly, how much of his practice does the chief conduct in the hospital in which he is responsible for the residency program?

2. How many of the obstetrics and gynecology staff appear qualified to instruct residents in obstetrics and gynecology? How soon out of their own residencies were members of the staff certified by the Board? How much of their practices do the better qualified members of the departmental staff bring to this hospital?

3. Is there an outpatient clinic service which would be a source of an adequate number of inpatient ward service cases for the residents to regard the clinics not only as a responsibility but also as a source of their inpatient services as well?

4. How much experience as first assistant in major gynecologic operations has the individual resident received before he has assumed the responsibilities of the "chief operator"? Are assurance of instruction as well as the opportunity to operate both considered to be important?

5. In how many major operative procedures has the resident been listed as the chief operator? Is there a desirable variety of operative experience in the resident's list of cases? How does the resident's list of cases operated compare with the hospital's record of the number of ward patients dismissed from the service during the same period?

6. Is there evidence of continual self-appraisal by the department? Particularly, is there evidence of the preparation of collective reviews of the management of problem cases, regularly scheduled reviews of complications, of perinatal morbidity, etc.?

The importance of these factors may not seem to have been emphasized in the information and directives available to the service chief and hospital administrator *before a residency is surveyed.* But I find it difficult to believe that a service chief would fail to anticipate the likelihood of the importance of such factors and questions. Before his residency is inspected, he should consider what he would look for if he were surveying a hospital that was seeking approval of a residency program.

Characteristics of a Good Residency

I shall make a few additional comments to suggest what might be characteristic of a good residency in obstetrics and gynecology.

The residency must provide an educational opportunity and not be designed primarily to provide hospital service.

The size of the hospital is neither a guarantee of the quality of the care given patients nor an indication of the educational opportunity for the resident. There is reason to believe that a volume service is of more importance in the obstetrical phase of a program because of the infrequency of pathology in almost every type of obstetrical service. There is also reason to believe that the best obstetrical experience occurs where the number of deliveries per day, per month, and per year is such as to require the presence of experienced personnel for anesthesia on the floor at all times. This means perhaps 3,000 plus deliveries per year. In such a labor-delivery service, paramedical, nursing, and resident personnel are likely to handle obstetrical emergencies often enough so that their behavior sets a good example for the new residents. A demonstration of the competent, efficient management of an obstetrical emergency is difficult in a hospital department that delivers less than 100 patients per month unless the incidence of obstetrical pathology is unusually high because of the selection of patients for the teaching service from a larger antepartum pool of obstetrical patients, most of whom are delivered in other institutions.

There can be no rule as to the number of cases per resident, either in the obstetric or the gynecologic phase of the program. The resident's experience can be made valuable where only a comparatively few patients are managed. Some of the poorest clinical obstetricians can be found where the residents are too busy delivering babies to have time to think of the significance of what they see. This sort of inattention to other aspects of the obstetrician's responsibilities can easily become a matter of habit, a danger where there are too many cases for a good learning experience. Too few or too many residents in a program can be equally undesirable, and the Review Committee now specifies the number of residents approved for each program.

The resident's experience must provide an opportunity to acquire progressive responsibility for the care of patients. This is particularly true in gynecologic surgery, where no amount of assisting is a substitute for the responsibility of deciding that surgery is advisable, conducting the operative procedure, and managing postoperative care. Nonoperative gynecology as well as the antepartum and postpartum care of obstetrical patients are no less important than operative experience. The hospital's lack of provisions for the care of outpatients is not infrequently the explanation for disapproval of a residency program.

While the qualifications, interests, and abilities of the chief of the program are perhaps of the greatest importance, the abilities and interests of his staff really determine the quality of the educational opportunity that can be provided in a residency.

All residencies strive to maintain a balance between clinical experience acquired through patient care and knowledge gained as a result of the educational activities of the department program. An impressive schedule of rather didactic teaching conferences "for the residents" usually suggests a lack of a truly teaching atmosphere. Staff and residents should share in the consideration of daily problems and in mutual effort to keep abreast of concepts offered in current literature and the reports of current research.

It is not essential that all residencies adopt the same program, nor is it desirable to attempt to maintain a rigidly uniform sequence of experience for each resident in the program. Approved residencies are encouraged to arrange for more than the minimal 36 months of progressive experience now required, but such additions should not dilute the minimal requirements. When longer programs have been arranged, the trainee must usually complete the entire residency as approved by the Residency Review Committee in order to fulfill the requirements of the Board.

CONCLUSION

It is my personal opinion that the work of the Residency Review Committee—helping to assure an increasing number of *good* residencies in obstetrics and gynecology—is being done in an effective manner.

It is also my opinion that more cannot be expected of the Residency Review Committee until the requirements of the American Board of Obstetrics and Gynecology are so altered as to require better preparation of the individual for the practice of obstetrics and gynecology. It should be noted that the minimal requirements of the American Board of Obstetrics and Gynecology have remained essentially unchanged since the Board was organized in 1930. Many of us are pleased that within a year or two our present concepts of an adequate residency experience for the obstetrician and gynecologist in training may have changed considerably. I am confident, however, that any such changes, as well as the continued work of the Residency Review Committee, will help assure a larger number of better residencies in obstetrics and gynecology.

II. DISCUSSION

By E. Stewart Taylor, M.D.

E. Stewart Taylor is professor and chairman of the department of obstetrics and gynecology at the University of Colorado School of Medicine. He is also a director of the American Board of Obstetrics and Gynecology. He received the M.D. degree from the State University of Iowa and is a diplomate of the American Board of Obstetrics and Gynecology.

Dr. Randall has presented a very complete description of the concept and content of a good residency program in obstetrics and gynecology. Of the necessary elements for a good program, the resident himself is the most important. A bright, energetic resident will turn out well even in a poor to mediocre program, for self-learning is a very important part of a resident's education. The resident must, however, have his work subjected to regular critique and review.

Since responsibility is a valuable teacher, a resident must be given increasing responsibility. He must have patients for whose welfare he is responsible. It should be possible for the resident to have some patients whose illness he follows from beginning to end. Although there is value in complementing his learning through teaching and responsibility with private patients; the value is limited because the resident is not the responsible physician. It is my opinion that a residency program should provide at least 15 free beds for resident education in obstetrics and gynecology if there are three residents in the program (one for each of the three years of progressive training). The resident can then admit a representative group of patients to his own service. His medical, obstetrical, and gynecological care of these patients will be supervised by the attending staff under the chief of service. Such a service should provide operative experience of at least 100 major obstetric and gynecologic procedures.

49

The Future Training for Family Practice

I.

By Francis L. Land, M.D.

Francis L. Land is a general practitioner in Fort Wayne, Indiana, where he has served on the executive committee of Lutheran Hospital. He received the M.D. degree from the University of Indiana. He has held many offices and appointments in organized medicine and is past president of his county medical society. He is a delegate to the American Medical Association, a member of the AMA Council on Medical Education, a member of the AMA Residency Review Committee for General Practice, and a member of the Ad Hoc Committee on Preparation for Family Practice. He is vice president and a member of the Board of Directors of the American Academy of General Practice and has served as a member and chairman of the AAGP Commission on Education for nine years.

(ED. NOTE: *The material in this chapter is presented by four men who have long been active in the field of medical education and who have a special interest in the future of family practice.*)

This subject is probably one of the most widely discussed subjects in medical education today. To my knowledge, there are at least six committees or groups studying the problem in depth. Some of these are:

1. The American Medical Association Ad Hoc Committee on Preparation for Family Practice including three representatives from the American Medical Association Council on Medical Education, two represent-

461

atives from the American Academy of General Practice, one represent-
ative from the American Medical Association Section of General
Practice, and three representatives from the Association of American
Medical Colleges.

2. The Citizen's Committee on Graduate Medical Education.
3. The American Academy of General Practice Commission on Education.
4. The Coggeshall Report.[1]
5. The American Medical Association Internship Task Force.
6. The President's Commission—National Community Planning Association.

In discussing the future of anything, we must first review the past. Dr.
John Nunemaker has traced the history concerning the establishment of
general practice residencies, and recalls some interesting facts in his section of this chapter.

I believe it is obvious that neither the family practice nor general
practice pilot programs have been a howling success. The reasons are
manifold and varied and include factors such as lack of participants,
poor training programs, and so on.

I believe that there is no reason to establish new types of training
programs unless other changes are made in the entire medical curriculum.
Among those changes are such things as training programs which will
lead to certification in Family Practice. The Congress of Delegates of the
American Academy of General Practice approved the principle of
certification in April of 1965. The Commission on Education of the
American Academy of General Practice believes that the minimum
training for certification should be a basic two years after medical school
with an optional third year. They also feel there should be continuous
training in the care of ambulatory patients.

Since we are postulating the future, let us consider certain definite
trends which, in my personal opinion, appear to be evolving. First, there
is a definite place in the medical spectrum of practice for a physician to
do family practice. Second, in order to develop this concept, medical
schools must reorganize their curriculums to include the family physician
as an integral part of the health care team.

II.

By R. Neil Chisholm, M.D.

R. Neil Chisholm is a general practitioner in Denver, Colorado. He received the M.D. degree from
the University of Colorado, and he is a clinical

instructor in the division of general practice of the department of medicine. He is a member of the education committees of the Colorado Heart Association and the Colorado chapter of the American Cancer Society, a past chairman of the Colorado Academy of General Practice Education Committee, and a member of the Commission on Education of the American Academy of General Practice. He is past president of the Colorado Academy of General Practice.

At the present time, many committees of the American Academy of General Practice are working diligently to organize the great volume of knowledge that has derived from numerous conferences with medical educators and much research. We want to define the core content of family practice and use this to develop a training program that will produce the general practitioner of the future.

In the meantime we have applied for a board certification mechanism which we feel will be the ultimate reward for successful completion of an adequate training program.

III.

By Edward C. Rosenow, Jr., M.D.

Dr. Rosenow is the executive director of the American College of Physicians. He received the M.D. degree from Harvard Medical School and was a fellow in internal medicine at the Mayo Graduate School of Medicine. He is a diplomate of the American Board of Internal Medicine. He was in private practice in Pasadena, California, for 17 years and was clinical professor of medicine at the University of Southern California School of Medicine and is presently the adjunct clinical professor of medicine at the University of Pennsylvania. He has held many important offices, being past president of the Los Angeles County Medical Association, the Los Angeles Society of Internal Medicine and the Los Angeles County Heart Association. He was chairman of the Committee on Postgraduate Activities of the

California Medical Association and editor of Audio-Digest.

Any physician doing family practice should be capable of being a
"first contact" physician who is qualified to see that the patient gets
comprehensive and continuous care, including appropriate referrals to
preventive, diagnostic, therapeutic, and rehabilitative services. He should
consider the care of the family as a unit.

Obviously general practitioners are ideal family practitioners. Internists with pediatricians offer an excellent team for a family. Groups
of specialists in multi-disciplinary clinics are also capable in the field.
Many other specialists do fairly adequate family practice to a greater or
lesser degree.

There is no strong attraction for a young man to strive for any training
which is not specialty oriented. If there were any strong trends in the
direction of general practice, the total number in this field would more
nearly replace men who die, who leave general practice for specialty
training, or who retire.

There should be no conflict between specialists and generalists. There
is a feeling somehow that the specialist is not warm, friendly, or devoted
like the old-time family general practitioner. This may be partly true, but
it does not condemm the specialty, only the specialist. Unquestionably
we need to pay much more attention to education in behavorial sciences
by all physicians. More study needs to be devoted to methods of effectively using specialists in all ways to meet the needs of patients. Our
profession should stop being defensive in answering the public's question,
"How can I get a doctor?" and begin to educate the public on how they
should satisfy their medical needs. The public expects two basic things
from the profession: knowledge and availability of such knowledge. After
all, until the patient calls, he is his own doctor.

Many of us feel that attempts to set up educational standards for
family practice as a discipline are bound to fail even if such idealized
training might lead to certification by a board of family practice. Medical
scientific knowledge is too complicated and too rapidly expanding for
any one man to keep up in everything. Hence most men feel more
comfortable in taking on less than the whole. If family practice education
is oriented in too many directions, the man so educated will become
primarily a referral center; and this will inevitably make him feel loss
of status.

A word must be said about the tendency to think the main difficulty in
this area is centered in the small remote communities of our country.
Nothing could be more misleading. It is just as difficult for the patient
to find immediate answers to his medical emergencies in large urban

centers as it is in rural communities. Much more effort must be made to satisfy these needs, or the profession will lose its place of leadership in health matters.

Finally it must be recognized by all physicians that a physician is developed and trained for the patient. The physician's ability must be extended to care for larger numbers of patients. One way in which this may be done is in the training of ancillary personnel who can do certain repetitious, time-consuming duties which are now done by physicians. Computers will be increasingly used to help doctors become more efficient. There is little doubt that the physicians of the future will rise to these many challenges.

IV.

By John C. Nunemaker, M.D.

John C. Nunemaker is the associate secretary of the Council on Medical Education and Hospitals of the American Medical Association. Prior to taking this post in 1958, he served as director of the Education Service in the department of medicine and surgery of the Veterans Administration from 1952 to 1958. He received the M.D. degree from Harvard Medical School, and he is a diplomate of the American Board of Internal Medicine. He is also a lecturer in medicine at Northwestern University Medical School.

(ED. NOTE: *This paper was presented at the Second Regional Conference of the American Academy of General Practice at Hartford, Connecticut, January 29–30, 1965, and was published in the Compendium of reports for this conference.*)

In searching back through our records to establish the birthday of the present general practice residencies, I came across some very interesting historical facts which are worth recalling.

The first recorded instance in which the House of Delegates referred to the Council on Medical Education a resolution to "encourage the designation of the practice of general medicine or 'family physician' as a distinct and dignified specialty" was in June, 1919, and the resolution came from California. This is almost 50 years ago, and I imagine most of us are quite unaware of this fact.

In 1941 the House of Delegates disapproved the establishment of a new Section on General Practice but approved an experimental "session" in the Section on Miscellaneous Topics. Also in 1941 a resolution from Indiana recommended the development of "standards and means by which certification may be given in recognition of special training, experience and fitness, and special qualifications for general practice," but this resolution was disapproved by the House of Delegates.

In 1944 a resolution was introduced from Michigan, recommending the establishment of a Board of General Practice, but the House of Delegates disapproved this resolution because of lack of jurisdiction and referred it to the Council for transmission to the Advisory Board for Medical Specialties.

At the December, 1945, session, the House of Delegates finally approved the establishment of a Section on General Practice. One year later a resolution was approved by the House of Delegates encouraging the establishment of general practice sections in hospitals and containing the interesting statement that such a section should not per se prevent approval of a hospital for the training of interns and residents. This resolution was transmitted to the American College of Surgeons, the American College of Physicians, the American Hospital Association, the Protestant Hospital Association, the Catholic Hospital Association, and to every hospital in the country.

In 1947 the House of Delegates recommended that the Council proceed with the development of a program of utilizing smaller community hospitals not directly associated with medical schools as training institutions for general practitioners.

In 1948 a resolution was introduced from New York that two-year rotating internships especially designed for training in general practice be set up as rapidly as possible. This same resolution has been introduced almost annually from New York state since that time.

In that same year, 1948, the Council did establish a new category of approved residencies in general practice and reported in 1949 that the response from hospitals interested in establishing such residencies had been gratifying. By 1953, the Section on General Practice had requested that there be fewer approvals of specialty residency programs until the residency program in general practice had been properly augmented. To this the Council responded that for the previous year only 40 per cent of the established general practice residencies were filled, and it would not appear that there was any immediate need for the establishment of additional residencies of that type. It was further pointed out that many graduates entered general practice after taking residency training in other specialty areas and that the number of residents in general practice residencies is no measure of the number of graduates planning to become family physicians.

Pilot Programs

In June of 1957 the Council reported the formation of a committee, with representation from the Council, the Association of American Medical Colleges, and the American Academy of General Practice, "to objectively analyze and make recommendations as to the background preparation today for general practice." The report of this committee was accepted by the House of Delegates in June of 1959 and was the basis for the establishment of pilot programs which I shall discuss briefly. The title of their report was, "Final Report on Preparation for Family Practice," but we must remember that the term "family physician" was used 40 years earlier in the House of Delegates. These pilot programs were designated "family practice" programs and were called neither internships nor residencies even though they embraced the initial two years after graduation from medical school. The 24-month period was to contain 18 months of medicine and pediatrics in a very broad sense and an elective 4 months of obstetrics; but a formal assignment to the surgical service was not required. At least eight resolutions were introduced to the House of Delegates in 1960, directing the Council to consider other two-year programs in general practice which did incorporate obstetrics and surgery. With acceptance of these resolutions by the House of Delegates, the Council identified these aditional programs as "general practice" and included them in the pilot group of 20 programs to be established and evaluted on a long-range basis. It was the intent of the Council that as wide a variety of situations be identified as possible—urban, rural, affiliated and non-affiliated, north, south, east, and west, in tax-supported and non-tax-supported institutions, in hospitals with and without other competing graduate programs, and even in an appropriate group practice situation if one could be found. It was the policy of the Council to use the "soft sell technique" in the belief that a program would be more aggressively supported by a hospital staff if the impetus for the program originated with the staff rather than from the Council staff or some other outside agency using a "hard sell technique."

In the 1964 *Directory of Approved Internships and Residencies,* we have listed these pilot programs at the end of the list of approved internships. To the eight family practice programs and the 11 general practice programs we can add the final one on which both AMA and AAGP officials have worked and consulted for several years, bringing the total number of programs to 20. This last program is entitled the "Charity Hospitals of Louisiana General Practice Program" and involves three of the Charity Hospitals outside New Orleans as well as New

Orleans Charity Hospital and has the active sponsorship of both medical schools in New Orleans.

As for very recent history, at the June, 1964, meeting of the AMA House of Delegates, a recommendation from the Council was accepted for the creation of another committee with composition similar to that established seven years earlier, to be known as the *Ad Hoc Committee on Education for Family Practice.* Perhaps it is significant that the Council staff member for this committee has primary responsibility in the area of undergraduate medical education rather than graduate medical education. While this committee has just begun its work, it will unquestionably consider many of the problems now being considered by the Citizens Commission on Graduate Medical Education (under the chairmanship of Dr. John S. Millis, the president of Western Reserve University), as well as many of the matters already considered by a Task Force on Internships which will make a report to the Council at its spring meeting. The very existence of these various groups, all considering the initial medical education of the future physician, is eloquent evidence of the unrest and the concern with the present state of affairs in this field.

In support of its recommendation for the new ad hoc committee, the Council submitted data in June, 1965, indicating that there were four different programs besides the one-year internship which were directed at the preparation of the general or family physician. The oldest program is the two-year internship, which goes back at least to the first list of approved internships published by the Council in 1914. It is of interest that in this list some of the specialty hospitals offered internships of from three to six months' duration. The great majority of general hospitals offered internships of at least one year, but many listed 18 months and 24 months, while Mount Sinai Hospital in New York listed its internship as 30 months.

The general practice residency, of course, is a two-year program following a one-year internship, and the general practice and family practice programs are two-year programs following graduation from medical school. We summarized the filled positions in each of these four programs from 1960 through 1963 and found that the general practice residencies which were 69 per cent filled in 1960 were only 47 per cent filled in 1963. The general practice and family practice programs, which by 1963 offered slightly over 100 total positions, were only about 30 per cent filled. The hospitals approved for internships of longer than 12 months' duration offered 261 positions, and these were only 64 per cent filled. All four programs filled 583 positions in 1960, 548 in 1961, 536 in 1962, and 539 estimated in 1963. It was clear to the Council and convincing to the Board of Trustees and the House of Delegates that these programs were not obtaining trainees in the numbers desired. It must also be recalled that of the 370 general practice residencies filled over

50 per cent were filled by foreign graduates who were using them probably as way stations while they searched for something better. Thus we demonstrate again that a horse which is not thirsty is no more likely to drink out of four different watering troughs than he is out of one.

The Residency Review Committee for General Practice is composed of equal representation from the Council and from the Academy of General Practice, and this committee has become increasingly concerned and dissatisfied with the current status of general practice residencies. *It encourages voluntary withdrawal of programs which are completely unsatisfactory,* either because of total inactivity or because of poor organization and non-support by the staff. This is because the very low percentage of filled positions and the very high percentage of vacancies is not an attractive advertisement for the field. In the period between June, 1963, and November, 1964, 14 new applications for general practice residency programs were approved; but during the same period, 31 programs disappeared from the approved list. Of these 31 programs no longer on the list, only 10 were disapproved by the Review Committee while 21 were voluntarily withdrawn by the sponsoring hospitals. Thus, 68 per cent of the programs were withdrawn from the approved list voluntarily by the hospital staff.

Another item which has concerned the Review Committee for many years is the *tendency of many of the trainees to refuse a second year of residency training.* This resulted in the tendency of the program sponsors to attempt to incorporate into the first year of residency training a full rotation on the four major services, especially including surgery and obstetrics which are supposed to be reserved for the second year of residency. The committee has been told repeatedly that many of these trainees who have completed one year of internship are willing to complete only one more year of residency either for economic or other reasons; therefore they request more experience with obstetrics and surgery. There are even some instances in the record where individuals have resigned their residencies upon completing their surgical training. It must have been for this reason that the present standards require that obstetrics and surgery be restricted to the second year of the two-year residency program. The Review Committee always welcomes an application for a three-year residency in general practice, but such applications are extremely rare.

A further study of the data reported in the 1964 *Directory,* relating to the status of filled general practice residencies as of September, 1963, gives some interesting confirmation of the unpopularity of the second year of this residency, particularly in non-affiliated hospitals. Of the 165 programs reported, only 20 were in hospitals affiliated with medical schools. There were 432 total positions offered with 370 filled. When we break down the data for the filled positions according to the first or second year, we find that there were 241 filled in the first year and only 129 in the second. When we break this down according to medical school affiliation, we find that the affiliated hospitals filled 30 positions the first year and 34 the second; the non-affiliated filled 211 the first year, but only 95, or less than half, in the second year. To express it in percentage figures, for the affiliated hospitals 53 per cent of all the general practice residents were serving at the second year level, while in the non-affiliated hospitals only 31 per cent of all the residents on duty were serving at the second year level.

In our universal concern and interest in the problem of attracting physicians into family practice, it is even difficult to find reliable figures on the number of men actually practicing family medicine or general practice. Dunphy has commented on the number of general surgeons actually doing family practice on a neighborhood basis, presumably on their friends and neighbors.

Much of the criticism directed at the Council on Medical Education as well as at medical educators and medical school faculties in general blames the unattractiveness of general practice on the lack of exposure of medical students to general practitioners.

While there are numerous preceptorship programs for medical students, and while they may be popular and appreciated by students generally, one former medical school dean whose school had had a preceptorship program for many years reported to this writer the following: while the students enjoyed and valued their preceptorship experience, they returned generally convinced of one thing, namely, that they *did not want to go into general practice.*

I sincerely believe that a solution to the problem of attracting men to general practice lies not in simple exposure to general practitioners during the undergraduate period nor in the creation of innumerable new designs for training programs; rather it lies in a redefinition and reorganization of the pattern of training of all members of the health care team and the reidentification of their relationships to one another. In most of the established training programs today, the resident in the general practice programs is regarded as a second-class citizen or as a junior member of the team and carries less responsibility than the other trainees in the institution. Nowhere in undergraduate education or in graduate education in hospitals is it clear to young trainees that the general or family physician has a job just as vital in the total health care program as that of the professor of neurosurgery. While the proper base of operations of the family physician may be more in the office and in the home than in the hospital, this in no way lessens the importance of these functions. *The problem is that he is not recognized as an effective member of a total team operation.*

In the postwar years, we have become increasingly aware of the necessity for lengthening the shadow of the physician through his participation in a team effort in which he may be the captain or the director; but many of the things formerly performed personally by him will now be performed by others. In other words, while he may be the key to the health care program for his patients, he cannot be the lock in the door. The long-gone image of the grand old general practitioner was both the key and the lock in the door. While those days are gone, we now face the dilemma of many keys fitting many locks in many doors, all relating to health care.

One of the problems confronting graduate medical education in the other specialties as well as in the field of family practice is that of preparing the trainees not only for the scientific side of medical practice but also for the administrative aspects. When this is incorporated into graduate training programs today, it is usually by accident and not because of any overall national concerted plan. It has been suggested that residency training in hospitals is actually training in group practice. However, there is no requirement on the part of the Council and no concerted plan on the part of any group of hospitals to include in the training of residents their relationship to each other in terms of their own practice when their training is completed. Far too little effort is made, either in affiliated or non-affiliated hospitals, to set up situations in which the house officers can actually participate in a situation truly mimicking private practice on ambulatory patients.

One of the pilot programs in general practice was designed to permit the trainee to function under careful supervision in a group clinic and to follow his patients in the hospital and back to the clinic, all the time learning to relate himself and his practice to the other members of the group team which cared for these patients.

Several years ago, I stated that I felt the future of the general practitioner lay with group practice where the family physician and the specialist work side by side as members of a team in a position of mutual trust and harmony, each with his own responsibility and each contributing to the continuing education of the other as well as to the more comprehensive care of their patients.

Several years ago, a respected member of the AMA Board of Trustees visited the Council offices, and in the course of discussing family practice he raised the question as to whether all specialists should not have the philosophy of caring for some families regardless of their own particular specialty interests. This was to us a radical thought, and we gave him a rather strong argument. However, many specialists do in fact carry on a family practice to one degree or another.

In this connection, Dr. John H. Hunt, Honorable Secretary of the British College of General Practitioners, wrote, "In many countries, some of the surgeons, obstetricians, specialists in internal medicine, and anesthetists had started in general practice, and still like to do a certain amount of it themselves. *They have a perfect right to do this;* but if they do so, they cannot expect other family doctors *who are not their partners* to send them much special work." [2] [Italics mine.]

Dr. Edward Liston of the Palo Alto Medical Clinic stated at the American Association of Medical Clinics meeting in 1964 that the general practitioner in a multi-specialty group is readily accepted by other specialties, particularly the surgeons and orthopedists; but his difficulty is in establishing rapport with the internists. The point is that there is an important place for these men in groups and clinics, and the importance will increase as group practice increases, I am sure. For this reason, I believe most of our present training programs in family and in general practice are deficient in not preparing their trainees for effective team relationships with other physicians, and *I believe the other specialty residencies are equally deficient in this regard.*

These ideas were supported strongly by Dunphy in his address before the Student AMA in May of 1964. He stated that teamwork between the family physician and the specialist is essential, that the family physician must become the central figure in a new pattern of medical care, and that he should no longer practice solo but work with a team of other men in some type of group practice. While Dunphy pleaded for the establishment of training programs involving experience in internal medicine, pediatrics, psychiatry, and surgery and the establishment of pilot studies, he did not recognize the existing efforts that have been made in this direction.

CONCLUSION

Dr. John F. McCreary, the Dean of the Faculty of Medicine of the University of British Columbia, delivered the Donald Frazer Memorial Lecture before the Canadian Public Health Association on June 2, 1964.[3] In this delightful paper, he indicated that the problems in this country regarding family practice are identical in Canada, and he devotes considerable space to the problem of the declining number of general practitioners, changes in medical education, a new concept of the general practitioner, and the physician and the health team. I must confess that his remarks have done much to solidify my own thinking; and I would hope his remarks could find wide distribution in this country. He emphasizes that medical educators and practitioners have failed to solve these disturbing problems because we have not yet decided what our pattern of health care is to be.

I shall conclude by quoting from his remarks since they are so pertinent to the problem we face in producing all manner of health personnel generally, and physicians in particular, for the future welfare of the public.

Although the teaching of comprehensive medicine may have changed the attitudes of some students, it has done little to make prospective doctors conscious of the contributions which can be made by other members of the health team. True they worked with social workers and public health nurses, but they were still separated from other members of the team.

I do not believe that we will achieve a truly functioning health team until more fundamental changes are made. As long as dentists, pharmacists, physicians, social workers, dieticians, clinical psychologists, rehabilitation therapists, and the others are educated in their own cells on the campuses of our universities, each group with its own teachers, each developing its own sense of importance, and its own vision of its own separate goal, we will not develop a health team. Instead, we shall continue to see artificial barriers arise between the groups, which will interfere with their functioning together. It seems possible that the next development in the education of physicians will be to educate the doctor along with the others who will work with him in providing health care. When all these groups are taught together by the same teachers, on the same patients and in the same environment; when the combined student body of all faculties and schools in the health sciences study together, eat together, and examine the future together, then we may have a chance of welding a functional unit from its disparate parts.

BIBLIOGRAPHY

1. Coggeshall, L. T.: "Planning for Medical Progress Through Education," Association of American Medical Colleges, Evanston, Ill., 1965.

2. Hunt, J. H.: General Practice in the World Today, *GP*, 30:203–223 (Nov.) 1964.

3. McCreary, J. F.: Education of Health Personnel, *Canad. J. Public Health*, 55:424–434 (Oct.) 1964.

Epilogue

PROFESSIONAL EXCELLENCE AND THE PATIENT

By Rev. John J. Flanagan, S.J.

The Reverend John J. Flanagan, S.J., has served as the executive director of the Catholic Hospital Association since 1947. He received the A.B. and LL.B. degrees from Creighton University and the M.A. degree from Saint Louis University. After serving as assistant dean of arts and sciences at Saint Louis University, he became dean and later president of Regis College in Denver.

Father Flanagan is an honorary fellow of the American College of Hospital Administrators, and he holds honorary membership in the American Hospital Association. In 1964, he was named "Health Association Executive of the Year," an annual award of *Hospital Management*.

The second conference for Hospital Chiefs of Staff is all but over. Many are asking if it is as good or better than the one which was conducted so successfully last year. Only time and follow-up will really decide this. I visited many hospitals in the course of the last 12 months, and I was greatly impressed by the number of physicians and administrators who reported that representatives of their institutions had been at the Conference in Denver and that as a result a new philosophy was being experienced in the hospitals. Never have I known of a medical or hospital meeting which produced so many favorable results and brought about so much direct influence.

I have asked myself why this happened. It is true that the meeting was excellently organized, and the program and speakers included many of the most experienced men in medical administration. But these factors are not altogether new.

I am convinced that in these conferences for Hospital Chiefs of Staff a new type of medical forum has been developed. Perhaps this is one of the few times when intelligent, sincere practitioners of medicine could assemble in an environment which was entirely free of the usual pressures of typical medical meetings and could discuss their favorite topic in which they glory and excel—patient care. Perhaps for the first time they received a clear and authoritative message on the values of medical staff organization in terms of patient care and received it from medical men who could speak from experience and with authority.

In the course of this conference you have heard presentations on the component elements of good medical care in hospitals and have discussed procedures and techniques of delivering to patients the quality of care to which they are entitled in this decade in the United States. Excellent as these presentations have been, dependent as the hospital is on the role of an organized medical staff, *there remains the problem of effective implementation*. This conference can go down in history as another noble gesture toward excellence; it can go into the archives as a memorial to sterile academic rhetoric and medical polemics unless we can invoke the necessary mechanics of implementation.

Medical and hospital history will report for the 1950s and 1960s the great phenomenon of record-breaking numbers of meetings on health; it will bear witness to the flowering of hundreds of brilliant ideas. But it will also record the great blight of inertia and administrative frustration which caused great ideas and fond hopes to deteriorate on the recording tapes.

Two groups bear the primary responsibility for the improvement of medical care in the hospitals of this country. They are the complementary forces which must unite in a crash program for excellence. They are, of course, the organized medical staff in the hospital and the policy-making and executive forces of the governing board and administration.

Although I wish to speak primarily about motivation, attitudes and values, I wish to stress the paramount importance of mutual understanding, cooperative planning, and the joint responsibility of these two groups.

It appears to me that *our first duty is to fully realize the meaning of the enlightened age in which we live*. The horse and buggy days of medicine had their own glamour and their own achievements, but also their built-in limitations. The greatest achievement in those days was the rugged even heroic men who did the very best they could with the resources available to them. This attitude we could imitate: where they were hampered by deficiencies, we luxuriate in the richest resources. We have more, and more is expected of us.

Dr. Tom Dooley could boast that he practiced nineteenth century medicine in Laos because it was an infinite improvement over nothing and was the best he could do. We are not in Laos, and we should not be paid for hospital or medical care that is even of the 1940 or 1950 vintage. Dr. Schweitzer could plead that he must adjust his practice to a level which his people could accept and that he must conform to the environmental influences in which he functioned. We dare not in our modern hospitals thus excuse ourselves. We in the hospital field and you of the medical profession are privileged to live in the most enlightened era of medicine. Our medical schools and our research centers progressively enrich our knowledge and develop new procedures; the American people, either through taxes or donations or fees, have provided us with the most complete buildings and efficient equipment with which to work. We hold these gifts in sacred trust for the citizens who made them possible, and we have a moral responsibility to return to them not nineteenth century medicine, not the medicine of the frontier and the missionary countries, but the best medicine and hospital care which is being developed today and for which people are paying.

From time to time we wake in the clear cold dawn, and see ourselves in relationship to our neighbors and the good God Who gave us our talents and Who has blessed and enriched this nation. In these moments, do we ask ourselves for an accounting? In these moments, do we look beyond the Cadillacs in the parking lot and the impressive hospital structure and see the men and women and children who are dependent on us? They are not looking for mediocrity, not the ordinary, but the extraordinary measure of care which we can, if we will, give to them. Our riches of money, resources, and buildings attain their greatest value when translated into services to our fellowmen.

What are the further implications for hospitals? We must exercise to the fullest our legal responsibilities; we must be most sensitive to our moral responsibilities toward our patients. We boast of the legal rights invested in us by our corporate charters and by the decisions of the courts. But we sometimes shrink from the legal and moral responsibility of providing resources and facilities for improved care; we hesitate in taking strong policy and administrative stands against the various establishments when the best possible patient care is at stake.

In the very best tradition we are willing to delegate to a medical staff the organization and supervision of medical services. But when deficiencies appear or when the organized staff defaults in self-discipline and fails to advance the quality of care, hospital governing boards must take appropriate steps to improve the situation. This means that the administrator and the board must have some mechanism for evaluation—ideally this is self-evaluation by the staff itself and follow-up reporting to the administrator and the board. When this fails, the board must seek outside assistance. This may be an outside medical auditor who will evaluate and report; it may be a medical director who will establish a system of supervision and discipline, and initiate programs of continuing education for physicians. As in other areas, a governing board can delegate specific responsibilities, but it can never delegate final accountability.

Medical practitioners and hospital administrators are at a crossroads today. They must choose, and rather soon, to identify voluntarily themselves with excellence or to lapse into the cataegory of second-rate institutions, satisfied with mediocrity, willing to compromise with excellence and dedicated to the philosophy of "not rocking the boat" or disturbing the sacred status quo.

To discharge their responsibilities, governing boards of hospitals must better understand their jobs. No longer can they concern themselves only with fiscal problems, brick and mortar, and parking lots. Administrators must help them to understand what the primary function of a hospital is; must help them to learn what constitutes good care; must develop in them an appreciation of the difference between a good hospital and a poor one. And the boards must insist on a reporting system which tells them about quality of care rather than be satisfied with financial reports. They must understand the patient care values of education, research, and accreditation. After that they must learn to use all approved techniques of implementation. Hospitals also must undertake the task of educating the public to an understanding of what good care is.

I am told again and again that most physicians want to practice good medicine. I am willing to subscribe to that, but that does not mean that the good physician does not need help, that he does not need stimulation; it does not mean that we must excuse and close our eyes to individuals who are lazy, lax, grossly incompetent, and unscrupulous.

We think in recent years that we have *awakened in Catholic physicians and Catholic hospitals a better understanding of ethical values.* Priests and Catholic moral theologians, because of their limited contact with medical practice, created the impression that all medical morality centered around the reproductive systems. So vehemently did we condemn birth control and abortions that people, including physicians, were led to believe that if a physician did not distribute birth control literature, did not tie tubes, and did not produce abortion, that he was a model Catholic physician. We now insist that medical and hospital morality also depend upon quality of service to· people. Every professional act of a physician, every activity within the hospital is a matter of our moral concern, because we are bound in justice to give to the patient care which at least meets minimum standards. This is not a change of principle or policy, but it is perhaps a re-emphasis of basic principles which may have been forgotten or overlooked.

I hope enlightened hospital governing boards will be instrumental in helping physicians *shake off certain shackles which seem to have inhibited them and which have been barriers to progress.* Has not the time come to interpret the vaunted personal relationship between patient and physician as something more than the privilege of rendering a bill directly to the patient? It should involve courtesy, compassion, and an active interest in giving each patient comprehensive and thorough attention and the depth of treatment which each case demands.

When there is a question of strengthening a service or giving better care or when a salaried physician can better do the job, we should boldly break with the traditional subterfuge of resorting to a fictitious interpretation of ethics and pay the person a just salary for a professional job. Ethics in the true sense of the word deal with morality and are intended to protect patients, not to be subordinated to the petty whims of vested interests.

I think that very soon there should be some thorough investigation of what we mean by the corporate practice of medicine. A continued reliance on legal and medical cliches which were developed many years ago to cover abuses of another era leads only to misunderstanding, confusion, and to a certain degree of hypocrisy. I think there are certain medical values which must be protected from institutional encroachment; I think there are definite areas pertaining to medical judgment, the professional dignity of a physician, and freedom of choice which must be protected in the interest of good medical care. Once this essential area is defined, the medical profession can take a determined and intelligent position. Once this is accomplished, hospitals should and will support medical men in preserving values that are truly in the interest of good patient care.

Under these circumstances ethics become meaningful. We can no longer rely on methods of payment as a sole criterion.

Hospitals must take a fresh look at their objectives and review their services. They must determine if they are actually fulfilling their responsibilities to people in the community and to physicians who wish to move off a plateau of mediocrity and to go all out for excellence. We in hospitals can have a vested-interest philosophy, too. We can be primarily concerned about institutional stability and security when we should be responding to challenges.

Medical staffs and hospitals must quickly face the *problem of adequate and competent coverage of emergency service.* The failure of physicians to take responsibility for this is scandalous; the timidity of administrators and governing boards to take drastic action is equally shocking. Again we must not be frightened by the threat of the label of "corporate practice of medicine." In a Christian democracy the welfare of people is more important than outmoded, self-serving cliches behind which selfish and timid souls take refuge.

Physicians and officials of voluntary hospitals are concerned in this decade that *traditional practices long identified with the voluntary sys-tem are being threatened and that the basic values deriving therefrom may be jeopardized.* There is reason to be concerned. But both groups seem to forget their essential dependence on each other. There are the usual courtesy gestures toward each other but not enough understand-ing and trust in day-by-day relationships.

I am appalled at the growing chasm of misunderstanding, distrust and suspicion that is dividing health care in the United States. Good physicians feel that they have no voice in making hospital policies which affect their activities. Many are completely uninformed about routine hospital policies and have failed to understand the relationship between good management and good patient care.

To the best of my knowledge, voluntary hospitals do not wish to have a closed staff of paid physicians. They do resort in some instances to the paid full-time medical director or full-time chiefs of service, not to practice medicine but to carry out administrative duties which a busy chief of staff usually cannot assume and which are not appro-priate to a non-medical administrator. It is regrettable that this is not better understood.

Some administrators, on the other hand, are insecure and fearful of the strong, forthright physician. And sometimes they do not help the governing board to understand better the physician-hospital rela-tionship.

Too many good physicians become frustrated; they feel they are kept in ignorance of hospital policies and lapse into a sort of cold war of cynical indifference—a fatalistic coexistence with "city hall."

As part of their management function and responsibility, adminis-trators have a solemn obligation to change this picture. They must work with the medical staff, to think through and rebuild a better un-derstanding and better working relationship between the two groups. Together these two must preserve the voluntary system of health care. Administrators, with the support of governing boards, should help medical staffs develop self-government into a positive, constructive, statesmanlike force in the medical care complex of the hospital.

In theory the Joint Conference Committee is an excellent instrument; in practice however, it has failed more often than it has succeeded. It has been strongly recommended by the American Medical Association and the Joint Commission on the Accreditation of Hospitals. The ad-ministrator should take leadership in making it a more successful liaison. He should solicit ideas of individual members regularly. To these he must add his own broad perspective and weld these into an agendum that is vital, challenging, and provocative.

I look forward to a closer working relationship in our voluntary hos-pitals between medical staffs and governing boards so that physicians can exercise a responsible influence on all aspects of hospital planning, policy making, and administrative procedures. I hope that they shall become so involved that they will develop a better understanding of good and bad administration so that when they have objections and constructive criticisms they will be based upon sound and intelligent reasons and will not be wild allegations against a system which they fear but do not understand.

I hope also that governing boards and administrators will continue to grow in an appreciation of real patient care values and be courageous in supporting them and enforcing them.

I have spoken most frankly and most boldly today because of the values I see in this program; because of the great movement for improvement in patient care which is being launched here today; because of the confidence which I have in intelligent men and women of the medical profession when they are free to concentrate on their great vocation—the care of sick people. May God continue to bless you with an understanding of the potentials of your vocation and the courage to pursue it.

Appendix

QUESTIONS AND DISCUSSIONS

ED. NOTE: *The questions and discussion in this section have been selected and freely edited from the tape recordings of four panel discussions presented at the Hospital Medical Staff Conference, October 11–16, 1965. Because more than one speaker usually discussed each question, the discussion has been consolidated, and the identity of individual speakers has therefore not been made. The editor assumes full responsibility for all statements.*
The panels were as follows:

Medical Staff Organization
    Anthony J. J. Rourke, M.D.
    Robert R. Cadmus, M.D.
    Kenneth J. Williams, M.D.
    Karl S. Klicka, M.D.
    William W. Jack, M.D.
Hospital Privileges
    Stanley R. Truman, M.D.
    Ronald D. Yaw
    Kenneth J. Williams, M.D.
    Phillip T. Knies, M.D.
Disciplinary Problems
    Floyd C. Mann, Ph.D.
    Stanley R. Truman, M.D.
    John C. Leonard, M.D.
The Continuing Education of the Hospital Staff Physician
    C. Wesley Eisele, M.D.
    Kenneth J. Williams, M.D.
    Vergil N. Slee, M.D.
    James A. Campbell, M.D.
    Henry S. M. Uhl, M.D.

We have a small community hospital with four doctors on the active staff, one of whom is a qualified surgeon doing all the surgery in the hospital. Who should serve on the surgical and tissue committees?

You do not necessarily need surgeons to review tissues and to review surgery. In the first place, in the ordinary hospital you are not going to do a very sophisticated medical audit on neurosurgery, eye surgery, chest surgery, or open heart surgery. The three general physicians on your staff could do a splendid job on these committees, determining what you want to know. Did the surgeon take a history? Did he do a physical examination? Did he write his stop orders? Do the preoperative, tissue, and final diagnoses agree? What is his death rate? How many autopsies is he getting? Such questions would be enough of a brake on his surgery. In these committees it is not one physician sitting in judgment of another physician. The medical staff has established its own standards, and the committee merely sees that its associates maintain the standard which all have agreed upon. It is not a question of saying, "You used a different suture," or "You should have made a longer incision." These are not matters for the committee. Performance is evaluated against the staff's own standards, and in that light this question really takes care of itself.

Records of utilization and tissue committees are subject to subpoena. For this reason criticism made by the committee may be presented in a court of law. It has been suggested by some that records of cases should not be included in the minutes. What are your suggestions?

This is an old and very good question. First, although committee records might be subpoenaed, the chain of proof would generally be too tenuous to allow admission of the record as evidence. There is not a documented case in which any of these records have ever backfired on the committee. Secondly, we must recognize that all staff committees and functions are designed to improve the quality of care, and the purpose is educational and not policing or regulatory. Courts generally recognize this as being in the public interest.

Basically, I do not think names should be used in committee records, but unit numbers of patients are certainly permissible. If the committee looks at the staff work as a whole and uses the educational approach and if the meetings and minutes are directed in this way, then there is no problem about the committee records becoming a legal weapon against the committee, the hospital, or the physician.

Another speaker: First of all, there would be no need to record anything if we could be sure that all medical staffs across the country did their job, but this has not been the case. There have been many situations in which committees have not faced up to nasty situations.

Here is a method that has worked for us. In the tissue committee, for instance, we recommend that the results be divided into three categories. For the first, the minutes record that "the following records were reviewed, and the preoperative, tissue, and discharge diagnoses agree." A group of patient numbers are then listed under this statement, and that is all you say. In the second category, where the preoperative, tissue, and discharge diagnoses disagree but surgery was justified on the basis of the records, another set of numbers is listed. In the third category, preoperative, tissue, and discharge diagnoses disagree, but you do not say that surgery was unjustified because every man should first have the right to come and defend his actions. The patient numbers are listed, and the minutes state, "refer to the executive committee." When the matter gets to the executive committee, this physician should be notified that the committee wishes to discuss record 278934 with him. This gives him a chance to go to the record room, get out the record, and review it—not change it, but review it. When he comes in, the executive committee states that this matter was referred by the tissue committee and asks the physician if there is anything the committee does not know that he would like to bring to its attention. He may do one of three things. He may say, "I have no defense; and in hindsight it was a poor job, and I will never do it again." At this point the executive committee says in a sense, "Go, my son, and sin no more," and the matter ends there. The mere fact that he has been brought before his confreres in medicine is punishment enough; and the executive committee minutes record, "Case 278934 was discussed with the doctor of record." Or he may say, "Look, fellows, there is some information that I did not put down in the record. Here it is, and I can document it for you." The new information may change the entire complexion of the committee's judgment. Or he may do the last of three things, and the foolish thing— become angry and stubborn and try to defend a poor bit of medicine. In this case the committee says in effect, "This case is not at all impressive. In our judgment and in the judgment of the tissue committee, this was poor medical practice. Don't let us see you again soon." If the committee does see him repeatedly, then the necessary steps must be taken to control the situation—remove privileges, demand consultations, or insist on regular supervision in the operating room. When the matter is handled in this manner, the records may be subpoenaed without threat to anyone. Keep in mind that the lawyers already have the name of a plaintiff; they do not have to find it in your records. And what is there in the minutes? There is evidence in the minutes, for the man who is subpoenaed or the man who is being sued, that everybody in that hospital is standing behind him. We do review our records, and we are witness to good medicine. Now if the doctor is out in left field and has pulled a blooper, your committee records are not going to change it. This evidence is in the lawyer's hands already. I am not quoting law to you; I am describing a method that has worked for us and seems to answer the problem.

A speaker referred to senior physicians, junior physicians, and physicians holding subordinate positions. How is such an order of seniority established? What are the criteria? How is it established in the hospital with an open staff?

In discussing this general principle of doctors supervising doctors, we must first of all set certain bench marks. When a young physician who is well trained and worth his salt takes care of a patient with a coronary occlusion, he will do almost as good, if not just as good, a job during the first few years of his practice as somebody with hair as gray as mine. But I think there are other areas where he probably cannot do as good a job as I can, and these are in the areas of interpersonal relationships and supervision of other people. For a youngster to have supervisory responsibility over my practice, which I have been at for a long while, would heckle my feathers more, even though I need it, than for a more mature person to do the same. So the senior, junior, and subsidiary physician is a matter of hospital development and "coming up through the chairs." I take my hat off to the younger physician who is well trained and who is doing a fine job, whether it be in family practice or in the specialty of cardiology. But in the practice of medicine he should not be doing anything which he is not doing well. In the hierarchy of medicine, the committee work, the supervision, and the seniority positions come with experience, which he can only get by living longer.

Discuss the organizational relationship between the departmental chief of service and the executive committee. The departmental chiefs serve on the committee, and to what extent should there also be members-at-large?

Almost everything that we do should be done on the basis of common sense and local satisfaction. Rigid rules should not be set down in a dictatorial fashion, but the cloth should be cut to fit your own institution. In many small hospitals, the whole staff does the work of every committee; there is no reason for an executive committee nor for a complicated organization. But in larger institutions, I cannot see how an executive committee can really work unless it is fully represented by the departments concerned. That is, in a fully departmentalized hospital, every department should be represented on the executive committee. Certainly there should also be representation by elected members-at-large. How many depends to some extent on the assignments and functions given to the executive committee. But by and large, if everybody is happy about the amount of representation he gets, it does not matter whether it fits a specific standard. The pattern in the next community may be a different one. The representative-at-large may not necessarily be a member of the committee to make his great contributions; he may be there just to prove to the staff that there is no trickery or maneuvering going on.

Another speaker: This idea of local satisfaction is not always the whole answer, for there is a very basic principle involved here. We must regard the executive committee as the cabinet of the medical staff organization. If this is going to be the governing body of the staff, then I agree that you must have on it the clinical chiefs and also representation from the general staff. Recently, I visited a hospital in which a council composed of seven elected members from the staff had been superimposed over the executive committee of the clinical chiefs who had to answer for the quality of care. The executive committee was answerable to the elected council. I think you can have only one governing group, and this is the executive committee. All of our efforts should be directed toward building this committee into a stable and durable structure—one that will outlast the chief of staff, the medical director, and anybody else.

Cannot the chief of staff be responsible to both the staff and the governing board? Their objectives are the same, are they not?

In the small hospital, because of a small number of physicians on the staff, the chief of staff I think must wear these two hats. Of course, the objectives are the same, but we as physicians, by virtue of our training, tend to resent having a "boss." Nevertheless, these two lines of responsibility must be delineated. You have got to know who is the boss—he is the chief of staff. There may be a real danger in trying to demarcate too closely whose man is whose, but we must accept the basic principle that the chief of staff is the board's man. The staff must also have its own man, the president of the staff, and the two must work together in harmony for common objectives.

How often are the hospital privileges of general practitioners curtailed simply because they are general practitioners and without regard to their competence or ability?

This question was raised in our seminar yesterday. There was only one man in the group who indicated that this had happened in his hospital. This means that our group was not a representative one, for we know this situation has occurred in many hospitals. It is certainly not a legitimate way to curtail privileges, and it is not a legitimate or realistic way to raise standards, although this is usually the motivation given for such action. Usually this action is taken when there are one or more general practitioners on the staff who are "old-time fellows," men who have great prestige in the community but whose standards of practice have fallen behind. The whole staff, including the majority of the general practitioners, want to curtail the privileges of these few grand old men. But no one has the courage to stand up and tell them that they are falling behind, going beyond their capacities, and not practicing up to expected standards, simply "now that you are 72 years old, you should reduce your activities and limit yourself to things you can do well." In almost every instance that I know where across-the-board restrictions were imposed upon general practitioners, it has been under these circumstances. If one is going to be fair and if a high level of practice in the hospital is going to be maintained, curtailment of privileges should always be done on an individual merit basis and never as a blanket restriction on a group or class of practitioners.

Many hospitals give some practitioners "major" privileges and others "minor" privileges, and they give general practitioners "minor" privileges only. But no one has adequately defined which are major and which are minor procedures. A more effective method is to ask each member of the staff to list the privileges that he thinks he should have, and it is then up to him to justify his list to the credentials committee. This puts the shoe on the other foot and puts the burden of proof on the physicians requesting privileges.

Another speaker: I think we all agree that the real purpose of delination of privileges is to assist and guide the physician to practice within the scope of his capabilities and training in the interest of better patient care. It is one thing to delineate privileges; but many of our hospitals then fall down in supervision, and I am pointing particularly at the chief of the department. In the hospital with which I have been associated, every new member on the staff receives a letter from the executive committee stating that his work will be supervised and that the chief of his department will submit a report on his work to the executive committee at six-month intervals. This means that the chief of the service must go into the operating room, must look at his records, and must evaluate the quality of his work. This is difficult, and many chiefs do not like to do this. The bylaws should specify the process in detail so that the individual coming on the staff knows that this supervision is required and will be given, and the chief knows that he must do it.

When one speaks of restricting staff privileges, he usually refers to the privileges of general practitioners. What about delineating the privileges of specialists?

It is a common practice to grant an American Board diplomate full privileges in his specialty, and he is allowed to proceed pretty much as he pleases with any procedure in his specialty, regardless of his depth of experience, unless it becomes evident that he cannot do the procedure properly. This brings up one of the most important mechanisms for quality control. *Restriction of privileges should be imposed at the time the physician first comes on the staff and not later when privileges already granted must be rescinded.* Rather than delineate privileges according to a long list of procedures, every new staff member, regardless of board qualifications, should serve a *probationary period*, preferably for a year or more, during which time his work is carefully observed and supervised. Since less and less surgery is now being performed by general practitioners, it becomes increasingly important for the work of specialists to be adequately supervised.

Another speaker: It has been stated repeatedly that no physician should be appointed to the staff or given specific privileges solely on the basis of American Board qualifications or by membership in specialty societies, and I think that this is generally true. At the same time, it seems to me there is no reason why these qualifications—board certification, board eligibility, associateship or fellowship in the American College of Physicians or American College of Surgeons or similar organizations—should not be considered as evidence of some degree of personal and professional qualification. Perhaps professional qualifications are better defined by the American Boards, and some of the personal characteristics of an individual may be attested to a little more by fellowship in a college. Nevertheless, an individual can be a poor physician and a scoundrel and still wear the badge, but I believe these instances are unusual. Consequently, the personal characteristics of the individual, how he works with the staff, and how he accepts obligations on the staff must all be taken into account. Quite obviously this usually cannot be done effectively before he becomes a member of the staff. Therefore, in view of the special difficulty and the various legal entanglements in getting a physician off the staff of the hospital, it seems wise to establish a *provisional status of staff membership* which has an automatic termination. This appointment may be for six months or in most instances for a year, during which time it may be possible to assess his work, his personality, and how he cooperates in his staff work. The provisional status might be extended into a second year in the case of some specialties in which the work a new man might do within the hospital during one year is not sufficient to allow an adequate judgment. At the end of the provisional period, it is not the responsibility of the staff, nor the trustees, nor the administrator to take action on the continuation of that individual's appointment. His provisional appointment terminates; and if he does not apply for regular appointment, usually with courtesy staff status to begin with, he is dropped. Perhaps his activities may have become concentrated in another hospital in the city, and he is no longer interested. It is wise to remind him a month or two before the termination that in 12 months his provisional appointment is over, otherwise he might honestly forget it.

Another speaker: Psychological, emotional, and personality qualifications, or lack of qualifications, are not sufficient justification in themselves for giving or withholding staff privileges. This has been affirmed by high courts.

Another speaker: Again, we are stating that privileges should be granted on an individual basis and not categorically. Recently, in one of the hospitals in the Bay area, the staff approved a regulation that in the future no physician who is not board certified could be appointed to the obstetrical staff of this hospital. Of course, this again was aimed at a few general practitioners who were not providing good obstetrical care. They put in a grandfather clause, unfortunately, and ended by having the American Academy of General Practice, the San Francisco County Medical Society, and the California Medical Society oppose their action. After a year, the staff reconsidered their action and reaffirmed this regulation. Now the Medical Society, the California Medical Association, and the American Academy of General Practice are anxiously awaiting the day when some well-trained, competent general practitioner or obstetrician who is not board certified applies to this staff for obstetrical privileges and is denied them. The attorneys of the county society and the state society are all set to fight this hospital. This is a tragic situation, and it does not solve their problems. I can give you a list of board certified obstetricians who have been dropped from hospital staffs because their qualifications and their capacity to perform was inadequate. It is a great misfortune when a hospital tries to raise its standards by means that absolutely will fail to produce the desired results.

Does provisional appointment obviate the need for a legal hearing or any other procedure at the end of the term?

The need for a legal hearing at the termination of a provisional appointment is obviated if the bylaws are properly written and applied. I quote the following from the constitution and bylaws of the medical staff of our hospital; both the constitution and the bylaws have been approved by the staff, the hospital council (board of trustees), and the hospital attorney.

> Provisional Appointment: New appointees to the staff for a period of one year following initial appointment to permit mutual evaluation of the desirability of regular appointment, or previous members of the staff placed in provisional status as a disciplinary measure in order to permit evaluation of the desirability of continued appointment. It is understood and agreed by the administration representing the Council and by the appointee in accepting the appointment that provisional appointment may be terminated by the hospital at its convenience and will in any event terminate after the designated period of one year. Appointment to the staff will then terminate unless regular appointment has been granted on request initiated by the provisional appointee during the last quarter of the provisional year.

The provisional appointee signs the bylaws, and thereafter the bylaw provisions are binding without a legal hearing or any other legal procedure.

Another speaker: We have a very small hospital in an outlying area that does a very similar thing, and it is working beautifully. General practitioners and specialists alike have found it a very excellent means of functioning.

Restrictions of privileges usually refer to surgical or obstetrical privileges. Is it not equally important to restrict privileges for internal medicine? How is this done?

I have been waiting for some inspiration from this and previous meetings on the answer to this question.

The definition of privileges for internal medicine has been a very difficult problem, and I am not sure that I know an equitable way of determining it. Here is one way in which this has been done. The internist who is recommended for staff appointment to the board of trustees should have had appropriate training and should be able to attend to most of the work that comes within the scope of internal medicine. However, in recent years certain other specific qualifications have been added, such as knowledge of electrocardiography. The specification of privileges for the official reading of electrocardiograms was perhaps the first differentiation of staff privileges in internal medicine. More recently, with the advent of the artificial kidney and transperitoneal dialysis, it has been possible to designate one or two or three individuals on the staff who have qualified themselves in this area. Endoscopy is not always carried out by surgeons, some of it, for example, sigmoidoscopy, gastroscopy, bronchoscopy, and peritonoscopy, rather characteristically is done by internists. Fluoroscopy may also be added to an internist's privileges if he has qualified himself in that particular technique. All of these special procedures require additional specific training, and I believe that some specification of advance qualification can be determined in granting specific privileges in internal medicine.

Another speaker: Privileges in internal medicine for general practitioners are easily managed in the hospital in which I am most accustomed to work. When a general practitioner attends a medical case such as pneumonia, diabetes, or a cardiac problem, he does so on the medicine service. He belongs to the department of general practice, which is an administrative department, but his professional work is done within the appropriate clinical department. Those groups of medical cases can be followed and evaluated by the department of medicine.

The bylaws specify that it is the obligation of the chairman of the department to require consultation when he feels it is necessary. The problem is, how does the chairman of the department learn that some work may not be satisfactory? There are several channels. One may be through the house officers, particularly the residents, who by this time have a pretty fair idea of what is good and what is not. Also, I think the department chairman should give some attention to the morning reports of the nursing service. Quite obviously the chief of medicine cannot supervise 87 internists and 135 general practitioners by personal attendance of all their cases. There is an obligation, in my opinion, for the administration to bring cases of questionable propriety or competency to the attention of the department chairman, and there should also be a regular, systematic review of *all* the work in the department.

Is there any workable answer to having both limited and unlimited categories of privilege in internal medicine such as we have in surgery and obstetrics?

I think there is not. I do not know how to determine whether a patient is a severe diabetic or an unstable brittle diabetic who can change within an hour's time. I do not know how to specify degrees of severity of any illness, and such specifications would be necessary to adequately define privilege categories.

Should a small hospital have an official reader of electrocardiograms?
Yes, I think it should.

How are privileges to be reviewed? Are they to be considered static, or should they be changed?

Certainly, they must change. Physicians who develop special qualifications should call them to the attention of the credentials committee. Every department should maintain a personnel file for each staff member to which data may be added from time to time, including publications, addresses, or other participation in scientific meetings. Attendance at major meetings and postgraduate courses should also be recorded. The official recognition of the changing qualifications of a physician should be brought to the attention of the entire credentials committee by the departmental or section representative on that committee.

When an intern, resident, or nurse complains about a patient's care, does the department chairman examine the clinical record and the patient before requiring an attending physician to get further help?

The answer has to be very definitely yes. In many instances the chief of service, acting with tact and diplomacy, may not need to examine the patient at all. But he most definitely should feel free to do so if he thinks it necessary after examining the clinical record.

Do lay board members have a legal privilege of studying patient charts?

As I recall, Mr. Southwick cited a case in which a court in New York held that they do have such a privilege. As a practical measure, I would feel that they certainly should not have this privilege, for in my opinion this short-circuits the entire staff organization. I feel that they may properly bring their questions to the joint conference committee or to the chief of staff. This is not what the law says, and I disagree.

A radiologist employed by the hospital is incompetent. The staff recognizes this but feels reluctant to act. What is the best method of handling this situation?

I would like to go back to the first sentence: "A radiologist employed by the hospital is incompetent." Such a statement might be based on the prejudice of a small group; therefore, there would have to be some rather detailed and objective proof that the statement is true. "The staff recognizes this but feels reluctant to act." After having gathered adequate data, the chief of radiology should be approached by the chief of staff with this information; and at this point the administrator of the hospital should be brought in so that discussion or action will not go on without his knowledge. The matter should then be brought before the executive committee of the staff. Finally, if it cannot be settled to the satisfaction of all at this point, it should be taken to the joint conference committee.

When a nurse calls a physician regarding a patient and his need and the physician chooses to ignore her request for help or guidance, is the hospital relieved of its responsibility for providing adequate care?

The answer to that question is positively no. The Goff case in California, the Darling case in Illinois, the Bing case in New York—all would answer that question no. We can easily imagine a situation in which a nurse knows, in her professional judgment and competence, that the patient needs immediate attention. Her first act, of course, is to call the attending physician. He tells her over the telephone or personally, "I do not believe the patient needs attention." If the physician chooses to ignore her request for help, what should the nurse do? If she, in her professional judgment, thinks the patient does need immediate attention, she should report the matter to her superior at once. The nursing supervisor in turn reports to the administrator or to the chief of staff, who then provides for the safety of the patient. This raises some important questions and issues and implications. No nurse has the right, if she thinks the patient is endangered, to stand by and let the patient die. This in fact did happen in the Goff case in California.

Where does the utilization committee and its members as individuals stand in regard to liability from suit by patients and doctors? Where does the hospital stand in regard to liability from action of the utilization committee?

These two questions refer to an action in which the utilization committee has urged or pushed another member of the medical staff to dismiss his patient. Often the patient and the doctor are upset. From a legal point of view, if a doctor or a hospital prematurely discharges a patient who is in need of further attention, there can be liability for damages. The test of law is reasonable care under all the facts and circumstances, and the hospital must not act unreasonably under all the facts and circumstances. Now therefore, lawyers would generally advise that hospitals discharge patients only on the written order of the attending physician. Conservative lawyers, and I would be among them I think, would say that a utilization committee should not actually discharge the patient, because to do so might invite a law suit by the patient or the doctor. Still, suppose for a moment that you have a case where the utilization committee, in its professional judgment which is documented by medical records, takes it upon itself to actually discharge the patient over the objection of the attending physician. Even though this happens, it is very difficult for me to see how there could be liability as long as the committee exercised reasonable care under all the facts and circumstances that can be documented with expert testimony. I draw the conclusion that there is no, or perhaps minimal, legal risk in serving on utilization committees as they are now constituted and as they now operate. I would not for a minute hesitate to serve effectively on a utilization committee for fear of legal liability as long as reasonable care is exercised under all the facts and circumstances—you could not then be held liable.

How do you get staff physicians to come and listen to an educational program?

Not being a medical educator and being basically involved in medical administration, I justify my interest in hospital educational programs with the knowledge that there first must be an effective medical staff organization to make such programs successful.

Another speaker: I do not think there is any question that the internal medical audit can be one of the most effective and rewarding educational activities carried out within the medical staff. Physicians cannot very well escape participation in a medical audit or avoid the impact from it if they are going to maintain a position on the medical staff. This, of course, occurs only if the medical staff is organized in an effective manner. There is just no substitute, in my opinion, for reviewing one's own practice; and this will require a review of current medical thinking, the best medical information of the day. To find that one's own practice has not quite measured up to the standards of care one thought he was providing can be most stimulating for personal study. There is also a certain amount of feedback to the staff, which can be used for more formal educational programs.

Another speaker: The attending medical staff of a hospital usually conducts its medical audit as a medical staff function for the attending or the permanent staff. There is little or no effort made to teach interns and residents that they should plan to do this the rest of their professional lives, that they should carry out self-evaluation procedures and pull themselves up by their own boot straps. They must be taught how to look at their own practices critically and continuously from here on.

Another speaker: We have extended the analysis of patient care and a regular review of the type of patient care given to the outpatient department so that the house staff will be involved in self-evaluation. Such programs have been reviewed by W. Randolph Tucker and Joyce Lashoff (W. R. Tucker et al., Implementing Improvements in An Outpatient Department, *Arch. Environ. Health,* 11:22–27 (July) 1965). The house staff identifies rather strongly with the outpatient group, and I certainly agree that the time to inculcate critical introspection is at the house-staff level if not before. I would like to see such activity in medical school, but I think that this is probably impossible at present.

Consumer demand is not generated spontaneously. Public relations personnel are well aware of this and have resorted to the subliminal as well as the direct pressure approach. Does medical school faculty opinion have anything to do with consumer demand, either with the direct or subliminal approach?

I think the answer undoubtedly would be that faculty opinion has something to do with consumer demand if this is with reference to medical students seeking house officer positions. My contacts with faculty have indicated that they are almost as human as people who are not members of the faculty and are subject to the same pressures and the same drives. There is no question but that faculty will try to influence students, interestingly enough, to study harder and to learn more. This they have tried by both the direct and subliminal approach, if I understand this. I think they tend to be successful with either technique. I would like to remind all of us that *the people who are seeking postgraduate instruction are the same people who have been seeking undergraduate instruction.* I know nothing about continuing education; but as you would suspect, I try to get all kinds of data and then make very positive statements. Some data which interest me greatly are the motivational studies and the emotional and learning studies made by the Liefs of Tulane. Yesterday, at our three discussion sessions, we asked why anyone would want to put up with the heartaches and the headaches of a graduate education program such as an internship or a residency. Inevitably one of the primary and almost unanimous reasons stated was the continued education of the staff. These programs are devices whereby the staff educates itself with more enthusiasm, more effectiveness, and more consistency. I think this concept is something we can very well accept because of the results in the study by Lief and Young (V. F. Lief, et al., Academic Success: Intelligence and Personality, *J. Med. Ed.,*

40:114–124 (February) 1965) on the reasons students go into medicine—their motivation toward medicine. They tested and interviewed two groups of roughly twenty students each from two medical school classes; one group was made up of the ten top students in each class, the other made up of the bottom ten students. In the top group, intellectual curiosity was the most significant drive of all, with status and the opportunity to work with people tied for a close second. In the lower group, the motivational drives were different, the most notable difference being the sharp decreases in intellectual curiosity and in the opportunity to work with people as motivational drives. But status remained high on the list of drives in the lower group. In our discussion seminars yesterday on "Problems of the Internship," I was personally fascinated by the reasons given by the group of hospital staff leaders for being willing to put up with all the headaches and heartaches of an internship because the reasons very closely paralleled those which motivated the group of top undergraduate medical students—intellectual curiosity, expressed as the desire for effective continuing education of the staff; the desire for status, personal status on the part of the medical students and hospital status on the part of the staff; and the desire to work with people, in the case of the hospital staff with young people in the traditional Hippocratic teaching role.

Does intellectual curiosity date back to high school days for a particular student or intern, or is it something that can be developed during college or medical school?

The data of Lief, Lief, and Young are only from the time of entering medical school and at the end of medical school and do not predate entrance. I think this is a very important point, and it gives rise to another critical question.

I feel very strongly that unless there is an active educational program aimed at the staff physician, and with a measure of discipline for those who do not attend the programs and functions, unless you have this, it is quite futile to try to offer house staff training programs. If the practicing doctor does not keep up to snuff, I do not know how you can have a proper milieu for house staff training.

Another speaker: There is a very interesting article entitled "Why Teachers Fail," by B. F. Skinner of Harvard University, in the current issue of the *Saturday Review*. Our whole educational system, from the time the youngster goes to kindergarten to the time that he graduates from medical school or any other professional school, is based on the philosophy that the student must continually be threatened if he is going to do his work. This may be the basis of one of our problems in postgraduate medicine. Perhaps by the time the physician has finished his last specialty board examination and has survived his last ordeal at the hands of educators and examiners, he has consciously or subconsciously decided that he is going to enjoy the fruits of his labors for the rest of his life; and he is not going to bother with education and learning again unless it suits him and when it suits him. I do not know whether this is an important factor in effecting motivation or not, but it deserves serious thought. The practical approach to the problem, it seems to me, is to organize our hospital staffs so that the physician will be rewarded for his participation in education; rewarded by promotion, advancement, reappointment, and perhaps by some priority in the assignment of beds for admission to those who contribute most to the hospital's educational program.

Another speaker: I raise a philosophical point. Did I gather that you thought that we should not threaten physicians in any matter? If we should relate promotion and appointment and bed allocation to educational participation, then if this is not a threat, I do not know what is.

Reply: We should keep in mind that a position on a hospital staff is essential today in the practice of medicine. We do have something that doctors want, namely a position on the hospital medical staff, and this can be a reward and can be used as a motivating factor.

JOINT COMMISSION ON ACCREDITATION OF HOSPITALS: STANDARDS FOR HOSPITAL ACCREDITATION

(ED. NOTE: *These Standards of the Joint Commission on Accreditation of Hospitals are in effect as of June, 1966. Revision of these Standards is currently under way, and it is expected that this will be published in 1967. Copies of the revised Standards may be obtained by writing to the Joint Commission on Accreditation of Hospitals, 645 North Michigan Avenue, Chicago, Illinois 60611. Explanatory Supplement to the Standards for Hospital Accreditation is also available from the Joint Commission at the above address. Another useful publication is the Hospital Accreditation References, 1964 edition, available from the American Hospital Association, 840 North Lake Shore Drive, Chicago, Illinois 60611.*)

INTRODUCTION

The Standards for Hospital Accreditation of the Joint Commission on Accreditation of Hospitals have been adopted by the Board of Commissioners.

These Standards have evolved from years of experience and observation of those hospital practices which have proved consistent with high quality patient care. To accredit and recommend a hospital to the public, the Commission considers it essential that the hospital meet these Standards.

The Standards which are fundamental for the accreditation of all hospitals are stated as Basic Principles. The implementation of these basic principles is outlined in Standards of Procedure. The methods used to achieve the Standards of Procedure may vary with the type and size of the hospital; but to be accredited, the hospital must carry out the functions implied in the Standards of Procedure.

The Joint Commission on Accreditation of Hospitals is a voluntary organization, supported by its member organizations. Upon written invitation, the Commission will survey a hospital if it has at least twenty-five beds exclusive of bassinets, has been in operation for at least twelve months, and has been accepted for registration as a hospital by the American Hospital Association.

The four member organizations of the Commission pay the administrative costs of the program of accreditation. Each individual hospital is charged for the survey proper; the formula being $60.00 per hospital, plus $1.00 per bed (exclusive of bassinets), up to 250 beds. The latest edition of the Administrative Guide Issue of the American Hospital Association is used in determining the number of beds. Invoice will be sent to the hospital at the time of notification of impending survey. Payment must be made directly to the Commission. Surveyors are instructed not to accept payment from the hospital.

JOHN D. PORTERFIELD, M.D.
Director

BASIC PRINCIPLES

The following basic principles must be followed in order for a hospital to be accredited by the Joint Commission on Accreditation of Hospitals.

I. ADMINISTRATION

A. Governing Body

The governing body must assume the legal and moral responsibility for the conduct of the hospital as an institution. It is responsible to the patient, the community, and the sponsoring organization.

B. Physical Plant

The buildings of the hospital must be constructed, arranged, and maintained to insure the safety of the patient; and must provide facilities for diagnosis and treatment and for special hospital services appropriate to the needs of the community.

C. The following facilities and services must be maintained:

1. Dietary
2. Medical Records
3. Pharmacy or Drug Room
4. Clinical pathology and pathological anatomy
5. Radiology
6. Emergency care for mass casualties
7. Medical Library

II. MEDICAL STAFF

There must be an organized medical staff which is responsible to the patient and to the governing body of the hospital for the quality of all medical care provided patients in the hospital and for the ethical and professional practices of its members.

III. NURSING

There must be a licensed, graduate, registered nurse on duty at all times and graduate nursing service must be available for all patients at all times.

STANDARDS OF PROCEDURE

To implement the basic principles, the following Standards of Procedure are outlined. Experience and knowledge have verified that to insure safe patient care, these standards are essential. The methods used to achieve these standards may vary with the type and size of the hospital; but to achieve accreditation, the hospital must carry out the functions implied by the standards.

I. ADMINISTRATION

A. Governing Body

The governing body is legally and morally responsible for the conduct of the hospital. In the discharge of its duties, it places the responsibility for the medical care of the patient in the hospital primarily upon the medical staff. For effective performance the governing body should do the following:

1. Adopt bylaws in accordance with legal requirements.
2. Meet at regular stated intervals.
3. Appoint committees. There should be an Executive Committee and others as indicated for special purposes.
4. Establish a formal means of liaison with the medical staff preferably by a Joint Conference Committee.
5. Appoint members of the medical staff.
6. Appoint a qualified hospital administrator as the official representative of the governing body, who is responsible for the management of the hospital, and who provides liaison among the governing body, the medical staff, the nursing staff, and other departments of the hospital.
7. Provide a physical plant equipped and staffed to maintain the needed facilities and services for patients.

B. Physical Plant

The buildings of the hospital must be solidly constructed with adequate space and safeguards for each patient. The hospital shall provide:

1. Fire protection by the elimination of fire hazards; the installation of necessary safeguards such as extinguishers, sprinkling devices, and fire barriers to insure rapid and effective fire con-

trol; and the adoption of written fire control plans rehearsed three times a year by key personnel.

2. A sanitary environment to avoid sources and transmission of infections.

3. Facilities for the isolation of patients with communicable diseases, especially in obstetrical, newborn, and pediatric sections.

4. Facilities for the segregation of obstetric patients and newborn infants.

5. Emergency lighting in operating, delivery and emergency rooms, nurseries, and stairwells.

6. Adequate diagnostic and therapeutic facilities.

C. Services which must be maintained

1. DIETARY DEPARTMENT

a. There shall be an organized department directed by qualified personnel and integrated with other departments of the hospital.

b. Facilities shall be provided for the general dietary needs of the hospital. These shall include facilities for the preparation of special diets. Sanitary conditions must be maintained in the storage, preparation, and distribution of food.

c. There shall be a qualified dietitian on full time or on a consultation basis and in addition, administrative and technical personnel competent in their respective duties.

d. There shall be a systematic record of diets, correlated with the medical records.

e. Departmental and interdepartmental conferences shall be held periodically.

2. MEDICAL RECORD DEPARTMENT

a. Administrative Responsibilities

1) There shall be a medical record maintained on every patient admitted for care in the hospital.

2) Records shall be kept inviolate and preserved for a period of time not less than that determined by the Statute of Limitations in the respective state.

3) Qualified personnel adequate to supervise and conduct the department shall be provided.

4) A system of identification and filing to insure the rapid location of a patient's medical record shall be maintained. The unit number system is preferred.

5) All clinical information pertaining to a patient should be centralized in the patient's record.

6) The Standard Nomenclature should be used as a nomenclature.

7) Records should be indexed according to disease, operation, and physician and should be kept up-to-date. For indexing any recognized system may be used.

b. Medical Staff Responsibilities

1) The medical record must contain sufficient information to justify the diagnosis and warrant the treatment and end results.

2) Only members of the medical staff and the house staff are competent to write or dictate medical histories and physical examinations.

3) Current records and those on discharged patients should be completed promptly.

4) Records must be authenticated and signed by a licensed physician.

c. The medical records should contain the following information:

1) Identification data
2) Complaint
3) Present illness
4) Past history
5) Family history
6) Physical examination
7) Provisional diagnosis
8) Clinical laboratory reports
9) X-ray reports
10) Consultations
11) Treatment: Medical and Surgical
12) Tissue report
13) Progress notes
14) Final diagnosis
15) Discharge summary
16) Autopsy findings

3. PHARMACY OR DRUG ROOM

a. There shall be a pharmacy directed by a registered pharmacist or drug room under competent supervision.

b. Facilities shall be provided for the storage, safe-guarding, preparation, and dispensing of drugs.

c. Personnel competent in their respective duties shall be provided in keeping with the size and activity of the department.

d. Records shall be kept of the transactions of the pharmacy, and correlated with other hospital records where indicated. Such special records shall be kept as are required by law.

e. Drugs dispensed shall meet the standards established by the United States Pharmacopeia, National Formulary, or New and Non-official Drugs.

f. Policies must be established to control the administration of toxic or dangerous drugs with specific reference to the duration of the order and the dosage.

g. There should be a committee of the medical staff to confer with the pharmacist in the formulation of policies.

4. LABORATORIES

a. Clinical pathology
   1) Clinical pathology services adequate for the individual hospital must be maintained in the hospital.
   2) Provision shall be made to carry out adequate clinical pathology examinations including chemistry, bacteriology, hematology, serology, and clinical microscopy.
   3) Facilities and services should be available at all times.
   4) Personnel adequate to supervise and conduct the service should be provided.
   5) Routine examinations required on all admissions should be determined by the medical staff. These must include at least a urinalysis and a hemoglobin or hematocrit.
   6) Signed reports should be filed with the patient's record and duplicate copies kept in the department.

b. Blood Bank
   Facilities for procurement, safe-keeping, and transfusion of blood should be provided or readily available.

c. Pathological anatomy
   1) The services of a pathologist must be provided as indicated by the needs of the hospital.
   2) All tissues removed at operation should be sent for examination. The extent of the examination should be determined by the pathology department.
   3) Signed reports of tissue examinations should be filed

with the patient's record and duplicate copies kept in the department.

5. RADIOLOGY

    a. The hospital must maintain radiological services according to needs of the hospital.

    b. The radiology department shall be free of hazards for patients and personnel.

    c. Personnel adequate to supervise and conduct the services should be provided.

    d. The interpretation of radiological examinations shall be made by physicians competent in the field.

    e. Signed reports should be filed with the patient's record and duplicate copies kept in the department.

6. EMERGENCY SERVICE

    a. There shall be a written plan for the care of mass casualties. This plan should be coordinated with the in-patient and out-patient services of the hospital and rehearsed by key personnel at least twice a year.

    b. If an emergency service is maintained:

        1) The department shall be well organized, directed by qualified personnel, and integrated with other departments of the hospital.

        2) Facilities shall be provided to assure prompt diagnosis and emergency treatment. There shall be adequate medical and nursing personnel available at all times.

        3) Adequate medical records on every patient must be kept.

7. MEDICAL LIBRARY

    a. The hospital must maintain a medical library according to the needs of the hospital.

    b. Facilities should be provided to meet the requirements of the services in the hospital.

    c. Basic textbooks and current periodicals should be available and catalogued according to the needs of the hospital.

    d. Personnel should be provided to assure efficient service to the medical staff.

D. Services which may be maintained

    1. OUTPATIENT DEPARTMENT

        The Outpatient Department shall be organized into sections (clinics) the number of which shall depend on the degree of departmentalization of the medical staff, available facilities, and the needs of the community.

        a. There shall be such professional and non-professional personnel as are required for efficient operation.

        b. Facilities shall be provided to assure the efficient operation of the department.

        c. Medical Records shall be maintained, and correlated with other hospital medical records.

        d. Conferences, both departmental and interdepartmental, shall be conducted to maintain close liaison between the various sections within the department and with other hospital services.

    2. REHABILITATION DEPARTMENT

        The organization of the Rehabilitation Department shall be comparable to that of other departments of the hospital.

    3. MEDICAL SOCIAL SERVICE DEPARTMENT

        a. The department shall be well organized, directed by a qualified medical social service worker, and integrated with other departments of the hospital.

        b. Facilities shall be provided which are adequate for the personnel of the department, easily accessible to patients and to the medical staff, and which assure privacy for interviews.

        c. Records of case work shall be kept. Such records shall be available only to the professional personnel concerned.

        d. Departmental and interdepartmental conferences shall be held periodically.

II. MEDICAL STAFF

A. Responsibilities

The governing body of the hospital must delegate the responsibility of medical functions to the medical staff, including recommendations as to the professional qualifications of all who practice in the hospital. The medical staff is responsible for the quality of medical care rendered to patients in the hospital. Maintaining high standards of medical care will depend upon the character of the staff and the effectiveness of its organization to carry out the following duties:

1. Selection of those recommended for staff appointments and hospital privileges.
2. Constant analysis and review of the clinical work done in the hospital.
3. Support of medical staff and hospital policies.
4. Maintenance of adequate medical records.
5. Procurement of autopsies (a minimum of 20 to 25 per cent of hospital deaths).
6. Holding consultations.

   a. Required consultations
   Except in an emergency, consultations with another qualified physician are required in:

      1) First caesarean sections.
      2) Curretages or other procedures by which a known or suspected pregnancy may be interrupted.
      3) Operations performed for the sole purpose of sterilization on both male and female patients.
      4) Cases on all services in which according to the judgment of the physician:
         a) The patient is not a good medical or surgical risk.
         b) The diagnosis is obscure.
         c) There is doubt as to the best therapeutic measures to be utilized.

   b. Consultant
   A consultant must be well qualified to give an opinion in the field in which his opinion is sought. The status of consultant is determined by the medical staff on the basis of an individual's training, experience, and competence.

   c. Essentials of a consultation
   A satisfactory consultation includes examination of the patient and the record. A written opinion signed by the consultant must be included in the medical record. When operative procedures are involved, the consultation note, except in emergency, shall be recorded prior to operation.

d. Responsibility for requesting consultations
The patient's physician is responsible for requesting consultations when indicated. It is the duty of the hospital staff through its chiefs of service and executive committee to make certain that members of the staff do not fail in the matter of calling consultants as needed.

B. Membership

1. APPOINTMENT

a. Procedure
Staff appointments are made by the governing body. Recommendations are made by the active staff and should be submitted prior to action by the governing body. Limited terms of appointment are recommended but not required. The prevailing custom is for a term of one year, with re-appointments continued so long as qualifications remain satisfactory.

b. Qualifications
Members of the staff must be qualified legally, professionally, and ethically for the positions to which they are appointed.

2. CATEGORIES

The privileges of each member of the medical staff shall be determined on the basis of professional qualifications and demonstrated ability.

a. Active Staff
Regardless of any other categories having privileges in the hospital, there shall be an active staff, properly organized, which shall perform all the organizational duties pertaining to the medical staff. These shall include:

1) Maintenance of the proper quality of all medical care and treatment in the hospital.
2) Organization of the medical staff, including adoption of rules and regulations for its government (which require the approval of the governing body), election of its officers, and recommendations to the governing body upon all appointments to the staff and grants of hospital privileges.
3) Other recommendations to the governing body upon matters within the purview of the medical staff.

b. Other Categories of the Staff

In larger hospitals, and in some smaller hospitals, the medical staff may include one or more of the following categories in addition to the Active Staff, but this in no wise modifies the duties and responsibilities of the Active Staff.

1) Honorary Staff

The Honorary Staff shall be former Active Staff, retired or emeritus, and other physicians of reputation whom it is desired to honor.

2) Consulting Staff

The Consulting Staff shall be recognized specialists willing to serve in such capacity. A member of the Consulting Staff may also be a member of the Active Staff, but only if the two appointments are made.

3) Associate Staff

The Associate Staff shall be those members who use the hospital infrequently or those less experienced members undergoing a period of probation before being considered for appointment to the Active Staff.

4) Courtesy Staff

The Courtesy Staff shall be those who desire to attend patients in the hospital but who, for some reason not disqualifying, are ineligible for appointment in another category of the staff.

C. Organization

1. OFFICERS

There shall be such officers as may be necessary for the government of the staff. These officers shall be members of the Active Staff and shall be elected by the Active Staff, unless this is precluded by hospital policy.

2. BYLAWS

Bylaws to govern and enable the staff to carry out its responsibilities in accordance with these Standards for Hospital Accreditation shall be adopted.

3. ADMINISTRATIVE FUNCTIONS

The effective discharge of the responsibilities of the medical staff will depend in great part on the clear assignment and full acceptance of each responsibility by the entire staff, its officers, individual members, committees, or other mechanisms formed to deal with the specific tasks identified in Section II A. above. The form and complexity of organization of the medical staff needed to discharge these responsibilities effectively is a determination which must be made by the medical staff of each individual hospital. They will vary substantially depending upon the size, composition and disposition of each staff. While committee establishment will be a common device, other methods will be acceptable to the Joint Commission *provided effectiveness can be demonstrated by the documentation of activities.*

The following medical staff functions are required:

a. Coordination of the activities and general policies of the various departments;

b. Interim decision making for the medical staff between staff meetings under such limitations as shall be set by the medical staff;

c. Follow-up and appropriate disposition of all reports dealing with the various staff functions;

(Commonly Executive Committee Functions)

d. Review of all applications for appointment and annual reappointment to all categories of staff and recommendations on each to the governing body, including definition of privileges to be granted in each case;

(Commonly Credentials Committee Function)

e. A formal and official means of liaison among the medical staff, the governing body and the administrator to provide a channel for medico-administrative advice;

(Commonly Joint Conference Committee Function)

f. Provision for keeping the entire medical staff informed concerning the accreditation program, the current accreditation status of the hospital and the factors influencing that status;

(Commonly an Accreditation Committee Function)

g. Surveillance of the quality of patient care provided in the hospital by the promotion and maintenance of the following elements:

i. Currently maintained medical records describing the condition and progress of the patient, the therapy provided, the results thereof, and the placement of responsibility for all actions taken in sufficient completeness as to assure transferable comprehension of the case at any time;

(Commonly Records Committee Function)

ii. Review and clinical evaluation of the quality of medical care provided to all categories of patients on the basis of the documented evidence;

(Commonly Medical Records, Tissue and Medical Audit Committee Function)

iii. Review of hospital admissions with respect to need for admission, length of stay, discharge practices and evaluation of the services ordered and provided;

(Commonly Utilization Review Committee Function)

iv. Surveillance of inadvertent hospital infection potentials and cases and the promotion of a preventive and corrective program designed to minimize these hazards.

(Commonly Infection Committee Function)

v. Surveillance of pharmacy and therapeutic policies and practices within the institution to assure optimum utilization with a minimum potential for hazard.

(Commonly Pharmacy and Therapeutics Committee Function)

These functions shall be carried out with sufficient periodicity to assure their objectives being achieved. Written reports shall be submitted for follow-up and disposition in accordance with item c.

4. STAFF MEETINGS

The improvement in care and treatment of hospital patients is the responsibility of the medical staff. To accomplish this, meetings of the medical staff are required to review, analyze, and evaluate the clinical work of its members.

a. The number and frequency of medical staff meetings shall be determined by the Active Staff and clearly stated in the bylaws of the staff.

b. Attendance requirements for all medical staff meetings shall be determined by the Active Staff. The requirements for each individual member of the staff and for the total attendance at each meeting shall be clearly stated in the bylaws of the staff. Records of attendance shall be kept.

    c. Adequate minutes of all meetings shall be kept.

    d. The method adopted to insure adequate evaluation of clinical practice in the hospital shall be determined by the medical staff and clearly stated in the bylaws. Any one of the following three methods will fulfill this requirement:

        1) Monthly meetings of the Active Staff.

        2) Monthly departmental conferences in those hospitals where the clinical services are well organized and each department is large enough to meet as a unit. Clinicopathological conferences may be substituted for a departmental conference provided an adequate review of the clinical work is covered by one or another of such conferences.

        3) Monthly meetings of the Medical Records and Tissue Committees where the quality of medical work is adequately appraised, action taken by the Executive Committee, and reports made to the Active Staff.

D. Departmentalization

Division of the staff into services or departments to fulfill medical staff responsibilities promotes efficiency and is recommended in general hospitals with 75 or more beds. Functional division for the medical staff into more than the minimal medical and surgical services is frequently desirable in larger hospitals. It is necessary that each autonomous service or department be organized and function as a unit.

1. MEMBERS

Medical staff members of each service or department shall be qualified by training and demonstrated competence; and shall be granted privileges commensurate with their individual abilities.

2. CHIEF OF SERVICE OR DEPARTMENT

The chief of service or department shall be a member of the service or department best qualified by training, experience, and administrative ability for the position. He shall be responsible for the administration of the department, for the general character of the professional care of patients, and for making recommendations as to the qualifications of its members. He shall also make recommendations to the administration as to the planning of hospital facilities, equipment, routine procedures, and any other matters concerning patient care.

3. CONFERENCES

In those hospitals where the review and evaluation of clinical practice is done by committees of the medical staff or by monthly meetings of the entire staff, departmental meetings are optional. In those hospitals where the clinical review is done by the departments, each service or department shall meet at least once every month. Records of these meetings shall be kept and become part of the records of the medical staff.

E. Departments which may be maintained

1. ANESTHESIA

The organization of the Department of Anesthesia shall be comparable to that of other services or departments. There shall also be required for every patient:

    a. Pre-anesthetic physical examination, with findings recorded, by a physician within forty-eight hours of surgery.
    b. Anesthetic record on special form.
    c. Post-anesthetic follow-up, with findings recorded, by an anesthesiologist or a registered nurse-anesthetist.

2. GENERAL PRACTICE DEPARTMENT

The Department of General Practice shall be an organized segment of the medical staff comparable to that of other staff departments.

    a. The responsibilities of this department shall be administrative and educational. If desirable, it may be made responsible for conducting the outpatient department in whole or in part.
    b. Since the Department of General Practice is not a clinical service and no patients are admitted to the department, the members of the Department of General Practice shall on recommendation of the Credentials Committee have privileges on the clinical services of other departments in accord with their training and experience. On any service in which any general practitioner shall have privileges, he shall be subject to the rules of that service and subject to jurisdiction of its chief.

3. DENTAL SERVICE OR DEPARTMENT

According to the procedure established for the appointment of the medical staff, one or more dentists may be appointed to the dental staff. Where more than a few dentists are so appointed, a dental service may be organized. The organization of the Department of Dentistry shall be comparable to that of other services or departments. Whether or not the dental service is organized as a department, the following requirements shall be met:

    a. Members of the dental staff must be qualified legally, professionally, and ethically for the positions to which they are appointed.

    b. Patients admitted for dental services may be admitted by the dentist either to the Department of Dentistry or if there is no department, to an organized clinical service.

    c. There must be a physician in attendance who is responsible for the medical care of the patient throughout the hospital stay. A medical survey shall be done and recorded by a member of the medical staff before dental surgery is performed.

III. NURSING

A. Responsibilities

Safe nursing care for all patients is a primary responsibility of the Department of Nursing Service. To be accredited, the following are required:

1. The selection of individuals qualified by education, experience and demonstrated ability for the positions to which they are appointed.
2. A well organized departmental plan of administrative authority with delineation of responsibilities and duties of each category of nursing personnel. This deals not only with patient care, but also with the educational responsibilities of the nursing service.
3. Well established working relationships with other services of the hospital, both administrative and professional.
4. Constant review and evaluation of the nursing care provided patients. This necessitates written nursing care procedures and written nursing care plans for patients, either on an individual or nursing unit basis.

B. Personnel

1. There must be an adequate number of licensed, graduate, registered nurses to meet the following minimum requirements:

    a. Director of the Department.

    b. Assistants to the Director for evening and night services.

    c. Supervisory and staff personnel for each department or nursing unit to insure the immediate availability of a graduate, registered nurse for bedside care of all patients at all times.

2. Ancillary personnel in sufficient numbers to provide nursing care not requiring the service of a graduate nurse.
3. Adequate nursing personnel for the surgical suite, delivery rooms, clinics, and other services of the hospital in keeping with their size and degree of activity.
4. Nursing personnel assigned to care for obstetrical patients and newborn infants must not have other duties which may create danger of infection being carried to these services.

C. Conferences

Meetings of the graduate nursing staff shall be held at least monthly to discuss patient care, nursing service problems, and administrative policies. The pattern for meetings may be by clinical departments, by categories of the staff or by the staff as a whole. Minutes of all meetings shall be kept.

Index

Accident toll, 310
Accreditation of hospitals, 179–195
  small hospitals, 294, 304
  (*See also* Joint Commission on Accreditation of Hospitals)
Accreditation committee, 509
Achieving an effective staff, 85–100
Administration, in disaster planning, 328–332
  vital interest in professional standards, 76–83
  (*See also* Administrator)
Administrative efficiency, 117
Administrative skill, 89, 167
Administrator, 106–107, 109–111, 117–118, 480
  need for security, 9
  relationship, to chief of staff, 37–38, 60
    to medical director, 48–50
    to medical staff, 111, 113–119
      in disaster planning, 327–332
      emergency service committee, 311, 322
      executive committee, 192–193
      joint conference committee, 198–200, 205
  in small hospitals, 292, 301–302
  and trustees, 106–108
  (*See also* Administration)
Advisory board for medical specialties, 407
Affiliation of, internship programs, 431
  small hospital with teaching hospital, 295–296
AMA (*see* American Medical Association)
Ambulance, personnel, 313–314
  and rescue units, 317–318
American Academy of General Practice, 174, 463, 467, 469
  Commission on Education, 462
American Academy of Pediatrics, 165, 444
American College of Obstetrics and Gynecology, guide for duties of chief, 156

American College of Surgeons, and the medical audit, 214
  survey of internships and residencies, 410
  trauma committee, 310
American Medical Association (AMA),
  Ad Hoc Committee on Education for Family Practice, 461, 468
  Council on Medical Education, approval of internships and residencies, 406–418
  definitions of kinds of internships, 426–427
  Essentials of an Approved Internship, 421
  and family practice, as a specialty, 465–471
  studies on, 461
  House of Delegates, *Essentials of Approved Residencies*, 407
  and family practice, 465–468
  and internships, 426
  Physician-Hospital Relations, 67–68
  Residency Review Committees, 409, 413
  Internship Review Committee, 412–413, 421–422
  Internship Task Force, 423, 462, 468
  National Voluntary Health Conference, 4
  Report on Physician-Hospital Relations, 3–4
Ancillary facilities, in small hospitals, 294, 304–305
  (*See also* Auxiliary facilities)
Anesthesia department, JCAH standards, 512
Appendectomy, justification, 243, 247
Appointments to medical staff, 70–76, 210
Attending staff (*see* Medical staff)
Audit, medical [*see* Medical audit; Committee(s), medical audit]
Autopsy rate, 231–233
  in pediatric residency, 448
  in surgical residency, 441
Auxiliary facilities, in disaster planning, 331